S0-AGY-222

Praise for
Sex Matters for Women

"The most comprehensive book on women's sexual health I have ever read. The clear, positive information and the suggested exercises cover all aspects of women's sexuality and offer ways for women to take charge of their sexual selves. The second edition features new information and resources, offered in a supportive and affirming manner, which will help readers develop sexual comfort, confidence, and satisfaction. A 'must read' for women of all ages."

—BEVERLY WHIPPLE, PhD, RN, FAAN, coauthor of *The G Spot* and *The Science of Orgasm*

"This book opened multiple doors for me as it helped me explore the story of my sexuality and reexamine sexual beliefs and misconceptions that I didn't even know I had. It is packed with factual, relevant information. It has also been an invaluable read for me as a mother raising a young daughter, who will have her own sexual story one day."

—ANDREA, Hawaii

"Coverage is comprehensive and accurate, with information about issues that are rarely addressed."

—*Library Journal*

"This is a book you can trust. The authors obviously know and care a great deal about helping women have fulfilling sex lives. The first edition was terrific, and the updated second edition is even better."

—PEPPER SCHWARTZ, PhD, author of *Prime: Adventures and Advice on Sex, Love, and the Sensual Years*

"This second edition takes a classic book on female sexuality to another level. It is comprehensive and grounded in research, yet fun to read alone or with a partner. With a focus on female sexual satisfaction and pleasure, this book is a 'must have' for women of all ages and backgrounds. I can't wait to share it with my daughter!"

—HILDA HUTCHERSON, MD, author of *What Your Mother Never Told You About Sex*

"The second edition of *Sex Matters for Women* will allow me to quietly retire my tattered and worn copy of the first edition. I have lent this superb book to dozens of the women I have treated."

—SHERYL A. KINGSBERG, PhD, Professor of Reproductive Biology and Psychiatry, Case Western Reserve University

"This is my favorite book on women's sexuality and sexual health! In the second edition, the authors respond to new research and deliver an up-to-date, even more enlightening book that emphasizes the positive. It's an empowering guide that you can fully rely on for accurate information and useful exercises for sexual growth. I especially love how the book celebrates female sexuality in its many diverse forms."

—PAMELA H. STEPHENSON-CONNOLLY, PhD, author of *Sex Life*

SEX MATTERS FOR WOMEN

Sex Matters for Women

A Complete Guide to Taking Care of Your Sexual Self

SECOND EDITION

Sallie Foley, MSW
Sally A. Kope, MSW
Dennis P. Sugrue, PhD

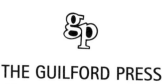

THE GUILFORD PRESS
New York   London

© 2012 The Guilford Press
A Division of Guilford Publications, Inc.
72 Spring Street, New York, NY 10012
www.guilford.com

All rights reserved

The information in this volume is not intended as a substitute for consultation
with healthcare professionals. Each individual's health concerns should be evaluated
by a qualified professional.

No part of this book may be reproduced, translated, stored in a retrieval system,
or transmitted, in any form or by any means, electronic, mechanical, photocopying,
microfilming, recording, or otherwise, without written permission from the publisher.

Printed in the United States of America

This book is printed on acid-free paper.

Last digit is print number: 9 8 7 6 5 4 3 2 1

Library of Congress Cataloging-in-Publication Data

Foley, Sallie.
   Sex matters for women : a complete guide to taking care of your sexual self /
Sallie Foley, Sally A. Kope, and Dennis P. Sugrue. — 2nd ed.
      p. cm.
   Includes bibliographical references and index.
   ISBN 978-1-60918-469-8 (pbk. : alk. paper) — ISBN 978-1-60918-999-0 (hbk. :
alk. paper)
   1. Women—Sexual behavior.   2. Sex.   I. Kope, Sally A.   II. Sugrue, Dennis P.
III. Title.
   HQ29.F65 2012
   613.9'54—dc23
                                                              2011030419

In the clinical cases reported in this book all names and identifying characteristics have
been altered.

To our clients and students:
you have approached learning with open hearts and minds
and taught us how deeply sex matters for women.

*   *   *

And to the loves of my life—Steve and our family.
—Sallie Foley

To Marty, my life partner, with all love, respect, and gratitude.
To the women in my life, all of whom are the soul of my wisdom.
—Sally A. Kope

For Cristina, Nicole, Angela, Megan, Shannon, Kelsey, Kelly, Diane,
and Abigail—remarkable young women who make me proud to be
their uncle. May this work support them and other women of their
generation in their quest for love, sexual health, and well-being.
—Dennis P. Sugrue (Uncle Denny)

Contents

Acknowledgments

When we wrote the first edition of *Sex Matters for Women*, the three of us believed that we could create a book that would be a comprehensive guide to women's sexuality. Our experience since its publication in 2002 has been deeply gratifying. Clients, students, and colleagues have generously shared their appreciation for our book, and many have asked for more information. The book you hold in your hands is the result of our commitment to write a completely updated second edition. It has been a lively collaboration, rich in both argument and agreement, and more dedicated than we could have imagined. We have profoundly influenced each other's thinking as the book has taken shape, and the book and the three of us are the better for it. Many colleagues have been generous in their assistance at every phase of the book's development. We wish to thank those individuals who so generously contributed their knowledge and skill.

For creating the illustrations to the book, we are grateful to Sally Kope. For reading and providing invaluable commentary on many parts of the manuscript, we thank Sheila Crowley, PhD; Dennis Hacker, MDiv; Sandra Jordan, PhD; Michael Kaplan, MSW; JoAnn McFall, MSW, RN; Anne Segall, MSW; Russell Stambaugh, PhD; Bernadette Sugrue, MA; Pat Warner; Beverly Whipple, PhD, RN; and Daniela Wittmann, MSW. For reviewing the manuscript for medical accuracy, our gratitude to Melinda Abernethy, MD; Evan Eyler, MD; Jessica Foley, MD; Hope Haefner, MD; Stephen Liroff, MD; Elisabeth Quint, MD; and Beverly Whipple, PhD, RN. We are grateful to Madeleine Amdur; Richard Balon, MD; Doug Davies, PhD, MSW; Lauren Foley, JD; Steven Foley, PhD; Meghan Gallagher, MSW; Martin Kope, MDiv, MS; Michael Kope, JD; Laura Nitzberg, MSW; Claudia Kraus Piper, MSW; Margaret Punch, MD; Caren Stalberg, MD; Peg Tewksbury, MS; Alice Um, JD; Aline Zolbrod, PhD; and our colleagues at the University of Michigan who provided countless hours of sound advice and listened patiently as we developed our ideas. For helping us add international resources to this edition, we are grateful to Arija Jarvenpaa; Pamela

Stephenson-Connolly, PhD; and Brad Waters, MSW. We are also indebted to our students and clients who have shared their experiences and trusted our guidance in better understanding the remarkable complexity of human sexuality. The book would not exist if it were not for our editors at The Guilford Press—Kitty Moore, for her amazing vision and organizational sensibility, Christine Benton, for her editorial incisiveness and insistence that we not stop till we got it right, and Anna Brackett, for her editorial agility, wise counsel, and sheer persistence.

Most of all, we are indebted to our partners—Steve, Marty, and Bernadette—and our families. They made the book possible because they not only loved us but also respected and believed in the importance of this work.

Introduction

Since the first edition of *Sex Matters for Women* was published in 2002, we've been gratified to receive volumes of positive feedback from both the general public and the professional community. Therapists, physicians, and nurses have told us they are grateful to have a book they feel comfortable recommending to their clients and patients. Women and men have written about their appreciation for the information and the respectful, empowering tone of the book, stating that *Sex Matters* increased their self-understanding and enriched their sexual relationships.

Many of our readers have also honored us with their personal stories describing how the book has affected their lives. There was the time, for example, when an acquaintance approached one of us who was gardening in the front yard. Speaking as though we were close confidantes, she revealed that her partner of 45 years had given her a copy of *Sex Matters for Women* and that after they had read and practiced the exercises together she became orgasmic for the first time in her life. She was in tears, even then, as she recounted what was obviously for her an important life experience. Then there was the mom who gave a copy of *Sex Matters* to each of her daughters as they left for college, confident that these young women would find guidance from a book that she described as "so accessible, so positive about female sexuality." And another woman—a survivor of childhood trauma—worked with her therapist to overcome the triggers that prevented her from having the pleasure of sexual touch and arousal. She asked her therapist to let us know that she had used *Sex Matters* to find her way back into her body and was now finding her way in connecting to others.

From across the street to around the world, women have shared their enthusiasm with us. One of our favorite comments came from a 40-year-old woman from Senegal, who reported with excitement and pride that she was reading the book with her friends and that for the first time they were discussing sexuality openly with each other. And as we are putting the final touches on this new edition of the book,

1

the first edition of *Sex Matters* is being translated into Vietnamese, which will make this book and the stories it inspires available to millions of women in Southeast Asia.

With this kind of success behind it, you might ask why we have undertaken a major revision of this book. In fact, many people have asked us what could we possibly add. The answer is, a lot has changed. There is new, substantive research about women's sexuality and sexual health. The first decade of the millennium has brought intriguing information about the sexual response cycle, the role of brain chemistry, and how willingness to be sexual can influence sexual responsiveness. We also now understand better that a woman's sexuality is influenced not only by her developmental phase of life, but also by what time period in history she came of age.

As we enter the second decade of the millennium, our view of women and sexuality has become one of empowerment and self-realization. In the first edition, fully a fifth of the book was devoted to overcoming sexual dysfunctions. We have now moved away from the somewhat protective, even defensive, tone of the original book, where we focused on the challenges women faced in being sexual in modern society. Yet, in our own defense, recall events around the turn of the 21st century: after the years of women pushing to be seen, heard, and taken seriously, sexually and otherwise, Viagra exploded onto the scene and shoved men's sexuality to center stage. Many women were concerned that their sexuality and the way that sex mattered to them, for so long marginalized or dismissed altogether, would be further set aside or, worse, reduced to a medical state in need of the pink version of that little blue pill.

Fast-forward almost a decade. We no longer view women's sexual response through the lens of men's sexual response, but instead validate the broad range of women's sexual experiences across several generations and in many cultures. In this new edition, we don't focus on overcoming dysfunction, but on how to facilitate sexual growth and satisfaction.

Sex Matters for Women: A Complete Guide to Taking Care of Your Sexual Self is still a self-help book with a unifying theme: sexuality is an essential part of every woman's identity. No matter what your age or cultural background, your sexual health and satisfaction require knowledge, self-awareness, and a willingness to embrace your sexuality. Through accurate information, examples from the lives of other women, and detailed self-help exercises, this book can help you. We use disguised composites of individuals and couples based on our many years of listening and learning.

In this book, we cover five important ways for you to take care of your sexual self:

• *Knowing your sexual story.* Your history influences your sexuality throughout your life. It has shaped your sexual attitudes and identity and affects how you respond sexually as an adult. Whether straight, lesbian, queer, or questioning, by understanding your personal story and the impact it has had on your sexuality, you're better able to take charge in the present. In Part I we discuss how childhood, adolescent, and adult experiences can impact your sexuality. We examine the era in which you came of age and the way it influenced your sexual development.

- *Understanding your body.* Understanding your body and how it functions helps you develop a positive sexual identity and gain greater comfort with sexual behavior. In Part II you'll find new research on women's sexual health and detailed, user-friendly information about anatomy, hormones, and sexual functioning.

- *Making peace with your body.* Body image has a dramatic impact on a woman's sexual identity. Cultural messages about the importance of being youthful, shapely, thin, or light-skinned can prevent a woman from feeling sexually desirable and, in turn, sexual desire. Learning to feel empowered by your physical appearance, coming to terms with your uniqueness, and feeling comfortable in your body can contribute to a healthy sexual identity. Accepting your body can be complicated if you've been sexually abused, have vaginal pain, contracted a sexually transmitted infection (STI), or live with a serious illness or disability. In Part III, whether single or partnered, you'll gain insights and learn strategies to help you move from hurt to sexual resilience.

- *Creating a better sexual relationship.* Most women are curious about ways to make relationships more meaningful. Regardless of orientation, women are interested in good sex with their partners, sex that both can enjoy. To create such a relationship, you will need skills in communicating, the ability to foster positive sexual experiences with your partner, and the savvy to avoid the pitfalls that typically beset long-term partnerships. If you're straight, you'll also benefit from understanding how your partner's sexual response may differ from your own. Part IV describes the steps that lead to a satisfying sexual relationship and provides suggestions to help you and your partner talk about your sex life together and experiment with ways to supercharge your lovemaking.

- *Developing sexual comfort, confidence, and satisfaction.* In Part V, the final section of the book, we discuss ways you can focus on your sexual health and relationship, giving advice and practical "go-to" exercises that put you in touch with yourself and your partner. You'll become more comfortable with touching, exploring, and enjoying your own body and that of your partner. Concerns about and causes of sexual problems such as low desire, lack of arousal, and inability to reach orgasm are discussed. Self-help techniques for overcoming these problems are provided, as is guidance for determining when sex therapy might be helpful and how to find a qualified therapist.

Sex Matters for Women is written by three sex therapists. We have worked with hundreds of women and their partners as they sought ways to take better care of their sexual selves. The stories we present in this book are composites of our clients' experiences. We think these examples are representative of the common themes we've encountered in our professional work. Above all, they reflect the remarkable effort that individuals take to make sense of their sexual lives.

Because the treatment of women's sexuality has not been one of the more cheerful aspects of human history, we've chosen to focus not on the discrimination, torment, and abuse that women have had to endure but instead on the stories of personal triumph, growth, and celebration of sexuality that serve as a testament to, and reminder of, women's resilience and strength. It's inevitable that we've overlooked or underappraised some aspects of women's sexuality, but we've tried to be sensitive to the many ways that women are sexual, to bring you the most up-to-date research, and to acknowledge the diversity of women's lives, orientation, and sexual choices. Although much of the book speaks of heterosexual relationships, lesbian relationships are discussed as well.

Writing this book has been an incredible experience for all three of us. We are grateful to many people for their support and inspiration along the way, especially the women who, over the years, have entrusted us with their care. Even for a writer there are some things that are very difficult to put into words. One of those things is the profound sense of respect that we hold for the people with whom we've worked. They've trusted us and allowed us to be part of their quest for greater self-understanding. In the end, it is they who have inspired us to write about women and sex. It is they who have taught us how much sex matters to them.

As you read this second edition of *Sex Matters for Women*, we encourage you to think about all the potential and possibilities for your sexual life. No matter your age, no matter your history or relationship status, the key to your sexuality is recognizing that it *matters* and striving to understand and grow comfortable with all *matters* in your life that are sexual. We hope our book inspires you to acknowledge and honor your own sexual story and to continue your journey of sexual growth.

PART I

Knowing Your Sexual Story

Are *you* comfortable with your sexual self? Many women instinctively answer "yes" until we ask more specific questions, such as: Do you feel at ease when you undress before your partner or stand naked in front of a mirror? Are you truly relaxed during lovemaking, able to focus on your body's sensations without distractions, worries, or guilt? Do you feel completely free to explore your sexuality, try new things, talk openly with your partner, and feel confident when educating your children about sex? Being comfortable with your sexuality means a lot more than just enjoying sex. It means all of the above and more. Discomfort, uncertainty, or confusion about any facet of your sexuality can have negative or limiting repercussions for *all* of your life, in all *parts* of your life.

In our experience, many women wrestle with myths and misconceptions about their sexuality and how it is formed. Today, at this very moment, your sexual attitudes, beliefs, and comfort level are the cumulative result of your past life experiences. How your early caregivers held you as an infant, how you made love with your partner last night, and countless experiences in between have helped shape how you now experience yourself as a sexual person. In addition to these life experiences, you have been continually exposed to mixed messages in your environment that have further shaped and influenced your sexual growth and development—messages that are shaped by your culture and the time period in which you come of age.

If sex matters to you, you may welcome the opportunity to review the sexual story that is such an important part of your life and to learn how other women have navigated the passages of sexual development. Upbringing that ignored sex or put it in a negative light, faulty sex education, confusing cultural messages about sex, constant exposure to media that foster dissatisfaction with real bodies, and double standards for men and women

5

are but a few of the challenges many women have faced and are still facing today. We have a lot to gain from the stories of women who have emerged from these challenges with a healthy, fulfilling sexuality.

If you have felt awkward, ashamed, distrustful, or inferior, coming to understand your sexual story can put you in a position to challenge the negative thinking that underlies these feelings. Realizing that your beliefs have been shaped by misinformation and cultural propaganda allows you to take steps to replace these faulty beliefs with accurate information. If you discover that sex intimidates you and that you hold back in sexual situations, you will be in a better position to experiment with new, more fulfilling behaviors. Once you know what is joyful, fulfilling, and inspiring to you as a sexual being, you will seek out similar ways to enhance your sexual growth.

To get from where you are to where you want to be, you need to know and understand your sexual story. In Chapters 1 and 2 we talk about how girls grow and develop sexually and common sexual experiences of adult women, both the challenges and the pleasures. We also talk about how different eras in history influence how a woman experiences her sexuality. Later in the book, in Chapter 13, there are exercises to help you reflect on your personal life story. We hope that these exercises and reflections will give you a clearer understanding of the factors that have shaped your sexuality and that, armed with these insights, you'll be able to make better use of the information and suggestions in the remainder of this book.

In Chapters 1 and 2 we look at common questions like these:

- "Is my attitude toward sex normal?"
- "Why do I keep making the same bad decisions about sex?"
- "At what age is masturbation normal?"
- "Why does it seem so much easier to *have* sex than to *talk* about it?"
- "Is there such a thing as too much sex education?"
- "Who decides what's sexy—me or my partner?"
- "How can I live by the values about sex that are important to me when everything around me says the opposite?"
- "Shouldn't the 'first time' be a romantic fantasy come true?"
- "How can I tell my daughter what's important about her sexuality when our generations seem to have such different priorities and values?"

ONE

Every Story Has a Beginning

Children are sexual beings from birth, and their adult sexuality is influenced by childhood experiences. In this chapter, we explore the common milestones of childhood and adolescence that impact a woman's sexuality. It's not our goal to write the definitive treatise on development and sexuality—entire books have been devoted to that theme (e.g., Zoldbrod, 1998). Instead, we want to provide you with the opportunity to reflect on how an important period in your life—the time between birth and young adulthood—influenced where you are today on your sexual journey so that you can better decide how you want to live your life now and in the future. The knowledge you gain may lead to a greater understanding of how you arrived where you are. It may also lead to your own sexual growth as a woman and greater satisfaction and pleasure in your life.

WHEN DOES THE STORY BEGIN?

Annie raced back home after playing with Jack and Sean. She dumped her things in her fort, a place she had constructed of plywood and old junk. She tried not to step on the tiny row of lilac bushes her mother had planted in front of the fort in a futile attempt to disguise her daughter's shack.

Eight years old today, Annie sat down and rested under the pine tree. Her shirt felt sweaty and sticky; she pulled it off and leaned back on the rough bark, scratching a few choice places as she relaxed. Just last summer her mom had made her start wearing a shirt all the time. Jack and Sean didn't have to wear shirts on hot summer days. But Annie's mother had told her that girls were different—they had to cover up their chests once they were in grade school because girls were "developing."

Annie didn't want to "develop." She wanted to move on hot summer days like the boys did. After all, she could run faster and climb higher than

Jack and Sean—why wasn't she allowed to be just as free? Annie decided that when she grew up she would live where she could take off her T-shirt whenever she wanted. Annie sighed and looked around her. This pine tree fort was Annie's favorite place in her backyard, and late afternoon was her favorite time of day. Drawing her knees up to her chest, she wrapped her arms around them and rested her head there. She breathed in and smelled the piney smell, then rubbed her face across her forearm. She thought how much she loved her body. She liked how her skin was so taut and smooth across her bones. She examined those tiny hairs that grew on her arms. She rubbed her cheek against them, feeling her skin's smoothness underneath that soft, fuzzy hair. Then she smelled her skin. More than anything, Annie loved these private, special smells of her body. She thought the skin on her forearm smelled the best: a clean, sweet smell that was all hers. She slid her hands along her legs and arms, scratched where a pine needle poked her in the neck, and then stood up and rubbed her hands over her body, making her feel cool and shivery. She looked down at her chest. There, too, her skin was smooth. There were few hairs to see, and her nipples were flat and round and pink and interested her.

Looking down at her body, Annie felt for the bones just under the skin and watched as her breath made her stomach suck in and out. Her ribs disappeared and reappeared. The muscles on her chest seemed to spread all the way out to her arms. She tightened her fist and flexed her arm like a strongman. The muscle bulged. *Boy, I'm strong!* she thought.

Annie was an 8-year-old girl, an explorer, and at that moment, a person at peace with her body and herself.

When does a woman's sexual story begin? The first time she makes love? The moment she discovers orgasm? Puberty?

A woman's sexual story starts in infancy and continues throughout her life. Early childhood experiences that most people would never consider sexual are, in fact, fundamental to being a sexual person. Young Annie, reveling in the wonders of her body, is learning to become a sexual person because she's learning how to live in her body, how to be at peace with herself, and how to find pleasure from her senses. Each of these discoveries is part of a lifelong sexual journey.

EARLY CHILDHOOD

Even during the first years of life, a girl's sexuality is being shaped and scripted. Biology assigns her gender, but it is people around her who quickly assign her the role that is supposed to go with that gender—a role that will influence how she views and values herself and how she will relate to others for years to come. During these earliest years she also will learn whether she can trust other people to love her and to respect her body and her emerging sexuality. The foundation for bonding and trust is established even before a child takes her first steps. Finally, as an infant and toddler, a girl will make important discoveries about her body that will influence her self-acceptance and her capacity to experience pleasure well into her adult years.

It's a Girl!

Sociologists have studied the reactions adults have to newborn babies. By the time babies are 1 minute old, they are treated differently depending on their sex. Think about the observations that people make: "Look at those delicate fingers." "Such big, strong hands!" "Check out the size of those feet!" Actually, most newborns look remarkably alike. But right from the beginning, people viewing a newborn will respond differently depending on the baby's gender. Parents will hold a girl more gently and speak to her more softly than with a baby boy.

This pattern continues as a baby girl grows into a toddler and begins exploring her world. If a little girl takes a tumble while running, she'll be consoled more quickly and allowed to cry about it longer than if she were a little boy. She'll be held more often than a boy toddler. And girl toddlers are often encouraged to be gentler and less aggressive than boys, and to get along and resolve conflicts quickly.

While the seeds of many wonderful attributes—such as sensitivity, nurturing, and an orientation toward cooperation and constructive problem solving—will be implanted by the age of 4 or 5, so will the seeds of characteristics that conform to the dictates of cultural sexism, myths, and double standards—such as the emphasis on being "nice" and "good," pretty and thin, and using clothes, jewelry, or makeup as a way of drawing attention. These characteristics may make it difficult to separate self-worth from personal appearance. They may also make adult relationships more complex because a woman's traditional gender role and identity may conflict with her attempts to gain autonomy, be assertive, and act competently. They may make the natural desire to enjoy sexual passion difficult because "good girls don't do that." Perhaps you can relate to what one woman told us:

> "Sometimes when I get really turned on during sex, I want to moan and thrash about because it feels so great. But I don't—I keep hearing my mom's voice saying, 'That's not what classy women do. That's trashy.'"

Peekaboo: Where Trust Begins

An important part of our sexuality is how comfortably we relate to a partner. The abilities to bond, to trust, and to freely touch and be touched are essential for a successful sexual relationship, and the foundation of these abilities is established in infancy. Even before a baby girl can speak, she's spoken to. Even before she can hug, she's hugged. Children's earliest experiences are shaped by their adult caregivers. When the child is hungry or in distress, she cries. If a parent or caretaker responds and tends to the child's needs, a foundation of trust is formed. If parents treat a baby with love, nurturance, and respect, the baby receives important information not only about trusting others but also about self-worth. Because her needs are met, she feels important and valued. And by feeling valued by others, she learns to value herself. Without early nurture and loving touch, a girl may grow up wary of trusting others, uncomfortable with physical contact, or feeling unworthy and unlovable. One woman recalled:

> "My parents came from the 'old school' of parenting—let your child cry herself to sleep, don't hold a baby too much, make a child independent as quickly as possible. They never touched or hugged me. It's made it hard for me, as an adult woman, to feel comfortable being in close contact with other people. I cringe when friends hug me, and even though I like sex, I don't like cuddling before or after."

Junior Scientists in Action

Our bodies are the epicenter of our sexuality. It is by means of our bodies that we experience sexual pleasure and connect with other people. This relationship between our bodies, pleasure, and connecting with others begins within minutes of birth. Sucking is the child's first experience of satisfaction. Whether breast-fed or bottle-fed, the child derives pleasure from her mouth, and this pleasure is associated with close physical contact with the parent or caregiver. This association between physical contact with another person and pleasure derived from the body becomes the basis for all future sexual relationships.

Later, a girl makes further discoveries about her body's ability to produce pleasure. During early childhood, children are junior scientists. They love to learn and explore. They are naturally curious about themselves and their world. One woman recalled:

> "When I saw a woman nursing her baby, my mom did a great job of explaining breast-feeding to me. But when I came home and tried to get my baby doll to suck my breast, she freaked out."

This curiosity includes their bodies. After all, children spend an enormous amount of time trying to learn how to do things in their bodies, from potty training to tying shoes, from skipping to whistling. It's normal and natural for children, girls and boys alike, to explore their own bodies with all their senses: sight, hearing, touch, taste, and smell. Part of that exploration will include their genitals. They will touch themselves for the pleasure of it. This isn't sexually stimulating in the erotic way that adults might think of it. Rather, it is a normal expression of interest and an experience of pleasure in a part of the body that feels good when touched. Many women remember playing in the bathtub as little girls and touching and looking at their genitals.

"Look What I Found!"

Little girls are at a disadvantage compared with little boys in developing long-term familiarity with their genitals. Little boys have "outies"—their penis is right there for them to explore, stroke, and tug. If a small girl attempts to probe her vagina in an exploratory way, her parent will most likely interrupt her and make it clear that she shouldn't do this. Little girls are far less clear about the source of their plea-sure because they have "innies." They probably have no idea that the pleasure they feel when rubbing their vulva comes from their clitoris, a part of their body largely unseen and, in all likelihood, unnamed. They may have been told that they have a vagina, but that's a part of their body they don't have ready access to, and it will be years before it will become fully biologically functional.

She may not know what to call it, but free of parental shaming or restrictions, a little girl will quickly learn that touching and rubbing her vulva can be very pleasur-able. It's natural and normal that she will want to reproduce these pleasant feelings, especially for the purpose of self-soothing or pleasant sensation. She may touch herself to settle into sleep or when she is nervous or bored.

> "Even now, in my 60s, I can still remember the pleasure I got from mastur-bating as a little girl. I would go to bed and tuck my hand between my legs and rock back and forth until I fell asleep. Before sex was arousing, it was soothing."

When this natural curiosity and self-pleasuring is allowed to occur without shame or embarrassment, the child has a fairly good start toward developing a healthy sexuality. Unfortunately, a girl can receive a message that her body is shame-ful and that genital pleasuring is bad at the same time she is discovering that it feels good to touch her vulva. All too often these messages are carried into adulthood and influence many women's sexual experiences.

Where do these messages come from? How does a little girl pick up negative attitudes about her body and genital pleasure?

"Shame on You!"

> "I remember I was watching TV and idly rubbing my vulva because it felt good. My mom came into the room, saw me, and screamed. I thought some-one had died. What 'died' was my interest in pleasuring myself."

Consider what happens when a little girl is caught rubbing her vulva or exploring her vagina. All too often parents react with anger or embarrassment. Not surprisingly, the girl associates touching her vulva with upsetting people and doing something wrong. All children rely on adults for love, and if faced with the fear of displeasing her parents, a young girl will readily give up the good feelings that come from touching herself so that she can hold on to parental approval. She will deny her own pleasurable experience because she's too young to determine that her parents are wrong; her connection to her parents at this stage of life is stronger than her connection to pleasuring her body.

Sometimes parents' reactions aren't meant to shame but to protect. Children must learn that orifices—ears, noses, vaginas, and anuses—aren't meant to have things put into them. But some parents go overboard by promoting a "hands-off" approach to the genitals. It's normal for a young child to ask questions about sex, to explore her genitals, and to be curious about other children's genitals. Because masturbation is a healthy part of development, forbidding or punishing self-pleasuring makes no more sense than forbidding a child to read books or punishing a child for eating healthy food.

What's in a Name?

Do you remember the names you were given for your genitals? Were they even *remotely* close to the accurate names for the vulva, clitoris, or vagina? Girls pick up negative attitudes about their bodies and their sexuality in a number of subtle ways. When parents refer to a girl's genitals as her "wee-wee," "tinkle," or "place down there," a girl is left wondering, *Why don't people like talking about that part of my body?* It's a small leap from this kind of thinking to *My body must be shameful or bad because no one mentions it.*

It isn't just that adults aren't comfortable teaching children the accurate names of genitals, but that most wouldn't know what to do if the children were to start using them.

> "When I was three, my mom told me all the names of my genitals. I was so proud I wanted to tell everybody. I showed my genitals to my friend Evan, pointing and naming. Then he showed me his, and we named them together. I still remember the feel of his penis when I touched it. When Grandma came over later in the day, I enthusiastically asked her if she had a vulva just like mine!"

Even adult women struggle to have open conversations with each other or their healthcare providers regarding questions or comments about their vulvas and vaginas. Recall that Oprah Winfrey playfully created the euphemism "vajayjay" on her daytime talk show and many women enthusiastically embraced the term, relieved to finally have a shared cultural slang term that is neither childlike ("pee pee") nor shadowed with disrespect ("cunt").

"Don't Forget to Wipe!"

Most of us don't remember toilet training, but we do have our "habits" in the bathroom, habits that often got an early start. Little girls are usually toilet trained differently from little boys. They miss out on the thrill of arching their stream at a floating target but instead are expected to sit quietly and to take thorough steps to wipe themselves clean afterward. The strong emphasis on staying clean after voiding can reinforce a notion that there must be something dirty about their genitals. One woman remarked that every time she got aroused, her underpants would get wet with discharge, and she'd feel embarrassed about "messing her panties." Another woman reported feeling like she has to thoroughly wash her genitals before sex with her partner, afraid that her natural smell is "dirty."

Private Property

As children grow, so does their need for privacy. While 3-year-olds want to show off what they did in the toilet, 7-year-olds want to be alone in the bathroom. There is a natural, increasing desire to be private about one's body. Most of the time this is what kids also see modeled in their homes. Mom and Dad request privacy for toileting, bathing, dressing, and other personal times. A child initiates her own need for privacy as she grows. Women recall very different experiences.

> "I was a wild, intense little girl, very high-spirited. My parents had to work with me to close bathroom doors. I'd masturbate in the living room 'til my mom helped me finally understand the difference between 'public' and 'private.'"

> "I was a painfully shy girl. I'd undress in my closet because I didn't want anyone to see me in my underwear. Annual trips to the doctor's office were agony. I could only get through them if my mom stayed right with me the whole time."

> "I live on my own, and because of a physical disability, I have a personal attendant to help me with toileting and bathing. As a girl, my mom did all that. You have a different relationship with your mom when you're arguing about whether you can watch *an R-rated movie* at the same time she's wiping your butt and changing your menstrual pad."

It's important for a child to learn about privacy and modesty, but often the lesson can go too far and a girl learns to associate nakedness with shamefulness. Some women report that they can't undress in front of their partners because they feel ashamed of their bodies; too flat, too fat, too tall, too short. Other women say they don't want to let anyone, not even their partner, see their vulvas; too "ugly."

Caught in the Act

Did you ever have the experience of walking in on your parents while they were having sex? Those moments when a child catches the parents in the act of lovemaking can also reinforce negative ideas about sexuality. It's not that the child sees the parents naked but that the parents' reaction to being discovered can confuse and frighten the child. If the parents react with panic and anger, such as diving under the covers and yelling for the child to leave the room, the child could conclude that her parents are up to no good.

Notice in the examples above how negative attitudes were reinforced not by abusive parents, sexual trauma, or emotionally impoverished environments but by normal parents relying on common, almost universal, child-rearing practices. Most parents do the best they can, and they too are products of a culture that views sexuality with suspicion and wariness. As a result, this suspicion and wariness is passed along to children at a very early age.

PREPUBERTY: THE AGE OF MASTERY AND MYSTERY

A school-age child knows there is a whole world beyond her home and family, a world in which she is not the center but only one of many players, and in which people other than her parents—teachers and peers—are important influences. She must figure out how she fits into this bigger world and how to thrive in it.

This is the age of mastery: "What can my body do?" "How fast can I run?" "Can I ride a bike?" "Do I know all my 'times tables'?" "Do the other kids like me?" At school, there are countless opportunities for testing mastery by comparing and contrasting. Fitting in is the all-important quest; being excluded or feeling different or inferior can be traumatic. If things go badly, a young girl may feel she did something wrong—even if the circumstances are out of her control. Because she failed to master the situation, she feels responsible. This is especially true if a girl is sexually abused. She may feel she is responsible for the abuse, that it was somehow her fault. This may also occur if a girl is teased about her size or how she looks. She may feel that she is a failure.

Long after they've grown up, women remember the painful experiences of childhood when they felt responsible yet utterly powerless. Instead of mastery, they remember misery. This may affect how they feel about their sexuality as adult women.

"When I was young, my older sister made me dress up and 'model' all my school clothes each year. Then she critiqued how I looked. It was agony. To this day, I hate to shop."

"At family reunions, our older boy cousins would grab us little girls and feel our bottoms and flat chests. We'd scream and everybody else would laugh. I still hate to be held."

"Because I was heavier, I got teased a lot at school. I couldn't run very fast in gym, and the kids called me 'chubbette' and 'tiny.' I've never stopped being sensitive about weight. I don't like to be naked during sex because I don't want my partner to see my body."

"That's Gross; Tell Me More"

For the most part, during the early school years girls are not very interested in the mystery of sexual behavior. Sexual feelings and curiosity are largely submerged, with an emphasis instead on accomplishment and social skills. This does not mean that sex is entirely ignored. School-age girls masturbate and can be orgasmic. Mild same-sex play is not unusual or abnormal, and many women remember some "show and tell" games or peeking at each other's changing bodies. You may remember being curious about sex and feeling dissatisfied with the sex education you received at school. Perhaps you prowled around your parents' bedroom looking for information about sex, or eavesdropped on the conversations of your older siblings, or got online and onto sex sites on the web.

> Nine-year-old twins Ruth and Hannah giggled as they looked at their parents' book on sex. "It looks like a hairy mouth," Ruth whispered, pointed to a drawing of a woman's vagina, then burst into nervous laughter.
> "You think that's weird, look at the man's thing," Hannah said, flipping through the pages, then stopping to stare at the drawing of a couple having intercourse.
> "I would never do that to have a baby," Ruth declared.
> "Me neither," answered Hannah, "but let me show you the picture of their butts. . . . "

Girls may react to sexual information in many different ways before entering puberty. Some women remember feeling uninterested or annoyed by this intrusion on their childhood. Others thought sexuality was fascinating and exotic. Some women recall that they were upset by the information and mourned that, as girls, their bodies would have to change, that menstrual periods would be monthly, and that they'd have to grow up and have "sexual relations." If the subject of sex was treated differently from other family topics, some women, mimicking their parents, learned never to discuss sex or confront sexual issues.

Unfortunately, for some girls lessons about sexuality don't come from innocent curiosity or parental instruction but from terrifying firsthand experience. One of every four girls is sexually victimized in childhood. For many of these girls, their victimization will sensitize them to sex in disturbing ways. Some will desperately avoid sexual talk and recoil if anyone attempts to touch them. Others will become sexually preoccupied and provocative, reenacting their own exploitation. They may say sexy things excessively or persistently masturbate in public areas of the house. They may be too sexual in their play responses with other kids.

If a woman was sexually abused as a girl, knowing her own sexual story will require grieving and courage. Most adult survivors of childhood sexual abuse find counseling an important part of healing. Chapter 10 may help you address any childhood losses related to sexual trauma.

PUBERTY: A GIRL FROM THE INSIDE OUT

By the time hormonal levels begin to change, a girl in her preteen years has come a long way from her junior scientist days of exploring her world with abandon and her fourth-grade days of trying to master everyone's social schedule. She will head into puberty approximately *24 months* ahead of the boys in her class. With the onset of puberty, she begins a phase during which she's more aware of herself as being separate from others. On the surface, she has friends and loves school and all the social activities. But under the surface, she is discovering more about herself and is trying to come to terms with the changes taking place in her body.

Invasion of the Body Snatchers

The time period from 10 to 12 years of age covers a lot of territory in a girl's development. As she begins to undergo changes in her hormones, her body will change also. Pubic hair may appear. She may have breast buds as early as age 8. The onset of menstruation can be as early as 9 or 10 or as late as 16 or 17. The average age is 11 or 12 years old.

The first period is called *menarche*. Typically this is experienced as a rite of passage, marked by pride mingled with some anxiety. Cultural slang like "being on the rag" can create negative attitudes about a girl's body. It is within this context that a girl faces the challenge of learning to relate to her body and her sexual parts in a healthy manner.

A woman may remember not only when she started her period but also where she was, what she was doing, and her first immediate rush of feelings. She remembers whether her mother and other women prepared her for this first period. She may feel sadness if she was not helped with this entry into puberty. Perhaps she remembers feeling confused, even angry, with her body for betraying her into adulthood.

> "I was at my friend's at a sleepover when my period started. I had no idea what was happening. My mother never spoke of menstruation and acted angry when I showed her my stained underpants."

> "I remember when my period started, I was at summer camp. I looked down and saw the brown spot on my bathing suit. Fifty years later, I can still recall that I felt a rush of excitement and thrill. But I was scared because it seemed such a permanent change."

> "When my period started, I wanted to avoid the whole thing. I went around ignoring it for three days, wadding up my bloody underwear and stuffing them under my bed. My mom had to come and talk to me. The whole thing made me anxious."

A girl may feel out of control because of all that is happening to her body. Although there may be pride and excitement about physical changes, she may grieve that her body is no longer familiar to her. Breasts can be so tender that it hurts to be bumped or jostled. Menstruation can be accompanied by painful cramps. Oily pores and hair need constant attention, and acne can seem like leprosy. Some girls become plump and round, while others appear all feet, elbows, and limbs.

Mothers and daughters face an important milestone at this point. A mother's discomfort with her own body and menstruation may cause her to react with disgust when her daughter enters menarche. Researchers are now studying these negative attitudes toward menstruation and how they can create a disconnection between mothers and daughters, a disconnection that hurts a girl's sexual health and development (Stubbs & Costos, 2004).

Unfortunately, peers can also ridicule, and teasing—about large breasts or small breasts, being too thin or not thin enough—can be so cruel and unrelenting during this vulnerable stage that, years later, a young woman may still hate her body due to these early experiences. Embarrassment and self-criticism over body changes during puberty can impact a woman's self-image well into adulthood. A mother's, aunt's, or grandmother's positive reassurance is extremely important to a girl's development.

"Leave Me Alone"

With puberty comes a heightened interest in sexuality. Girls may experiment with smutty jokes and vulgar language, often as a way of drawing attention from others. In the privacy of their own rooms, many girls masturbate during these years. Self-discovery, self-pleasuring, and even orgasm are normal parts of this stage of development. Finding time to be alone and explore their bodies is important.

Tamecca liked to be alone in her room. She'd lock her door and, in total privacy, touch herself. Using a mirror, she'd look at her genitals. She liked to rub her clitoris, especially when she lay on her stomach. She would place her hand cupped against her vulva and rub back and forth. Sometimes while rocking like this she would feel more excited and tension-filled. She'd rock harder until she had a tingly, pulsing sensation in her genitals. She didn't know that what she was doing was called *masturbation*—she simply thought of it as her special, private time.

Sometimes Tamecca thought about a famous movie star when she was touching herself. She was beginning to fantasize, and imagining herself grown up and involved with him made her feel even more excited when she masturbated.

Tamecca thought her genitals were lovely. She liked all the colors of her skin in her vulva. When she pulled back her labia, she could see her vagina, making it open and close by tensing her muscles.

When changing clothes, Tamecca noticed that her underpants sometimes had dried white mucus on them. Her mom explained that it was normal and called it "discharge." The next time she was alone, she reached her finger a little way inside her vagina and felt the wetness; it was moist, like the inside of her mouth. She pulled out her finger and brought it to her nose, breathing in the musty, comforting smell of her vagina. When she tasted the wetness on her finger, it was a little disappointing, a little chalky and bland. Nevertheless, she felt that she had the most interesting body ever made.

Leaving Childhood

As a girl enters puberty, she may alternate (sometimes rapidly) between extreme sociability and intense solitariness. In the years to come, she will no doubt learn how to handle her own unique emotional coloring. In her current daily life, however, she has had no prior experience with such intense moods, no language yet to describe what she is feeling. Physiology seems to have taken over what was once a familiar mastery of her body. She may feel that she fits in neither the world of children nor that of adolescents. It is a time in between the two, and some girls feel nostalgia for childhood even when they still seem like children.

On a quiet summer day just before seventh grade, Annie headed to her fort. The lilac bushes, now taller than Annie, partially hid the old fort's warped and weathered boards. Annie crouched and ducked under the branches, surprised that she could no longer stand in her old hiding place. How small it seemed.

Reaching out, she pulled on the boards closest to her; they came apart with only a little tugging. Knowing it was time, Annie solemnly took the fort apart, her strong arms easily stacking the lumber aside, until only the branches of the pine tree sloped vacantly to the ground. The emptiness made her nervous, and she wanted to get away from what had once been her sanctuary.

Young girls approaching their teen years are becoming biologically mature and capable of reproduction. Their gender role and identity have been established. For better or worse, they are imbued with attitudes and beliefs about sexuality that will influence their sexual comfort and satisfaction for years to come. What they do not have is the life experience and the emotional maturity that will help them integrate their biology, gender role, and sexual beliefs into a balanced, wholesome sense of being a sexual person. Much of this necessary experience and the time to mature further will occur in their next stage of life—adolescence.

ADOLESCENCE

We are fascinated by adolescence. This stage of life is the subject of countless books, the focal point of hundreds of movie and TV plots, and the topic of constant commiseration among parents. Perhaps this is because adults look back on this period as a poignant time in life. Teens need reminders that their struggles are not unique, and preteens look forward to the excitement of this major turning point. It is during these years that girls (and boys) make startling discoveries about sex, struggle with self-esteem, develop crushes, and are crushed by rejection. It is a time that helps define who we are, how we relate to others, and how we experience ourselves as sexual people.

An adolescent girl is a young woman, and she quickly learns that sex can be incredibly complex and perplexing. Some young women are cautioned against any partnered sexual exploration and warned that, if they get pregnant, they'd better not come home. Some hear this threat so young, they don't even know how pregnancy occurs. Young women are told that looking sexy means they're "asking for it" at the same time that fashion proclaims bare midriffs and spandex are the "it" clothing. Some young women are sexually abused by family members who claim they asked for it. Some are told they will burn in hell if they feel any sexual urges. But they're *not* told what they're supposed to do with the strong, hormone-driven sexual feelings they are already having in their bodies.

A complex matrix of factors defines adolescent sexuality. Internal and external forces interact with a young woman's sexual experiences in ways that can be both confusing and profound. These factors will influence how an adult ends up experiencing herself as a sexual person: whether she is comfortable, confident, and sexually satisfied. Most of us don't perceive this process as it unfolds and don't have any idea how we became the sexual beings we are today. Looking back on the factors at work in adolescent sexuality can help us see whether where we are today is where we want to be and, if not, which factors in our adult sexual lives we might address.

Biology

"I'm too tall and geeky looking."
"My boobs and hips are huge."
"Everyone hates me."
"No one thinks I'm pretty."

During adolescence, a young woman undergoes significant biological changes that affect her appearance, emotions, self-esteem, and self-confidence. Most young women's periods have begun, although it's still normal for menstruation to begin as late as 16 or 17. Breast development continues, height can shoot up, and oily skin makes life miserable. Sudden mood shifts only add to the inner turmoil.

Prior to puberty, children are curious about their bodies, responsive to pleasurable genital sensations, and aware of sexual taboos surrounding them. But during adolescence, sex becomes up-close and personal. A young woman is no longer merely curious about sex; she is often drawn to it, fascinated by it, afraid of it. She suddenly has physical sensations that go beyond mere genital tingling. She finds herself drifting into daydreams and fantasies that excite her. She finds herself so attracted to other people, both men and women, that at times she can't take her mind off them. These new experiences are very different from childhood ones of playing doctor, sneaking a peek at nude pictures, or giggling over new sexual information. This is the real thing—adult sexuality is becoming biologically hard-wired into a young woman's body *and* psyche.

This heightened sexual awareness has a disquieting impact on a young woman, especially in early adolescence, when self-awareness steadily increases. Nakedness becomes both fascinating and scary; a young adolescent woman in a bathing suit can be a mass of nervous energy—giggling, silly, and anxious. Because most early teens don't feel in command of their fluctuating sexual awareness and physical sensations, they often confuse sexual feelings with feelings of affection and love. As a result, one minute a young teen can hug Mom and Dad with abandon because she loves them, and the next minute she recoils from any touch because it feels weird. *Nothing* feels predictable anymore.

Self-Esteem

Barbara ducked into the school bathroom and squeezed her way to the mirror. Her thick, bushy red hair never seemed to lie flat. Next to her, Keisha wasn't any happier as she tried to tame a wandering wave of her own soft black hair. They both glanced enviously at Beth, who was smoothing her long straight blond hair over her shoulders.

I'd give anything to look like that, Barbara thought to herself.
Beth muttered under her breath, "I look like a freak."

"What are you talking about?" Keisha asked, dumbfounded. "Beth, you always look *perfect*."

"No, I have these bumps on my head where my ears stick out under my hair. Look, you can see it in the mirror." Beth tried to flatten her ears with her hands. "I feel like Dumbo."

The bell rang, and a dozen teens heaved their backpacks on their shoulders and left the bathroom for class, preparing to do another day of internal battle with their own critical voices.

Teenagers compare themselves to the standards of beauty they see in advertising and the media. Even with more than 40 years of accumulated benefits of Title IX and a plethora of strong female role models, many adolescent women still place more value on appearance than on competence, intelligence, or accomplishment. They struggle with self-scorn, convinced their bodies just don't measure up.

A young woman's self-esteem affects her sense of sexuality. As a child, a girl might have been comfortable in her body, touching herself and masturbating without awkwardness or discomfort. Now when masturbating, physical sensations have to break through a barricade of self-criticism. A girl rubs her skin and wishes it were darker or lighter. She slides her fingers over her vulva and is distracted, thinking other girls have prettier thighs than hers. If she looks at her breasts, she feels disgust over their size or shape. After this sort of once-over, it's a wonder she has any pleasurable sensations whatsoever.

Self-esteem can impact sexual development in other important ways. A young woman who lacks confidence and feels self-conscious about her body may pull away from opportunities to socialize and "hang out." As a result of her shyness, she misses out on opportunities to develop social skills, one of the building blocks for later success in relationships. A young woman struggling with self-esteem issues may engage in sexual behavior that is risky and beyond her ability to manage, believing that being sexually accommodating is the only way she can possibly land a boyfriend. Another young woman may be so worried about the feelings of attraction she is having for other females that she throws herself at guys in a frantic attempt to figure out her orientation. These young women run the risk of carrying into adulthood sexual attitudes marred by feelings of shame, confusion, and resentment.

The relationship between self-esteem and sexuality goes both ways. Not only does a young woman's self-esteem affect her sexual comfort and growth, but sexual experience also can influence her self-esteem. A lack of sexual information, a teen pregnancy, sexual victimization, or confusion over sexual orientation can lead to self-criticism and self-condemnation that follows a young woman into her adult years.

What does it mean to be a woman? Girls bring different notions of womanhood into adolescence, notions formed with the help of various models, both positive and negative. As teenagers, their understanding of what it means to be female evolves. The value of appearance learned in early childhood takes on new power. Young women know that being "hot" is power, but what does that have to do with their own feelings of sexuality, their own understanding of sexual satisfaction?

It's also during the teen years when cultural, ethnic, and other messages about female sexuality become mixed and complicated. On one hand teenage girls are told that women are powerful and competent, and on the other they learn the dramatic lesson that they are in danger simply because of their gender. Women have vivid memories of their first experiences with their sexual vulnerability.

> "At 16, I remember going to a pro basketball game with friends. In the parking lot, these drunk guys wouldn't leave us alone. They harassed us, calling us 'cunt' and 'sweet ass' and words I've never heard before or since."

> "I was at the mall by myself. In a crowded elevator, this man started rubbing my bottom. I was terrified but afraid to say anything. I know it doesn't make sense, but I thought I must have done something terribly wrong to be picked on by him."

> "I was dating this guy who got mean when he was drunk. One night he raped me. I didn't tell my parents because I was afraid they'd be mad at me for drinking, too."

There is a point in every girl's or woman's life when she feels bad about having a body that is noticed in an exploitative way. For some girls, it happens very young and may include sexual abuse. Although it is not her fault, a young woman feels ashamed of herself for being noticed. She thinks she must have done something wrong to "invite" this attention. Her sexuality seems wrong because it's noticed in a way that robs her of her control over her own body.

When women recall these events from their childhood, it's always with sadness. It is one of the reasons sexuality is far more complex, at a much earlier age, for women than it is for men. An adolescent girl may be told that sex is special and wonderful *and* that she must be on her guard against date rape and stranger rape. She may encounter adults who treat her lovingly, then turn around and slide their hands over her breasts and buttocks. It's a cruel discovery for young girls that they are vulnerable solely because of their gender. It's equally cruel that they will have to carry into their adult years a sense of vigilance and suspicion that can interfere with their capacity to love and experience life with a sense of abandon and joy.

As sex therapists, we often talk with women about their childhood memories of loss—the loss of innocence, protection, and the right to grow safely in their sexuality. These experiences are traumatic and can cast a dark shadow on sexual development. If these kinds of experiences happened to you, Chapter 10 may help you.

Gender Identity and Sexual Orientation

In recent years there has been increased public awareness about sexual minorities including "transgendered" and "intersexed" men and women, conditions in which a person's gender identity is different from the anatomical, genetic, and hormonal composition of her or his body, or when someone is born with both female and male chromosomal, anatomic, or hormonal characteristics. There are also individuals who do not believe that any gender or orientation should be used to capture their development and experiences, and they may prefer the term *queer* as a positive alternative to categorizing themselves. For more information about these gender identities, check the listings under "Lesbian, Bisexual, Transgender, Queer, and Intersex" in the "Suggested Resources" at the back of the book.

An important part of identity is sexual orientation. It's often during the adolescent years that lifelong sexual interests and sexual orientation emerge, although a woman may not acknowledge these interests or orientation until later in life. Many of the themes found in an adult woman's sexual fantasies originate during her teen years. It's in the adolescent's fantasies that she meets her desired sexual partner and experiences her ideal of romantic encounters. As a young woman explores her sexuality, first in fantasy and later in relationships, she becomes aware of the range and content of her sexual interests. These interests evolve over time. A woman's sexuality unfolds gradually and most often in the context of feeling connected to another person. This may be another woman.

Sexual Orientation and Sexual Fluidity

Interest in same-sex relationships is not unusual and can occur at any age. In the early teen years, many girls who go on to have heterosexual relationships are first attracted to and fall in love with a girlfriend. Some college-age women "come out" as lesbian or bisexual. For some this is indeed their sexual orientation for a lifetime, but other women may go through a time of being out as gay or bi only to settle into a straight relationship later. The opposite is just as common: A woman will be in a long-term straight relationship and after a breakup find herself falling deeply, passionately in love with another woman.

Lisa Diamond's research into women's sexual fluidity is an important contribution to our understanding of a woman's sexual identity. Her work cautions against assigning "cookie-cutter" categories to the complexities of sexuality and sexual orientation (Diamond, 2008). She reminds us that both women's experiences and their development may run the gamut from fixed and stable early on to varying throughout life. Because both women and sexuality are complex, she encourages us to conceptualize orientation with multiple ways of being rather than adopt a fixed, rigid categorization. Defining orientation is not as easy as the question "Are you gay or straight?" would imply (Diamond, 2005).

At 12, in the seventh grade, Sophie fell in love with Stephanie. They talked nonstop about school, their friends, and sports. Though they occasionally still spent an afternoon making up stories for their Barbies, they did this with a certain self-consciousness, aware that childhood was behind them.

Sophie and Stephanie listened to music for hours. Sometimes they stood in front of a mirror and danced together. They liked practicing and took turns being the "boy" for the slow dances. "Stephanie and Sophie, Sophie and Stephanie . . . Best friends," wrote Sophie along the edges of her notebooks.

When they slept over at each other's house, they talked through the night, hugging each other so close together that their voices were barely whispers between them.

"Let's pretend we're kissing," Sophie said and closed her eyes. They pressed their mouths together, bumped noses, and giggled.

"Come on, try again," whispered Stephanie. This time, eyes open, they kissed and kissed.

The kissing practice happened many times, but they never spoke of it the next day. During the day, Sophie would roughhouse with Stephanie, or giggle and gossip. Sophie knew she had never loved anyone as much as she loved Stephanie.

Years later, when Sophie identified as a straight woman with a husband she loved deeply, she would think back to those adolescent days and smile about her first passionate love.

Most adolescents and even young adult women have intense romantic feelings for other females—they quite literally fall in love with their girlfriends. The touching and hanging on each other, even the kissing, caressing, and fondling that occur, are not definitive statements about a young woman's sexual orientation. Instead, these are early forays into having strong attachments outside the family group. Usually the focus in these relationships is not so much on sexual activity but on the intense love and attraction one has for another person. Whether one is straight or gay, this is normal behavior and an important precursor for adult relationships to come.

Sometimes the experience of first love turns out to be true love. For lesbian teens, early feelings of affection for other girls turn out not to be fleeting and experimental. Instead these teens experience a growing and ongoing awareness that they are sexually attracted to women, not men. In a culture that is still largely intolerant of sexual diversity, this discovery often remains private during adolescence. A lesbian teen may feel isolated and seek out places where she can be comfortably "out."

A young woman can talk to many friends about concerns related to her heterosexual activity, but if she is questioning her orientation, thinking she might be more attracted to women than men, she often feels that she has no one she can talk to. Support from other lesbian teens and mentoring from older lesbian women can help a young woman gain pride in who she is as a sexual person.

"When I hear the words 'coming out,' I think of *brief*, like it happens quickly. But for me, coming out was a long process, sometimes filled with terror about being found out, alternating with terror that *I* wouldn't find out about myself. I got through it with the help of some close friends and a lot of reading that I did."

In adolescence (and continuing into adulthood), sexuality is influenced by cultural attitudes, biological development, peer influence, sexual experience, and relationships. For women, sexual orientation is a blend of biology and experience. Some women knew early in childhood that they felt "different" and didn't aspire to the heterosexual relationships they saw around them. Many become much more aware of an attraction to women—or to both men and women—in adolescence, when sexual interest escalates. For most girls, at least in our experience, orientation is so straightforward and self-evident that they don't question it. They just know they're attracted to guys, and the world around them confirms what they feel inside. But for those who don't feel that way, discovering their orientation can be a long journey, one that, if you are still struggling with this issue as an adult, might be aided by the orientation exercise in Chapter 13 under "Ways to Know Your Sexual Story." If you feel that you may be lesbian or bisexual and are confused or disturbed by this discovery, make a conscious choice to respect your feelings and your choices and trust that your decisions are right for *you*. A wealth of resources are currently available for lesbians and bisexuals. We list many of these in "Suggested Resources" at the end of the book. Websites are also plentiful, and we suggest you spend time checking them out.

"I love that I'm lesbian. I'm happy in who I am and what I do. It surprises others around me when they find out I'm lesbian because there are so many stereotypes. You can't fit me in a box or under a label."

Ethnic and Cultural Identity

It is in adolescence that many girls become aware of how they are different, and how their families are different, from what they see on television or at the local mall. Ethnicity and color exert a powerful influence on our self-identity, beliefs, and values as we grow and develop. From inside your community came one set of messages about how you, as a young woman, were perceived. Outside your community, people may not have seen *you* at all, only your color or your ethnicity. From inside and out, your ethnicity and color affect your sense of sexuality.

"Dating was always hard in high school. If I dated non-Asians, my parents weren't pleased, and I'd have to fight myths like 'All Asian women are sexually exotic.' The Asian guys I dated found me too American—because my family has been in America for generations. I felt like I didn't fit any-where."

"We moved here from India when I was 14. I wasn't used to seeing so much female nakedness and pretend sexual passion on television. In India, there was more censorship. You might see two flowers intertwining or two birds with their beaks together to represent a sexual image. I was uncomfortable seeing so much sex here."

"When I was growing up, seeing how women of color were portrayed in the media made a real impression on me. It seemed they were always shown as hookers or unwed mothers. It became a point of pride for me to keep my sexual urges under control—I was going to prove the stereotypes wrong. Unfortunately, I think I got too good at keeping my sexual side buried."

In some cultures, it is typical for families to exercise control, directly or indi-rectly, over young women's sex lives—perhaps by restricting dating or requiring a daughter to live at home until married. These forms of control may seem incon-ceivable to outsiders. Nevertheless, they are long-standing traditions within some groups and are not easily opposed.

"Other than church activities, I didn't do anything with guys as a teenager. In my African American family, it just wasn't allowed. Even when I gradu-ated from high school and began to date, the weekly grilling from my rela-tives hardly made it worth the effort."

If you were raised in North America but your ethnic heritage included the cus-tom of parental involvement in your dating and partner choices, you had to decide if, or how strongly, you would oppose this practice. Looking back on your adolescence, you may have wanted to honor your parents' wishes but, at the same time, were influenced by the images of dating and romantic love you saw all around you. Your sexual development occurred in the context of conflicting worldviews.

"Growing up in my ethnic community, we weren't supposed to have pre-marital sex. I was curious about sexual activity but thought I was wrong to have thoughts about it. I wanted to ask my older sister, but she said women in our culture discussed these things only after they were married, and then only with their husbands."

"I remember the statue of the Blessed Virgin Mary in our living room. Grandma would always point to the statue and say to me, 'Benita, you must be pure like our mother Mary.' But it wasn't very easy to be pure and popular at the same time."

To know your sexual story, it's important to understand and appreciate your ethnic and cultural identity. In Chapter 13 we give you a chance to ask yourself questions about your color and ethnicity. The questions are designed to stimulate your thinking about your childhood and adolescence and the messages you've internalized about your sexuality.

Peer Pressure

"Don't you want to do it? Everybody is," Brenda said, smiling smugly at Kelly. "We've been doing it for a long time. Sometimes we sneak out during lunch hour to fool around in the parking lot."

Kelly giggled uncomfortably. "Aren't you worried about getting pregnant?"

"No," Brenda said. "I know when my period is. Sometimes he pulls out, too. He doesn't like condoms. We're cool about it. Besides, it makes our relationship so special to have sex, and we really love each other."

During adolescence peers often have more influence than parents on a teen's attitudes and behavior. Peer culture often condones and even encourages heterosexual sexual behavior under certain conditions. In some teen groups, sexual activity verifies the boy's masculinity and the girl's femininity. A young woman may feel she has status in the eyes of her friends if she does "sexual things" with her boyfriend. A couple may be expected to be sexual once they decide to see each other exclusively. Sex may serve as a sign that the couple has an exclusive relationship.

Sometimes there's a fine line in teen culture between a young woman finding peer acceptance and suffering peer scorn. Despite a sexual revolution that occurred long ago, a double standard still exists. Boys who are sexually active are almost universally applauded for their conquests. Girls who are sexually active still run the risk of being labeled "sluts," "blow job queens," or "friends with benefits." Years ago young women, regardless of age, were usually stigmatized if they were sexually active. Today adolescent attitudes have changed so that the good-girl–bad-girl dichotomy more often applies only to young women in junior high and early high school. Starting at around age 16, sexual behavior is more tolerated and even respected among peers, as long as the young woman is monogamous and doesn't "sleep around." But young women who mix sex, drugs, and alcohol are vulnerable to sexual abuse, multiple sexual partners, and an increase in sexually transmitted infections.

Peer pressure can be a double-edged sword. It can influence a young woman to have sex before she is ready and comfortable. It can also crucify her mercilessly if she does have sex. For some reason she is judged "easy" or a "slut." Many adult women, remembering how impossible it was to figure out what amount of sexual behavior was acceptable, still carry emotional wounds and even trauma inflicted by their peers during adolescence.

Sexual Experience

In adolescence, young women engage in sexual activity for many different reasons—out of curiosity, for the thrill and pleasure of sex, to win or retain someone's attention, to prove love, or to express affection. Adolescents have a growing ability to love another person and feel intimate. In this context, it feels natural to become more physically involved—kissing, touching, and even having intercourse. A young woman's sexual exploration often progresses from holding hands, to kissing and French kissing, to breast fondling, genital fondling, masturbating her partner, oral sex, and finally intercourse.

There is tremendous variability in sexual interest and activity among adolescent and young adult women. Many young women are sexually active but have never themselves masturbated to orgasm. Interestingly, many young women tell us that they are happy to "go down" on a guy or manually stimulate him to orgasm, but they express discomfort with his interest in giving her oral sex or masturbating her to orgasm. They tell us that they aren't into orgasm for themselves, either through masturbation or sexual activity with a partner. They like the thrill or power of giving sexual pleasure but aren't looking for the commitment of being on the receiving end. Many young women need more time than young men do to feel comfortable with their bodies and their sexuality before they're really interested in, or ready to take ownership of what they want for themselves.

For most young women, in their home, school, or religion, sexual activity is center stage in their moral world. Sometimes they even watch the value of abstinence or the virtue of measuring sexual response with caution and responsibility being promoted in the media. The decision to be sexually active is burdened not only by fear of being caught, becoming pregnant, or contracting a sexually transmitted infection, but also by the weight of guilt and shame. Many young women feel caught, trying to reconcile their sexual actions with their self-image of being good. Many give lip service to one set of values while living on the wilder side.

Being sexually active involves a great deal more than just intercourse, but intercourse remains a rite of passage in most cultures. "Passage into what?" many women might add, aware that for young men intercourse is a rite of passage into sexual maturity, whereas for young women intercourse is a rite of passage into loss of virginity. For males, the opportunities may open up, but for females, the choices may shut down. In a national poll of teens regarding their sexual activity, 65% of girls and 57% of boys who had sexual intercourse wished they had waited (Albert, 2010). By the time they graduated from high school, 46% of all high school students had had sexual intercourse (Grunbaum et al., 2004).

A young woman's first experience with sexual intercourse is often disappointing. Many women report that their first sexual experience, in retrospect, was one in which they felt either physically forced or emotionally coerced by the intimation that they might lose the love of their partner (Laumann et al., 1994). The first time rarely delivers that expected thrill and ecstasy implied by media images of sexual abandon and passion. Many young women feel let down by their first sexual experience and wonder "Is that all there is?"

Some women remember feelings of anger, doubt, guilt, and shame after their first intercourse. Although some experience physical discomfort or pain afterward, many feel they cannot ask their parents for help for fear of rejection or anger for having sex in the first place. This fear usually increases feelings of isolation and loneliness. A teenager may also experience her partner as being selfish and uncaring after sex. Even if the first intercourse is consensual, some young women report being treated roughly, with a lack of caring during the experience, and feel traumatized by the experience.

So, instead of pleasure and satisfaction, a young woman may feel stunned or numb after intercourse. Language captures the culture's lack of respect for women by describing a woman's first coitus as "losing her virginity" and a young man's as "scoring." Although some young women believe their status in their social group temporarily rises as a result of having had intercourse, over time many describe the experience ruefully as "giving up virginity" to gain social acceptance. Ultimately, we create a lose–lose environment for women. They are considered either virgin or slut, or must deny they had sexual activity. The denial leads to disconnecting from one's own experience of sexual pleasure and from the belief that sexual satisfaction is an important part of sexual health.

Sex Education

Many young women learn about sex in confusing ways that have no contexts and no parameters other than "Just say no" (from their parents) versus "Everybody's doing it" (from their peers). Even little girls want to buy makeup to look pretty, and preteens are portrayed in the media as sexy and hip. Young women see images of sex and passion selling everything from rock songs to rocking chairs. The biology lessons in school aren't even remotely related to what they are feeling in their own biology.

> "I have a great mom who has explained a lot to me about sex, and she helped me get on birth control when I got active with my boyfriend, but now I'm having a lot of pain with sex. I mean it 'burns' down there. I can't talk to my mom about that!"

> "Sure I had great sex education. I mean my parents grew up in the 1970s, so they are totally comfortable talking about everything. But I don't know how to have an orgasm, and that is like so not something I would tell them!"

"When I was a teenager, I didn't know much about sex. But I would have died before I asked my parents. I was sure I knew enough to take care of myself."

Most young women have difficulty admitting that they know very little about sexual behavior. Their knowledge of birth control and STIs is often confused and misinformed. Sex slang is vague and usually holds multiple meanings, thereby rendering the terms useless. When describing sexual activity, many young women don't even know the names of their genitals, their patterns of sexual response, and sexy alternatives to having penetrative sexual activity with a partner. Sadly, many young women have no idea how to decide what is "right and wrong" for them in sexual relations or how loving couples should behave toward one another. If you're reading this book as a parent, you may wonder how to talk about sex with your own daughter. In the "Suggested Resources" section, we list books and websites that are helpful in talking about sex with children, teenagers, and young women.

If an adolescent is sexually active, she most often denies the possibility of unwanted pregnancy or STIs. Getting pregnant or getting herpes, let alone AIDS, is not a real possibility in her young world. The basic law of cause and effect is still being sorted out in adolescence, and it feels like life will go on as it is forever. Actions that have irreversible consequences seem as remote as old age. Bad things happen, but "not to me." Adolescents also use denial to cope with situations that are painful or beyond their coping capacities. If it can't be figured out quickly, many teens simply "tune out" because they don't like the helplessness of asking for help.

Parents often participate in this denial by turning their backs on adolescent sexuality. Uncomfortable or ambivalent about sex themselves, they haven't a clue how to discuss sex with their daughters (or sons). They may pass along a book or give a monologue about sexuality, but more often than not, they shy away from a face-to-face dialogue. Many "big talks" are one-time events, never to be repeated. Unfortunately, no single discussion can cover all the questions and choices that will arise daily throughout their daughter's adolescence. By avoiding ongoing conversations about sex with their daughters, parents fail to share their own understanding of sexuality and their own memories of teenage excitement and confusion.

Do you remember the fairy tale "Sleeping Beauty"? We think it's the story of a young girl becoming a woman. In the story, the evil fairy predicts that Sleeping Beauty will prick her finger on the spindle of a spinning wheel and die before she turns 16. A less powerful but good fairy commutes the sentence from death to deep sleep.

Sleeping Beauty's parents are heartbroken. In their grief and desire to protect their daughter, they have every spindle in the kingdom removed. They want Sleeping Beauty to grow up in a world without spindles so that she will never be exposed to them, won't even know they exist.

We all know what happens. Just before her 16th birthday, Sleeping Beauty (at least in the Disney version) finds the one spindle in the entire kingdom. Because she has never seen one before, she is fascinated by it and drawn to it. Because she doesn't know that it can hurt her, because she hasn't been taught to make choices about right and wrong, the good and the bad regarding spindles, she is in big danger.

Sleeping Beauty does what every fascinated junior scientist does: She moves toward the mystery to investigate it. She touches the spindle. The rest we leave to Disney.

Women often look back at their sexual adventures and misadventures during their teenage years and wonder, *Where were my parents? Why didn't they talk to me?* Like Sleeping Beauty, hiding the spindles didn't protect them either. Ironically, a woman may repeat this silence of denial with her own daughter because that is how sex was treated in her family and she still doesn't have a clue how to talk about sex, not with her partner, not with her daughter.

A teenager needs her parents' continual input about the normalcy and pleasure of sexual feelings and what's okay and not okay in their value system. Ideally, discussions about sexual feelings and behavior parallel and reflect a young woman's growing ability to love another person and to take responsibility for her actions. While reassuring her about the normalcy of these feelings, a parent can also help a daughter rehearse how to handle different situations before they arise.

HISTORY'S ARC

Women have not always had a place at the table. Cook the meal, serve it, wash it up, but no right to sit down and eat their share. Inequality and maltreatment continue in many parts of the globe in the form of human trafficking, prostitution, and the treatment of women as property. There are complex cultural, financial, and historical reasons for this injustice toward women, an injustice that exists in resource-rich countries as well as resource-limited ones.

"The arc of history is long, but it bends toward justice," said Barack Obama in his 2008 acceptance speech, paraphrasing the words of Martin Luther King, Jr., and earlier civil rights pioneers. And even in the relatively short lives of women still in their 20s, positive changes are occurring, from better survival rates for women in childbirth to more access to education and the freedom to make their own choices. Every woman today stands on the shoulders of the women who went before her.

Despite significant differences in the ways women now live their lives, many aspects of women's lives are remarkably similar over time. We are workers, caregivers, performers of multiple roles. Women may no longer bake the bread and pack it in a hand-woven straw basket, but every woman alive knows the experience of calling, sending a card, throwing together a meal, or stopping for take-out on her way to visit someone in need. This caretaking is part of the fiber of women's lives, regardless of country, orientation, or age. However, the expression of this caretaking is influenced by historical and cultural changes affecting each woman. Sociologists often refer to these changes as generational and describe groups born within a roughly 20-year span as a "cohort" sharing similar characteristics because they were influenced by the same social factors.

Generations

Lynne Lancaster and David Stillman describe these generational differences in the United States in their 2010 book *The M-Factor: How the Millennial Generation Is Rocking the Workplace* (Lancaster & Stillman, 2010). The generation born before 1946 are the Traditionalists, who were influenced by both the Depression and World War II— experiences that created hardship and required personal sacrifice and an emphasis on "the greater good" as a driving force for meaning. This group is responsible for voter rights and many of the women's rights and civil rights accomplishments in the 1960s. The group born from 1946 to 1964, some 80 million of them, are the Baby Boomers. Well educated and interested in individual rights as well as individualism, this group grew up in the context of civil rights and women's rights. They were influenced by the draft and Vietnam War as well as by the Kennedy/Johnson vision of a "great society." Boomers wanted to be seen and heard and to build social structures that would create change. The group born between 1965 and 1981 is called the Generation Xers (Gen Xers). Influenced by the roller coaster ride of tough economies followed by superheated economic bubbles and the changing social structure of having both parents in the workforce, the Gen Xers are less likely to believe that answers will be found in a single place or institution and emphasize that work must be balanced with "life" and with meaning that is highly personal. The group born between 1982 and 2000 are called the Millennials (also referred to as Gen Y, Tech Generation, or GenNext). Their numbers, currently 76 million, are expected with immigration to eventually surpass the Boomers. Millennials were raised by hands-on parents who spent more time with their children than any previous generation and viewed the parental role less as authoritarian and more as guide, ally, and supporter of their children. This close contact manifests in Millennials' unconcern about privacy and focus on connection by Internet and social networking. Millennials look to both work and relationships for more egalitarian and mutual involvement. The environment, social justice, and making a difference are familiar themes with an emphasis on working hard and contributing, but getting noticed and recognized for one's achievements.

Similarly, women's understanding of their sexuality and the importance of sexual satisfaction have been defined by their cohort. In high school, if you didn't think of yourself as influenced by peer pressure, or if you never wanted to be alone, it may be the result of an interesting mix of your family, cultural background, and generation cohort. If you never as a teen worried about getting AIDS, you may be a

Traditionalist or a Boomer, and if you never as a teen worried about getting pregnant, but worried a lot about sexually transmitted infections, you may have been born into the generations of Gen Xers and Millennials.

Discovering how her body responds; learning how the world views and reacts to her femininity; experiencing strange, wondrous, and, at times, confusing sensations—these are fairly universal experiences for every woman as she moves through her formative years from infancy to adulthood. These discoveries and experiences, often described as developmental milestones, do not occur in a vacuum, however, but within an historical context. World events (war, economic conditions, prevailing political and social philosophies, advances in technology) and the status of social institutions (the stability of family structure, the influence of religion, prevailing attitudes toward authority) can subtly and dramatically influence how sexuality is first perceived and understood by a child and how the child comes to experiment and react to sexual experiences.

Your cohort of peers, those who were born within the same narrowly defined era and share the same cultural influences specific to that point in history—your *generation*—can help you understand how your sexual story has unfolded. It is not only the developmental milestones described earlier in this chapter, but the generational influences that helped shape each woman's sexual attitudes, beliefs, values, and identity.

TWO

Adult Sexuality

A Lifelong Story

From the first days of life to the threshold of adulthood, your developing sense of who you are included what the world expected of you as a female. As you grew into your body and began to have sexual experiences, your values and your sexual interests emerged and your sexual story took shape. But your sexual story didn't end when you reached adulthood, and it doesn't close with marriage, divorce, menopause, or even old age. It is a lifelong story, made up of your ongoing discoveries about what it means to be a sexual person. No matter what your age, the ending has yet to be written.

You can spend your entire life capable of sexual response, pleasure, and enjoyment. To what extent, and in what ways, you fulfill the promise of your adult sexuality is up to you. You are the author of your sexual story, and if you are dissatisfied with any aspect of this personal narrative, you have the opportunity to revise the chapter you're living right now and supply your story with a new, more fulfilling ending. To do so, you have to review and reflect on the chapters you have already written from your childhood and the years of adulthood you have lived so far.

You may believe you know these chapters by heart—after all, you lived them. Just as reciting the words of a poem is not the same as understanding its many layers of meaning, being able to list the sexual experiences of your life isn't the same as fully understanding how they brought you to where you are today. Many women tend to take only a glancing look at their sexual past, moving on to other thoughts when their memories evoke a chiding response of *Girl, what were you thinking of?* or a wistful nostalgia for passion lost or an echo of pain at trust betrayed. Looking more closely at how your experiences, sexual and otherwise, have shaped your current sexuality is an important key to guiding your sexual growth in the direction that is best for you. Looking forward, anticipating how various life events might affect your sexuality, can also help you meet challenges and opportunities with an insight that will contribute to lifelong healthy sexuality.

The discoveries that women have shared with us about the events that influence their sexual growth are as individual and unique as their faces and personalities.

"The first time I ever had sexual intercourse, I was ready and the timing was just right for me. I felt this curious mix of being in charge and being utterly vulnerable. I thought everything would come naturally and that I'd be hot with desire, but it wasn't like that. I felt self-conscious because I wasn't acting like the women I'd seen having sex in the movies. Now I think that the newness and the unfamiliarity of intercourse made me self-conscious. Being lovers takes practice. I didn't know that then, but I wish I had."

"I learned about one sexual myth the hard way. It had been fed to me with my cereal and trotted out with my Barbie dolls. It was that there would be a perfect Ken for me. He would read my mind and know exactly what I needed sexually. Isn't this the age-old story? I got married before I knew who I was. For some inexplicable reason, I thought that loving him would teach me how to love myself. Sex was initially exciting, but I'm not sure I ever knew what I wanted sexually. It was all about him. Then the kids came and I was fed up with his needs on top of theirs. He was tuned out to all the daily demands. So I spent years withdrawing sexually and feeling resentful because he didn't even notice that sex wasn't working for me. We went to counseling, and I was smug at first, certain the counselor would join me in putting him in his place for being so checked out. Sure, she called him on being checked out, but it didn't stop there. She also pushed me to look at how little responsibility I was taking for myself. I had to learn to speak up and be clear about what I needed and wanted. Now I grieve about the years we lost because we cycled between resentment and blaming. Good sex takes work, but it's good work to do."

As you read this chapter, we hope you'll be moved to explore your sexuality in your present life as well as in your past. If you discover you have led your life as if sexuality were something you could shrug off like an unneeded sweater, we hope you will reconsider and find a prominent place for sexuality in your life. The women we know whose sexuality is an integral part of who they are and what they experience lead the full, vibrant lives that we wish for you.

"Over the years I've read many books about menopause. As a result, I grew to respect my body just as it is. I walk with a confidence that I never had in my youth. I am as sexual as anyone I meet. My body is far from perfect, but

I have lived and loved in it for decades, and I carry that with me wherever I am."

"I'm a nurse. I know the healing benefits of touch. I sometimes marvel at how wonderful hands are: They comfort, connect, reassure, and sexually arouse, too. To me all of these things are connected to my sexuality as a woman."

"It took some doing, but I got all three kids off to a sleep-over. Carlos and I had a whole night together—and it was terrific! Yes, it took planning, but so does everything else in a life as busy as ours. If we're going to have a sex life together, we have to be intentional about planning it. Wild abandon is not for a working mother with three kids—unless she schedules it!"

Unfortunately, even in our enlightened age, many women think of sexuality as a series of disconnected, discrete behaviors. Women *have* sex, they *act* sexy, and they *think* about sex at various times during any one day. But sexuality is not something we turn on and off, like a tap. We are sexual beings all the time, and the more we understand about how this facet intertwines with all the others, the richer our lives become.

Just as sexuality is connected to all that we are at any one time, it is also an important part of us throughout life's stages. Each stage of life comprises interlocking experiences and biological changes that influence sexuality. The burst of hormones you felt during puberty and adolescence transformed your childhood sexual curiosity into a strong fascination and a desire to explore all that is sensual. The emancipation you felt when you graduated from high school and moved out on your own led you to look for new relationships, including sexual ones. Your "biological clock" may have influenced your timing for having children. The physical and time demands of parenting may alter your sexual relationship with your partner. As the children grow up and move out, your relationship with your partner undergoes further changes. It may flourish, or it may break apart—either way, sexual activity and satisfaction will be affected. Divorce may impact your sexuality by depriving you of a partner or by opening you up to opportunities for better relationships and better sex.

During middle age, your body undergoes changes that can affect your feelings of both desirability and desire. The sense of mastery that comes from raising children successfully or succeeding in a career may infuse your sex life with new confidence and enthusiasm. Retirement may set you even freer to pursue pleasure in your body, including sexual pleasure. Failing health and widowhood may have a unique impact on your opportunities, desire for, and capacity to be sexual, but neither need derail your sexuality or sexual identity.

"Having breast cancer has affected my body on the outside, but it has made me stronger on the inside. I have even learned to love my scars. When I look at them, I see what I have come through and conquered. In a strange way, I've opened up more to sex than at any other time in my life. I like to savor all of my senses: I've never appreciated them as I do now. Now when I'm stroking my partner, I'm not just focusing on arousal; I'm aware of the wonderful feel of the soft skin moving beneath my fingertips and the intimate connection we have. Life is fragile, and making love seems more important than ever."

"My husband and I had a sex life that was more methodical than sensual. One night I talked him into renting a racy movie. It showed oral sex and was very arousing to me. Later in bed I really let my hair down. I got my courage up, pulled the sheets off, and started stroking and then kissing his penis. It seemed very natural to get into the rhythm of sucking him. I noticed that his diaphragm was shaking a little. I was feeling pretty shy, so I stopped and noticed he was giggling. 'What?' I asked. He said, 'Your boobs are bouncing up and down—you look like you stuck your finger in a light socket.' At that moment I knew that I'd never, ever again throw the bed sheets off with Theo. My eyes were wide open, and I realized that sex was just the tip of the iceberg of our constrained relationship. I found my courage again and got out altogether. It was the most freeing thing I ever did. It took a while, but I am in a new relationship, and the sex is a lot of fun."

Knowing your sexual story means understanding how life experiences have influenced how you accept your body, experience pleasure, and relate sexually to your partner(s). It also means knowing yourself well enough to anticipate how these experiences might affect your sexuality as they occur in your future. This is, sadly, no easy task for women today. Although, as a whole, we discuss sexual matters much more openly than did our mothers and grandmothers, we still don't share our stories and experiences with one another as freely as we could. We commiserate about menstrual difficulties, and pregnancy and childbirth seem to bring us together to share the most intimate physical details of this female experience. But when it comes to expressing worries about what are "normal" sexual feelings and activities or to sharing the joys and trials of our sexual self-discoveries, we often hold back. Women tell us, with deep sadness, how much they regret having been afraid to talk to others about themselves, including their sexuality. They cringe about their "dumb" choices when we ask them to explore their past. They seem visibly lighter when we help them see, for example, that women learn to reach orgasm with a partner and that it often takes time; or that for most women arousal doesn't come automatically, like flipping on a light switch. Overall, our knowledge has become more sophisticated, but many of our worries remain the same. By resisting thinking and talking about these concerns, we deny ourselves the full opportunity to learn from other women about the common experiences that impact many of us as we move across our lifespan.

We hope this chapter will help fill this gap. We describe what women have told us about their experiences with major life events, and we pose questions that will challenge you to think about your own sexuality in similar situations, whether these events have already occurred in your life or still lie ahead. We also make suggestions for finding additional information about each topic, either in a later chapter or from resources listed at the end of the book.

In Chapter 13, we provide exercises to help you take an even closer look at how your life events have shaped your sexuality. In addition, we include exercises to help you see how your ethnicity, sexual orientation, and the values you've learned from others have influenced your sexuality. The self-knowledge you gain from reading this chapter and doing the exercises in Chapter 13 will give you the springboard you need to better benefit from the rest of the book.

SEXUAL EXPERIENCES

What we call your "sexual story" is what psychologists talk about as your sexual development: the maturation of your sexual feelings, behavior, attitudes, and knowledge. As such, it is about far more than just your sex life at any one age or stage of life. Your sexual story is the product of all the events that occur at each life stage and how you respond to them. These responses, in turn, are shaped by your cognitive, emotional, moral, and social development. This perspective encourages you to explore and accept sexual feelings that might only confuse or worry you if you viewed sex and sexuality as one-dimensional and governed by one-size-fits-all rules and standards. The ever-broadening definition of what is sexually normal is liberating. Still, given how uniquely complex each woman's sexuality is, it's obvious that your sexuality not only *should* be defined by you but, really, can be defined *only* by you.

A large part of a woman's expression of her sexuality is, of course, the choices she makes about when to have sex and with whom. Years ago a woman's sexual choices were made *for* her. With certain cultural variations, she "saved herself" for marriage, giving her sexuality to her husband as part of her dowry, after which he could do with it—*her*—what he liked. A woman who was brought up to follow these rules might feel desperately bad just for *wanting* something different—much less for *doing* something differently. And a woman who didn't *feel* bad about having her own ideas and taking charge of her own sexual destiny was usually *labeled* "bad."

For many of us, all that has changed. Now we have choices about when to have sex and with whom. Unfortunately, those choices aren't always easy to make. Would you give in to desire and have sex with someone even though your family and religious values tell you to wait? Could you explore the possibility that you are bisexual without feeling as if you were violating a taboo? How would you feel about choosing to make love to your partner when you don't feel all that loving, just because it's easier than talking through your problems? Would having an affair sound the death knell for the two of you, or would you consider it just a brief fling? What if it were your partner who had the affair? Is it okay for you to have casual sex with someone you just met, but not okay for your 19-year-old daughter to do the same? If you finally ended your marriage because you could no longer live the lie that you are heterosexual, would you be able to have an active and open sex life as a lesbian, or would you remain celibate out of fear of shocking your friends and family?

As with all choices we make in life, sexual choices often present us with dilemmas—conflicts between two firmly held values, fine lines between wants and needs, mores versus manners, our needs versus someone else's, the benefits of planning weighed against those of spontaneity. How we resolve these dilemmas contributes to our sexual development. Not every sexual experience you have had or will have is transformative or momentous, but each sexual experience affects your ongoing experience of your body, your sense of yourself as a woman, your self-esteem, your sense of your place in the universe, and much more. When your sexual decisions are based on the personal values and external influences most important to you, your sexual experiences will generally feel emotionally comfortable and satisfying as well as physically pleasurable. If your sexual experiences today do not fit this description, it may not be your current sex life that's the problem but a pattern of past sexual decisions that contradicts your most important values and needs.

Time has a way of changing everyone's perspective; you need to take the factor of time into account when you reexamine the experiences you've had. Maybe you blush at your "stupidity" when you think about that person you fell into bed with in college when you were both drunk, but the erotic films that made your face flame then seem like a healthy part of a woman's sex life now—with or without a partner. For decades you might have lived by the precept that marriage is the only place for sex, but now, having fallen for someone 5 years after your partner's death, you think it is fine to be sexual without committing to each other. We know one woman who was unashamed of the number of people she slept with during her 20s but now reports unhappily, "I tend to keep a lid on in the bedroom because it's like I'm afraid that wild woman will reappear and mess everything up." We know many, many others who avoid intimate relationships altogether, pretending they no longer care about sex, when the truth is that they can't reconcile the less-than-perfect 40-year-old bodies they now own with their memories of the physical and sexual ideal they fulfilled 20 years earlier.

Development, sexual and otherwise, means *change*. If you can examine your sexuality today and say with confidence that you have matured and are where you want to be, then clearly your past decisions played a positive role—even if, in retrospect, it seems as if they must have been made by a stranger. If not, you can probably benefit from a closer look at why you did what you did in the past and why you're doing what you're doing sexually today. As to the future, forewarned is forearmed: Be prepared for the types of changes that women describe in the rest of this chapter!

Kinds of Sex: What Drives Your Choices?

In the movies, sex just happens. That's not the way it is in real life, even though our romantic notions sometimes trick us into believing that sex is just the result of two people getting carried away in the moment. Some sexual encounters do occur out of sheer abandon. Some are undertaken after a lot more conscious, deliberate thought than others. Each sexual circumstance is unique. Whatever the case, we've found that most women benefit from understanding their reasons for their sexual choices—if not beforehand, then at least upon reflection.

You made love with your best friend in an attempt to comfort each other over another close friend's death. Your best friend is married. How do you feel about the experience? How do you *think* you should feel? How will this experience affect your future decisions?

At a conference, you slept with a fellow physician you'd just met hours earlier. You're now chastising yourself for being unprofessional. Does that mean you shouldn't have enjoyed the sex?

You really liked him and hoped the relationship would go beyond friendship, but when he asked you to go to bed with him you knew it was casual—just for fun. And it *was* fun. But now you're really falling for him, and he's still just looking for fun—elsewhere. You're wondering if, for you, there is any such thing as casual sex.

All of our sexual decisions are complicated, even if they seem quite simple at the time. You may initiate sex for one reason but come out of the experience with an entirely different feeling. One partner in a sexual encounter may have an agenda, while the other is really giving in to the passion of the moment. The reason you give yourself for a sexual decision may turn out to be self-deception. The reason it's important to understand all this is to improve your capacity for self-determination in the future.

Loving Sex

A common reason for choosing to have sex with a partner is love. Loving sex is a powerful connection between two people who share a strong emotional bond; it's a way two people can say with their bodies, "I love you." Sex gains a new depth when motivated by love; love gains a new dimension of closeness when this profound emotion is expressed physically.

Loving sex is often depicted in movies and books and has inspired poems and paintings throughout history. For those who are in love, sex can at times be a powerful experience unmatched by anything else. At other times it can be a familiar and reassuring physical connector during the daily grind that can wear a couple down.

Unfortunately, loving sex does not always live up to its fairy-tale reputation. First of all, being in love is no guarantee of legendary sex. The earth does not automatically move for women just because they are having sex, not even when they are in love. Think about your first sexual experience. Even if you had been head over heels in love, it was not a guarantee that your bodies would move like "figure skaters together on ice." Whether you are looking for a few good tips or you seek the kind of powerful sex that poets write about, you will need to practice. See Chapter 13 for ways to understand your body and create better sex with your partner.

Second, for some people, having sex imposes pressure to declare love that may not be felt. No matter what age, some people will use "But I love you so much" as the reason to coerce a potential partner into having sex. Some women, especially young women, may even convince themselves that they love their partner as a way to assuage guilt brought on by the clash between a cultural or religious prohibition against unmarried sex and their growing sexual desire. Or they may simply confuse physical desire and emotional love. However it happens, when two people are mismatched in their reasons for a sexual encounter, the experience is bound to disappoint at least one of them.

We have met many women who, years later, were guilt ridden about a sexual experience or by an affair they'd had when they were dragging through the final months of an unraveling marriage. In cases like these, many women are greatly relieved to learn that it was perfectly natural for them to have sex motivated by sheer lust—or by many of the other forces discussed in the following pages. What's important is to gain perspective on why they did what they did in the past and how it may be influencing them, positively and negatively, today.

Casual Sex

Sometimes the motivation to have sex is pleasure, pure and simple. This is what many people call "casual sex." Nothing seems to inspire such heated debate as this form of sex. Is sex without love immoral? Is sex with different partners safe, in this era of AIDS and STIs? Is casual sex a normal instinct for men but abnormal for women? Is *casual* the equivalent of *irresponsible*? Conventional wisdom on this subject has varied over the years, and the answers to these questions will always vary depending on the speaker's cultural and religious background, life experiences, and other personal factors.

What does the phrase *casual sex* conjure for you? To some, it means any sex outside of an exclusive commitment. For others it may mean promiscuity. For still others, unfortunately, it may mean unthinking sex. What we mean is that casual sex includes any situation where two consenting adults enjoy physical pleasure with each other and the sex is responsible, nonexploitative, and mutually respectful. Perhaps a 28-year-old woman goes to bed with a man she met earlier in the evening; they are honest with each other and take precautions to prevent pregnancy and infection. Or a 50-year-old woman chooses to have sex with a woman she meets on vacation. Perhaps two residents of an assisted-living facility slip into each other's rooms at night so that they can be sexual. We believe the choices and direction shouldn't come from experts in such situations. Rather, they must be based on a woman's personal values, desires, and common sense. As mentioned earlier in this chapter, making the choice may involve reconciling conflicting values. One woman told us that although she has promised herself she'll have sex only when she and a partner have made a commitment to each other, sometimes she has sex with someone "just because it feels great." Another woman notes ruefully, "It's sometimes easier to have sex with someone than to talk with him about condoms."

Casual sounds easy, but responsible casual sex is anything but. As sex therapists, we tell our clients that casual sex, practiced safely, responsibly, and respectfully, falls well within many people's value systems—and for many other people, it does not. If you are going to make decisions you can live with, you have to think about which group you fall into ahead of time.

Biology may have a say in casual sex too, making it even more complex. More than at any previous time, we are now aware of the brain chemicals activated during sexual activity. Orgasm expands the brain's "banquet" of love chemicals, so the end result of what was to be casual sex *can* be propelled into closeness and connection—perhaps confusing the participants.

Sex as Solace

"I was halfway around the world when I got the call that my mother had died. I was devastated. David was a colleague and good friend, but certainly not my lover. I needed to talk that night, and he listened. I needed to cry, and he held me. I needed to feel close to another human being, and we made love. I'll never forget his tenderness. I'll never forget how powerful my need was at that moment to feel alive and cared for."

There are times when two people with no permanent commitment to each other have sex, and the act is anything but casual. Intense emotions can trigger a hunger or yearning to make intimate contact with another human being, even if the shared intimacy might be fleeting and short lived. Although some women later regret or feel embarrassed about having sex as solace, their self-judgment is too harsh. Sometimes sex occurs when a person's grief, isolation, fear, or shame makes her momentarily vulnerable and open to sexual decisions that she would not make otherwise. The woman connects with her body because it temporarily eases the emotional pain she is in; it feels good to be touched and to touch.

Sex as Conquest

If you are an adult in your 20s, 30s, or 40s, you may feel close to the cultural stereotype of sexual beauty. If you're in your 50s, 60s, 70s, or older, you may want reassurance that you are still attractive. Knowing that you've attracted someone through your beauty and sexuality is a powerful feeling, no matter what the age, and many women have engaged in what could be called "sex as conquest" at some point in their lives. Some women confine their power seeking to flirting, while others choose to have sex with men or women who then become their conquests.

Is there anything wrong with this? Not necessarily, as long as you and the other know what you're doing and how it makes you both feel afterward. Sex that is motivated by power seeking alone turns both you and your partner into objects in a power play, no longer real people seeking real contact with each other. Most women we have counseled say that the thrill wears off in time—or they lose their taste for sex as conquest once they have been the conquered as often as they've been the conqueror. One woman put it succinctly as "fun but limiting." Sex as conquest is the epitome of other-oriented sex. Eventually, sexuality has to be about what you like about yourself. For an expanded discussion of this topic, check out "Desirable versus Desiring—Enter Cognitive Distraction" in Chapter 6.

Agenda Sex

Women have always known that sex can be the route to any other goal or objective. Sex can be offered as some sort of unspoken barter, or it can simply instill the euphoria that makes a partner more amenable to giving a woman what she wants. This dubious feminine wile is rooted in the perception that women (as opposed to men) have little to offer besides their sexual favors. We call sex that is undertaken to manipulate someone "agenda sex." In general, it's problematic because it fosters uncertainty, resentment, anger, or all three.

Possible agendas for sex include proving something, bolstering the ego, feeling in control, manipulation, bartering, making up for some offense, and avoiding boredom. Some agendas are even well meaning. It's not uncommon for women to have sex with a partner to make him or her "feel better"—more loved, more attractive, more virile, and so forth. As an occasional gesture made out of love and compassion, this kind of agenda sex is not necessarily problematic. It's when sex is habitually undertaken without desire or love that agenda sex usually backfires in distrust and resentment.

"I don't really like sex with my partner," said one woman we know, "but he expects it at least once a week. He gets off, then rolls over and goes to sleep. I don't think sex with him could ever improve, so I just have it to keep him from bugging me." She is so busy keeping the peace that she may lose touch with her own sexual needs to make the sex better for *herself*. In the long run, satisfying a partner because a woman doesn't want to deal with the challenge of honesty will result in resentment and yearning; she'll resent her partner for his demands and oblivion, and she'll secretly yearn for a better lover who would be sensitive to her needs. Agenda sex always has a goal *other than* honest connection and intimacy.

Sex to Dispel Loneliness

One example of agenda sex that is so common and important that it warrants separate consideration is sex that serves as an antidote for loneliness. Young women away from their childhood home for the first time or older women out of the security of a long-term relationship may find living on their own lonely. A relationship soothes you when you're lonely or scared. Many women say they put up with sex in a relationship because it is the price they pay for being with someone—and it's the *being with* that is important, not the *someone*.

> "I never think about masturbating. I know about masturbation, but when I do it, I feel lonely and kind of empty. I like sex with someone because I like cuddling and sleeping together at night. It's not about sex; it's more about knowing someone is there."

If you always need to be in a relationship with someone, perhaps you use sexual connection to relieve loneliness or anxiety about being alone. If you are having sex primarily to avoid being alone, we suggest that you may not be ready to have a sexual relationship at this time. Your work lies in learning to soothe yourself, learning how to be in charge of you, and yes, even learning how to be alone. This is not to imply that loneliness is not a painful circumstance for many people or that you "should" never feel lonely. But if you are bargaining with sex to avoid confronting your apprehensions about loneliness or being alone, mastering the aloneness is the better solution.

> "I couldn't stand to be in my apartment alone. I would find excuses to crash at a friend's house. I invited Chris to live with me 2 weeks after we met. I knew we didn't have a chance of making it together, but I had sex almost without thinking about it, because I knew Chris would stay, and I wouldn't have to be afraid to be alone."

Experimental Sex

For many women (and men), sexuality is the most fascinating laboratory to which we have access. Because sex offers the possibility of seemingly boundless pleasure and limitless potential for human connection, some women engage in what we call "experimental sex." This may mean exploring the boundaries of erotica (see "Suggested Resources") or experimenting with heterosexual sex (for lesbians) or with lesbianism or bisexuality (for heterosexuals). Not everyone needs to explore their orientation or the boundaries of what's considered "conventional" or "acceptable," but for some women this exploration is vital to their identity. They don't want to be constrained by narrow definitions or locked into one orientation. Still other women find the thrill of the exotic or forbidden a compelling aspect of sex and enjoy experimenting.

Celibacy

Some women choose to remain celibate. Celibacy may be permanent or temporary; it may include masturbation or not. It may be a lifelong religious commitment, or it may be a choice to avoid sexual activity while not permanently partnered. A woman may view celibacy—sometimes called "being nonsexual"—as a means of increasing nonsexual intimacy in relationships or as a way of avoiding exposure to STIs. Celibacy is behavioral. It doesn't obliterate a woman's sexual identity; she is sexual whether or not she's having sex. That is true of asexuality as well, but women who feel asexual do not identify as sexual beings, nor do they have any interest in becoming sexual in their behavior. Although born into bodies that are capable of sexual response, asexual women do not care about sex. An asexual woman may engage in sexual activity, but it will not carry any significance for her.

Celibacy is different in that a celibate woman is aware of her sexual response, her sexual choices, and her sexual identity. A woman might choose celibacy in order to develop nonsexual relationships, to learn more about her own feelings, or to concentrate on a goal that she must attain in her work or personal life. Listen to what these women say:

> "Being celibate is a conscious decision. You still feel all your sexual feelings. You make decisions about celibacy continually; you work at it. Sometimes people say the most stupid things to me. They'll remark that because I'm celibate it must be so much easier because I never have 'those feelings.' What a flat, dull, two-dimensional view they have of me. I struggle with my celibacy, but I see what I gain by not seeking sexual connection with another. I feel that I am trying to deepen intimacy with others through nonsexual means—through friendship and honest dialogue."

> "Because I'm a nun, people don't think I have sexual feelings. How wrong they are! There are days when I get turned on watching the mailman walk by. You know, you just don't fall out of bed one day and become a nun. It's taken me years of prayer, work, and spiritual reflection to understand my spiritual path. But I do value nonsexual touch; this is vital to my life. And I know that, for me, the only real way I can show my love for God is by what I show in my love for others."

Sexual experiences are an important part of your sexual story. To better understand how they have impacted your life, reflect on the following questions:

- "Do my past sexual experiences feel the same to me now as I felt about them then? If not, what has changed? Do I like sex more now?"
- "How would I categorize my most fulfilling sexual experiences of the past: as loving sex, casual sex, sex as conquest, agenda sex, sex to dispel loneliness, or experimental sex?"
- "How would I categorize my most negative sexual experiences of the past: as loving sex, casual sex, sex as conquest, agenda sex, sex to dispel loneliness, or experimental sex?"
- "Is there one kind of sexual experience that predominates in my current sex life? Is it the same kind as in the past?"
- "How have I expressed my sexuality during a period of celibacy or abstinence?"
- "When I make a decision to have sex, what do I think of first: my own desires right now, the other person's desires, how I might feel later, how my best friend will react, or some combination?"
- "Do I usually plan my sexual experiences ahead of time or just let the moment dictate?"
- "Are any of my past sexual experiences still a source of embarrassment, shame, or guilt? If so, what are some possible reasons? Do these reactions impact my sexual experiences today?"
- "If I devised a set of rules for making sexual decisions, what would they be? Are these the rules I tend to follow? If not, why?"

Decisions you have made in the past are just that—in the past. Appreciate the decisions that have brought you joy or helped you to grow in sexual wisdom. Learn from the decisions that you now regret and try to move on. If you find it difficult to accept some of your past choices, refer to "Tell Me It's Not in My Head" in Chapter 15. In that chapter, you will find techniques to help you better understand and modify unfair and self-defeating thoughts and beliefs that can haunt you with feelings of guilt and shame.

Sexual decision making is as complex as any other set of life decisions. Some women wait to have sex until they're with their life partner. Other women have sex with someone they're with for the evening. You are always in the process of exploring your sexuality, because it is ever-fluid. We encourage you to ask questions, accept that there will be mistakes, take risks, and, above all else, be passionate about caring for your sexual self.

WHEN BEING SEXUAL HURTS YOU

We've been describing sexual experiences as choices—either ones you have made or ones you may make in the future. In reality, not all sexual experiences are choices, and some are hurtful. Sexual trauma can be so devastating that we've devoted a whole chapter to it; see Chapter 10. But even when a sexual experience seems positive, it can have a bad outcome, like getting an STI or having an unwanted pregnancy. Then there are those many experiences that leave women feeling guilty, ashamed, or confused. There is a big difference between the lasting effects of abuse or exploitation and the uncomfortable feeling that can follow a less-than-ideal sexual encounter, but all negative experiences call for self-care and reflection.

"We're all supposed to be so well informed these days that when I met Ian I thought he'd be like other guys I'd had sex with: up front about it if he had an STI. We cared about each other, and so I made assumptions I shouldn't have. I never thought about getting an STI from him, but now that I have herpes, I can't think about anything else. Whenever I even consider having sex with anyone, I think about herpes."

"I thought sexual harassment was something that happened only to dumb, naive women. In fact, I thought it was only dumb men who tried it. After all, there've been enough widely publicized negative consequences for it that I figured you'd have to be an idiot to try to get away with that today. Well, let me tell you, there are all kinds of harassment. I thought my coworker Matt was just being helpful when I started my new job. But his helpfulness was very controlling: For weeks no one else got near me, and he blocked my attempts to get to know others, especially guys. That's when I realized I was being harassed."

"When is a choice to have sex not really a choice? I'd like to tell my daughter just to *say* 'NO' loudly and clearly when that's what she means. But I remember once in college when I said no and no again, ended up sort of wrestling with the guy, and then just let it happen. After all, I'd slept with this guy before, it was the era of 'free love,' and it seemed silly to make a big deal of it. When it was over—which was pretty quickly—I didn't make anything out of it at all, but over the years I've felt ashamed. Why did I just give in if it was something I really didn't want? Maybe because it was uncool to make a big deal out of sex or maybe because I didn't even want to consider the other possibility—that this 'friend' of mine had exploited me and essentially raped me. Did I make a choice, or was the right to make the choice taken away from me? I don't really know, and that still bothers me."

As you look back on your sexual explorations, you may remember lonely, scary moments when you had to face sexual dilemmas like sexual harassment or discovering you had an STI. Perhaps there was a period in your life when you had to get drunk to have sex. Perhaps you entered a sexual relationship thinking that you were making an informed choice, only to discover later that you had been manipulated or exploited. You may remember being forced to have sex or being sexually assaulted. These are examples of when being sexual can truly hurt you.

There's an old phrase, "You play, you pay." Although being sexual can sometimes hurt you, it's not because sexuality itself is wrong, dangerous, or harmful. It's because of a lack of information and a culture that too often tolerates exploitation, coercion, and absence of choices.

As you read about the sexual misfortunes described below, take time to reflect on the following questions:

- "Have I experienced this problem?"
- "If I have, has it impacted my sexuality?"
- "Have I taken steps, such as confiding in a friend, reading a self-help book, or seeking counseling, to deal with the hurt?"

Sexual Assault

In any situation where you had sex because you were forced, drugged, drunk, or assaulted, you were sexually vulnerable and you were hurt. Sex wasn't lovely or fun; it was used to dominate and control. In fact, one out of every four women report having been forced to have sex at some time in their lives (Laumann et al., 1994). A woman's reactions to forced sex can range from tearfulness and distress to trying to deny it happened or treating it like it was no big deal. Because the range of reactions to forced sex is so wide, and because denying the event can lead to later problems with depression, low self-esteem, anxiety, or posttraumatic stress disorder, we encourage all women who have been sexually assaulted to speak to a mental health professional. Your nurse, physician, pastor, or community mental health clinic can help you arrange counseling.

Some types of sexual assault cause a trauma reaction of terror or deep shame and humiliation. Women can feel cut off from others, convinced that no one would accept them if they knew what had happened. If you have these feelings, we encourage you to read Chapter 10 to help you cope with the loss you've experienced.

Sexual Exploitation

"After I graduated, I started to sleep with my high school teacher. I was 18 and he was 30. I thought I was cool at the time—until he brushed me off for another woman. I felt ashamed then, but now I'm appalled at *his* exploitative behavior. How could he do that?"

At some point in your life you might have made what we call "sexually vulnerable decisions." Perhaps you had sex with a much older person or much more powerful person, like a boss. You thought it was consensual, two equal people at the time, but now you know you weren't in a position to make an informed choice. Perhaps you remember having sex while drunk or high, and now you can see that you were exploited even though you consented at the time. Just as rape and sexual harassment hurt a woman, so can experiences when someone took advantage of your sexual vulnerability. They can also have the long-term effect of eroding your confidence and trust in new relationships.

Women cannot and should not take sole responsibility for negative experiences, but in many cases their decision-making *did* play some role, and this may be a difficult fact to face. If you feel you have a history of repeatedly being in situations where you've been sexually vulnerable or a pattern of being sexually exploited, we recommend that you seek counseling to better understand your decisions and avoid further hurt.

STIs, UTIs, and Yeast

"I say I don't like to have sex on the first few dates . . . and then I make sure there are no later dates. Or I say I have my period and we'll have to wait. Or I just stay home and watch TV. The truth is, I have genital warts and don't know how to talk to men about the problem, so I just avoid sex. It looks like I'm going to end up spending the rest of my life alone."

Sexually active women are exposed to STIs. Physiologically, women are more vulnerable to these health risks during their early adult years than at any other time of their lives. In a woman's late teens and early 20s, her cervical cells go through accelerated changes toward physical maturation, which dramatically increases susceptibility to STIs (Greenspan & Nakashima, 1994; Kenney et al., 1998; Burchell et al., 2006). It's a sad irony but true that the riskiest time in a woman's life for contracting STIs coincides with the stage in which she is most apt to be sexually active in many different relationships. This is the ultimate double standard; there is no equivalent in male physical development.

A woman may also experience chronic yeast infections or chronic urinary tract infections (UTIs). These recurrent medical problems are often so painful and irritating that the woman loses sexual desire.

STIs and other infections can cause a lot of unnecessary shame. Contracting an STI does not rob you of the right to have sex for the rest of your life, though you'll certainly want to take steps to protect yourself in the future. For more information on coping with these problems, see Chapter 8 for information about pain, Chapter 9 for a discussion of the impact of STIs, and Chapter 15 for suggestions about overcoming low sexual desire.

Unwanted Pregnancy

"They say that no birth control method is 100% effective, and I'm living proof of that. I'm not even interested in this guy anymore, and I just found out I'm pregnant with his child. I can't believe I have to decide whether to have this baby or have an abortion."

Despite education, available birth control, and firm resolve, unplanned pregnancies occur. A woman's life is thrown into turmoil as she sorts out relationship issues with her partner and makes a decision about whether or not to terminate the pregnancy. Regardless of the decision made, sexuality and passion from that point forward may never feel the same. If this experience has happened to you, you may have difficulty enjoying sex. Sex may no longer feel carefree and liberating— memories of the emotional roller coaster that followed discovery of the pregnancy can cast a shadow on future sexual experiences. If you can't enjoy sex, you may find it helpful to read Chapter 15.

Sex and Alcohol

"I used to get drunk before having sex, then I didn't have to take any responsibility for it. My self-esteem got lower and lower, and the more I drank, the deeper the despair. I finally got counseling to sober up and help myself dig out of that pit."

If you have sexual inhibitions, alcohol and drugs can make it easier for you to have sex with a partner. The problem is that if you come to rely on substances to produce the desired state of arousal you're denied the opportunity to learn about your own sexual desire and arousal. Early on in your sexually active life with partners, even if you do not have a full-blown addiction problem but *do* have a pattern of relying on alcohol, you are holding back your sexual development by escaping (or so it seems) the social dilemmas and sexual decisions that you face. You let alcohol do it for you. Let us assure you: It doesn't get easier to go it alone (without mood-altering substances) later.

Some women with a history of sexual abuse or trauma tell us they will intentionally use alcohol to dissociate and disconnect from the experience. Other women tell us they'll use alcohol to "pump" themselves up for sex if they're anxious or depressed. Unfortunately, no amount of alcohol or drugs will make the underlying conflict go away or produce long-term sexual satisfaction.

Being in recovery from alcohol or drug addiction also requires new sexual awareness, since you may never have had a sexual experience without being high. In the sexual arena you will need to "begin at the beginning," taking time to explore your values, your history, your relationship to your body. Many professionals in the recovery movement observe that a person's sexual and interpersonal development stopped at the point where chemical usage began. If this is true, then you will need to have patience as you begin sobriety and the journey toward knowing yourself. The sexual exercises outlined in this book will provide you with tools to help you reconnect with your sexuality.

Most women either have had some bad experience with sex or know of a woman who has. If your sexual experiences have not been entirely positive, ask yourself the following questions:

- "Do I feel shame, guilt, or embarrassment about any of my past sexual experiences?"
- "If I were giving advice on sexual choices and decisions to someone I care about, such as a son or daughter or young friend, would my advice be consistent with the way I've made my own choices?"
- "Does recalling certain sexual experiences evoke different thoughts and feelings now than I had at the time?"
- [If you had a negative sexual experience:] "Have I gotten help from my healthcare provider with any physical problems it caused?"
- "Does having sex today bring to mind negative memories of past experiences?"
- "Does it take a lot of time and effort for me to trust my sexual partner?"
- "Do I tend to think of sexual activity as merely a means of physical release, unconnected to emotional attachment?"
- "Do I have a problem with low sexual desire and arousal?"
- "Do I have difficulty experiencing orgasm?"
- "Do I associate sex with immorality?"

If answering these questions makes you aware that you may have had a negative sexual experience that is still harming you, consider reading Chapter 10 ("Trauma") and Part V ("Developing Sexual Comfort, Confidence, and Satisfaction"). If these do not provide sufficient help, be sure to talk to your healthcare provider or consider seeing a therapist.

WHEN ONE BECOMES TWO

Most women enter into partnerships that include sex. Falling in love is a time when the world of one person suddenly becomes a world of two. In the early days of a partnership, romantic love unfolds. Most couples experience a wonderful preoccupation with each other, accompanied by intense physical feelings of attraction and arousal. A partner's strong points become exaggerated and weak points are nonexistent. Sexual passion is high, sexual activity frequent, and for a brief time, life can seem like a remarkable state of existence. But in all couples—heterosexual or gay/lesbian—that euphoric state gives way to the reality of day-to-day living. In Chapter 12 we discuss the challenges couples face as they make the inevitable transition from a sex life that seems effortless to one that needs attention.

You've "Lost That Lovin' Feeling"

"Something changed between us. When did fantasies inch him out of my dreams? We're happy together and we've got a million interests in common, but I just don't lust after him like I used to. He thinks I've got a sexual problem, but I think my feelings are normal—that after being married for a while, you just lose the passion. I don't think he really tries to be sexual with me either—he just wants to fall into sex before rolling over into sleep. I don't know where the passion went. I miss it, but it's too hard to figure out how to fix it."

Most couples experience a decrease in passionate feelings after the first or second year of partnership. You no longer exaggerate your partner's strengths, and you're left with a life-sized lover. Sex can take a nosedive.

The drop in sexual frequency can occur for many reasons. When a couple is together over time, the sense of urgency about sex drops. The novelty wears off and affection is more frequent than passion. Both Helen Fisher in her research on romantic love (*Why We Love*) and Esther Perel in her writing about couples in long-term partnerships (*Mating in Captivity*) address the changes that occur in many partnerships over time (Fisher, 2004; Perel, 2007). Although boredom may be part of the problem, there is also the reality that new relationships allow fewer distractions and often rely on sex to cement the partnership. Once you feel secure in a relationship, other demands—household tasks, career, family, and friends—require attention and create fatigue. Fisher points out that romantic love is like a reward system and, once attained, is followed by a shift in the relationship. Perel describes the dynamic tension between the comfort of intimate attachment and the unpredictability and tension of passion. Simply stated, if you want passion, you must expect the unexpected and not presume to know what will happen next. It is the tension and thrill of not knowing that drives passion, and it is the comfort and predictability that grows intimacy. Long-term relationships will need to create ways to promote both intimacy and passion. Barry McCarthy, in his book *Discovering Your Couple Sexual Style: Sharing Desire, Pleasure, and Satisfaction*, gives an excellent description of the different ways that couples may choose to be sexual (McCarthy & McCarthy, 2009).

Women often tell us how unsatisfying their sex lives have become. They wish their partners were better lovers or that they had more time for touching and getting turned on. They feel that if they weighed less, slept more, and had another 3 hours in the day, there would be time for sex and the sex would be better. Women tell us they feel more powerful and competent in managing their careers and household schedules than their love lives. Women claim they have bad sex because of a busy life, no life, or a lifeless partner.

Sexual problems like low sexual desire, sexual pain, anorgasmia (inability to have an orgasm), or sexual boredom can develop in any relationship. These problems can be the result of life stressors, tension in the relationship, or old fears and inhibitions reappearing once the intense passion and feelings of "new love" have subsided.

Every couple needs to take care of their sexual relationship by devoting time to creating fulfilling sexual experiences. Because sex is fun and pleasurable, we mistakenly believe we don't need to work at it. Women who have had satisfying sex lives with one partner over decades report that they conscientiously make a place for sex in their lives, not only by making time for sexual activity with their partner but also by masturbating. If you feel you've "lost that lovin' feeling" with your partner, Parts IV ("Creating a Better Sexual Relationship") and V ("Developing Sexual Comfort, Confidence, and Satisfaction") will help you take positive steps in your relationship.

> "I was beginning to trash my partner to my girlfriends, complaining that all he wanted was sex and all I wanted was chocolate. Then I realized how crummy this was, as if I'd decided to get my power from trashing sex rather than being sexual. So I decided to turn things around. I told my partner that Thursday nights were just for us—no phone calls, no e-mails. Because we won't have sex unless we get to bed at a decent time, I make an early meal. While he cleans up the dishes, I get in the mood for sex with a hot bath and some erotica. By the time he joins me in the bedroom, I feel more turned on and glad I set aside the time."

Arranged Marriages: Unique Challenges

In some cultures, forming a partnership presents unique challenges, especially in regard to establishing a comfortable sexual relationship. Arranged marriages are common in Indian as well as some Asian and Middle Eastern cultures. Women from these cultures may have their husbands chosen for them by their families. As adolescents, their exposure to sex education will be controlled and their knowledge of their future partner will often be limited. In an arranged marriage, sexual difficulties can emerge early in the relationship. The first sexual experience doesn't occur until the wedding night, and there may be family pressure to prove the marriage has been consummated. A lack of sex education and experience and not knowing each other can lead to problems with rapid ejaculation for men and painful intercourse and difficulty with arousal for women.

Many couples brought together through family arrangements report that, in time, they come to know, respect, and love each other deeply. As their relationship grows, so does their ability to explore and enjoy their shared sexuality. Some couples enhance their sexual relationship by openly discussing sex during their engagement and marriage. If they encounter problems, they seek advice, read self-help books, or work with a counselor.

> "I wanted to respect my family's wishes in an arranged marriage, but having grown up in North America, I was scared about marrying a complete stranger. My parents and I made an agreement: they would make a suitable match for me, but then I would date the person until I got to know him. I needed time to become friends and grow to love him."

Growing Together

Relationships go through different stages. At times sexual difficulties or lack of interest will correspond to a particularly difficult or challenging period of life. Yet many women also tell us that sex improved after they got through an especially trying time. Some women experience a stronger interest in sex in their 30s, others after their kids are born, and still others when the children leave home and the house, once again, is theirs. The sex you have in your relationship will be unique to the two of you, but certainly work, having children, aging, and illnesses will influence your sexual life together. The greatest asset to a good sex life is to remain curious and committed to growing together sexually.

If you are in a partnership, ask yourself these questions:

- "Do I care about being sexual with my partner? [If yes:] How have I demonstrated this through words and actions? [If no:] Is it because there are problems in the relationship, or am I feeling turned off by sex in general?" (Parts IV and V provide valuable information and suggestions.)"
- "When was the last time I made specific plans to be with my partner sexually? Did I follow through?" (If you can't remember making any such plans, or you've made them but never followed through, check Chapter 14 for helpful suggestions.)
- "Which one of us tends to be the prime mover in our sexual time together?"
- "How do I picture my sex life with my partner 10 years from now? Twenty years? Thirty years?"

If you're not currently in a partnership, take some time to reflect on the following questions:

- "How do I picture a long-term relationship altering my sex life? Would it be freeing or limiting?"
- "How do I maintain my feeling of being a sexual person even though I'm not in a sexual relationship?"
- "Would I like my future sexual relationships to be like any I have had in the past? If not, why not?"
- "What would my ideal sexual relationship with a partner look like?"

AND BABY MAKES THREE

Couples who partner during childbearing years face the decision about whether to have children. Answering in the affirmative will have a dramatic impact on a couple's sexual relationship because even in the process of trying to conceive, the focus can shift from passion to pregnancy tests. Other couples find the decision thrust upon them with an unplanned pregnancy. Either way, the drama intensifies as couples cope with coitus interruptus during pregnancy and childbirth or coitus interminable with the pain of infertility. These challenges are discussed in detail in Chapter 5.

When women with children recall their lives prepregnancy and prebaby, they often feel they were unaware of some important questions regarding their sex lives. If you are childless or considering having a baby, ask yourself the following questions:

- "How do I picture my sex life changing after having kids?"
- "Do I know any women who are mothers and with whom I can talk about the physical changes they felt during pregnancy and after childbirth?"

"Baby, Baby, Where Did Our Love Go?"

Kids bring life, quite literally, to a partnership, but they can bring death to sex. With babies, priorities don't just shift; they go through major upheavals. Some women fall so in love with their babies that their partners cease to exist. Their passion turns to nurturing their children.

> "I could go through the motions of having sex, even fake it. But if you really wanted to see me show passion, it was when my baby Jake clapped his hands and said, 'Mama.'"

Most women find that childrearing increases demands on both parents but primarily on themselves. There is less privacy, less (if any) time to be intimate, far more demands to meet, and far greater fatigue to bear. Current books on women, work, parenting, and homemaking document the grueling pace that has become characteristic of modern-day motherhood. A woman can be up until 1:00 A.M. every night doing housework after homework, then sorting laundry, prepping for the next day at the job, and finally firing up the slow cooker because tomorrow is another day of carpooling the kids after work.

> "Sometimes I look over at my partner, when we're all sitting together, and I think, *What a wonderful person!* I'll feel this surge of love that is sexual, too. The trouble is—the timing's *all* wrong. When we're alone together, I'm tired or busy with other tasks. If we're just hanging out, there are kids, and I have to attend to getting them ready for bed and the next day of school. My partner says I need to put that stuff on hold and just come to bed so that we can enjoy each other. Why can't I do that? How come I only put us first if someone else is taking care of the kids?"

On those rare occasions when women get together as friends, much of the conversation is about how busy and tired they are, as if fatigue were the primary bond that women share. So much for those sexy Saturday mornings in bed they so enjoyed when they were childless. Some couples may even think, *So much for sex, period!*

Women with children may feel overwhelmed by the extent of their responsibilities. They may also have ambivalent feelings about the changes in their post-pregnancy bodies and may resist being seen naked by their partners. They may feel resentment toward their partners, seeing them as unappreciative, uninvolved, and too demanding. It's not surprising that many women during this stage in their lives announce that they don't like sex and can live without it.

Because of the demands of raising children, sex often loses its place in the life of a couple. Some women simply resign themselves to becoming asexual; others refuse to relinquish this core part of who they are as sexual human beings but do little more than complain about their predicaments. Whether you have children or are thinking about having them, ask yourself these questions:

- "Am I getting together with friends to dump on sex and my partner? Have I thought about what I get out of these gripe sessions with other women?"
- "Is sex important enough for me to work on? If not, when will it be important enough?"
- "Do I complain about sex with my partner because I secretly fantasize that I could have a better sex life with some other partner?"
- "Do I believe that women have the power to create better sex lives for themselves, or are they helpless to make changes in themselves and in their relationships?"

If you don't want your sex life to end just because you're a mom, read Parts IV and V to identify strategies that will help you keep sex alive in your relationship and, more important, in *you*. In addition, the exercises in Chapter 13 will help you better understand the origins of your feelings of helplessness and anger.

> "We figured out that the house just wasn't a sexy place for us anymore; there's baby paraphernalia in every room. Some nights we have what we call 'take-out sex.' When the babysitter arrives, I'm out the door. First I stop for Chinese take-out, then I head to my office, where my partner meets me. We lock the office door and make love on the floor. I'm lobbying for a thicker carpet pad next time the office is redecorated!"

Being Single with a Baby

For a number of reasons, a woman may have a baby without a partner. Women who do so remark that their sex life is altered dramatically and that being single *and* a mother presents challenges.

> "It seemed that after I had the baby, I could meet only two kinds of guys. There were the ones who would run for the door as soon as they found out I had a kid and the ones who came on hot and heavy—figuring I must be desperate for sex. After a while, I pretty much gave up on sex and relationships."

This "giving up on sex" is not unusual. For a variety of reasons, women go through periods of their lives when they're not having sex. However, your sexuality is still part of you, and "giving up on sex"—meaning sex with a partner—does not have to mean giving up on the pleasure you can feel sexually. Find a place for sex through masturbation, fantasy, reading erotica, and taking time to be good to you. If you are considering involvement with someone, read "Endings and Beginnings" later in this chapter.

Whether partnered or single, children will occupy a big part of your life, but they don't have to take your whole life. The pleasure you feel in your own sexuality can bring you a deeper and fulfilling sense of all of who you are.

LOOKING 50 IN THE FACE

The greatest barrier to a woman's sexuality in midlife is the socially transmitted disease of *ageism*. The vibrant sexuality of women in their middle years is often socially invisible, obscured by our dominant culture's preoccupation with equating sexiness with youth. Nevertheless, women in their 40s and 50s continue to be sexually robust. Yes, your body changes; in life, change is certain. But by the time you are coping with the physical changes associated with menopause and aging, you are doing so with the advantage of lifelong experience with meeting and overcoming challenges.

> "We were heading out the door when my 16-year-old daughter turned to her friend Abby and said, 'Guess what! My parents are going out to celebrate my mom's 50th birthday.' Abby looked at me and exclaimed, 'Gee, that's great. And you don't look 50—in the face!'"

Our clients have taught us that women are sexual because they want to be and choose to be, not because they are young, in perfect shape, or gorgeous. Some of our stereotypically beautiful clients are the unhappiest because they have spent so much time obsessively striving to replicate the cultural standard that their view of themselves has shrunk to the single dimension of body appearance. They experience no inner peace or freedom in their sexuality. Conversely, many of our older clients describe an intimacy with their partners not possible in youth and a comfort with themselves unmatched in more youthful times.

> "I love sex in my 50s. During sex when I was younger, I tried to hide my thighs with my hands or insist on having the lights off. Now I don't care if my body's not perfect. I leave the lights on because every little detail of our lovemaking is erotic to me, and I don't want to miss a thing."

Passion That Isn't Skin Deep

Aging can actually be sexually freeing. Many older women report that the increased confidence of age and experience gives them the courage to be more passionate in their identity and in their sexuality. A passionate woman wears the clothes she wants to wear and looks people straight in the eye and smiles. Passionate women develop an attitude that says, *I'm delighted with this age and this body of mine.* Passionate women think talking about sex is important. Passionate women take time to have sex with their partners or masturbate regularly.

Perhaps you've noticed that you don't get the "looks" you got as a younger woman. You may be upset by the physical changes of aging and lament wrinkles in your face or increased thickness in your waist. Your hair may be thinning, to your dismay. If you are in perimenopause, the years before you stop having periods, there will be changes in your menstrual cycle, your metabolism, and possibly your energy level. You may find that your skin is drier and your muscles need more regular workouts to stay toned. Hormonal changes occur. Your sexual response may change. Read Chapters 4 and 5 for a discussion of the hormonal, physical, and sexual changes associated with aging.

Yes, these changes can be a challenge. You may judge your body's new shape and state as sexually unappealing, causing you to withdraw from your sexuality. This is a choice-point in your life. Will you continue to be sexual by finding a place for your sexuality and loving your body in all the shapes it will assume over your lifetime? In Part III ("Making Peace with Your Body"), we discuss body image, pain, illness, disability, and trauma and suggest ways to continue to be in touch with your body's remarkable ability to be sexual throughout your life, even in the face of change and challenge. Ask yourself these questions:

- "If I'm physically uncomfortable, am I seeing a healthcare practitioner, reading books, and talking with other women about adjusting to perimenopause?"
- "Have I spent time masturbating and enjoying my own physical sensations?"
- "If I'm feeling more depressed or anxious, or not sleeping well, have I considered this might be related to perimenopause?" (Discuss this with your healthcare provider.)
- "Do I continue to recognize myself as a sexual person? If not, am I prepared to take responsibility to change my negative thinking?

Looking 50 in the Face Together

If you are in midlife and in a healthy relationship, sex with your partner isn't skin deep. You're likely aroused by your partner's personality and your shared experiences. You may be less afraid of making sexual mistakes and more interested in making the most of your connection. Many times the early years of a couple's sexual experience involve intense, explosive, genitally focused sex. Sex in your middle years tends to incorporate the luxury of exploration, taking your time, and expanding the sexual act far beyond the scope of the fast and furious genital rubbing and penis-pushing of earlier times. For those who have worked to achieve it—be they straight or lesbian couples—sex and intimacy may be intertwined in ways that are possible only through time and trial in a relationship.

> "We took yoga lessons together. At first we felt awkward, but then I started getting turned on by watching my partner stretch. I suggested, 'Why don't we try tantra, spiritual sexuality?' We started going to workshops, learning about breathing, energy, and spirituality. Where have we been? This has fired up our sex life by teaching us new ways to be sexually alive."

Of course there is the possibility that your sex life with your long-term partner has become stagnant, predictable, and boring. Or perhaps a sexual problem has developed decades into your relationship. Maybe old preferred patterns of lovemaking don't "work" anymore. Sometimes the type of stimulation that used to feel wonderful now feels irritating or even painful. Perhaps you were always more "passive" to your partner's "active," but now your partner needs more initiation and physical stimulation from you to achieve and sustain the same level of arousal as in earlier years. Some couples take their sexual life together for granted. They have no language or experience for solving problems when they occur. One or both partners withdraw from the problem. Weeks drift into months or years, and sex is avoided altogether. Sleeping in the same bed with physical distance between you and your partner graduates to separate bedrooms, usually under the guise of other reasons (snoring, getting up too often during the night). See Chapter 12 for ways to talk about sex.

If you recognize yourself here, read Parts IV and V. Ask yourself these questions:

- "Have I 'checked out' sexually, settling for shopping and eating out as substitutes for passion?"
- "What happened to me during menopause? Did I stay in touch with my sexuality, or did I become so distracted with the sleep disruption and hot flashes that I 'checked out' of my body altogether?" (If your answer is yes, Chapter 5 may offer some ways to get back into your body and your sexual self.)
- "How sexually interested and supportive is my partner?"
- "Am I more turned on by fantasy—chick flicks, erotic novels, and the younger trainer at the health club—than by reality with my partner? [If yes:] Am I ready to stop escaping and address what's wrong with our sex life?"
- "Do I expect my partner to fix our sexual problems?"
- "Does my partner have an unaddressed sexual difficulty [such as difficulty with orgasm]? [If yes:] Are we avoiding the subject or even sleeping separately?"

Empty Nest

Looking 50 in the face often means also looking at a suddenly empty household. When children grow and go, it is often a mixed experience. At first your living space may feel different. Your relationship may feel different. You may feel different.

Elsewhere in the book we refer to *other-oriented* sex. This is sexual activity based not on what *you* feel, want, or desire, but on what the *other person* expresses, indicates, or desires. Life with children is certainly other-oriented, so your daily activities and sexual activities can mimic each other in ways that aren't particularly focused on you. By the time the children move out, some women turn their backs on sexuality because they have lived with other-oriented sex for too long, and they don't know how to be self-oriented in their sexuality (or perhaps in their empty nest). But many more women take a deep breath and relax, ready to embark on the adventure of sexuality (and time) for themselves.

Once children are grown, many times (hopefully) the child-rearing dramas go with them. Perhaps menopause and major work insecurities are behind you as well. You may have privacy for the first time in years. Although every stage of life presents us with unique and varied challenges, this stage, at least, may be freer of burdening responsibilities and time demands.

> "The first year or so after our youngest went to college, I felt torn when he would come home and leave again. I'd miss how his vitality would fill up the house. Then I began to notice a shift. After a while I'd enjoy his time at home, but my partner and I were getting used to our freedom and privacy, and we'd really miss that when he was back. Sometimes as we'd wave him off as he left again, I'd feel temporarily sad, but then we'd look at each other and make a beeline for the bedroom."

Looking 50 in the face is tough, but it is a wonderful tough. The "gift" of time beyond reproductive years is something our ancestors couldn't even have imagined. In fact, as we indicated earlier, as life expectancy continues to expand, you can look forward to having as many adult years postmenopause as you had during your adult reproductive years. You have been exposed to the myth—and it *is* a myth—that sex and sexual allure are for the young. Not so. That is true only if you allow it to be. Passion and sexuality come from the inside, and the secure sense of personal empowerment you may feel now that you are freed from the insecurities and uncertainties of youth can be the strongest aphrodisiac of all.

ENDINGS AND BEGINNINGS

In life one thing is certain: there will be losses. A woman's sexual life is inevitably affected by loss, whether it's in the form of her partner having an affair, the death of her partner, divorce, or desertion. Relationships tend to end either abruptly or slowly and painfully. In the case of an affair, the relationship may not necessarily come to an end, but the fantasy of unending love and total commitment does. In this section, we explore common *endings* that women experience in their adult sexual lives and the important *beginnings* that can, and often do, follow.

Ending a Fantasy: Affairs

In as many as 45% of marriages in the United States, one or both partners have sought sex outside the relationship (Atwood & Schwartz, 2002). There are many possible reasons for this pervasive pattern. People may be looking for what they think is missing in their marriage—be it passion, respect, or intimacy. They may be angry with their partner and want to "get even." The affair may be the product of a moment of vulnerability—an evening of too much alcohol or a time of inconsolable sadness. An affair may be an attempt to repair an old hurt of being ignored and unloved as a child. In recent years, a new phenomenon has emerged—Internet infidelity or "virtual affairs." A growing number of women and men are turning to online relationships for emotional intimacy and eroticism.

Affairs can signal the presence of a wound that will fester and tear the marriage apart unless it is healed. Affairs are often experienced as a violation of highly personal space, leaving the partner feeling a loss of pride and self-esteem. Trust may not be restored easily. Sex in the relationship can become strained or nonexistent because it serves as a poignant reminder of the hurt and feelings of betrayal. Perhaps what is most difficult is that an affair destroys the fantasy that the couple will enjoy a storybook life together—that they will "live happily ever after."

When an affair occurs, the question to be asked by the injured partner is not "How could you do this to me?" but "How could you do this to *yourself*?" For any chance of reconciliation, the person who has had the affair must grapple with this question. The partner has to ask similar questions: "What value does monogamy hold for me? What will be necessary to keep me in this relationship?" A couple who are committed to answering these questions honestly can best determine either how to repair what is broken or whether to bring the relationship to an end. They will make a commitment not to save the partnership at all costs but to be honest with themselves and each other about their goals and values. If promises are to be made, we recommend the partners make them to themselves and include these three:

"I won't tolerate [or have] an affair again."
"I won't be silent about my needs or disappointments."
"I won't settle for the kind of communication, sex, and intimacy we've had in the past."

Even when wounds heal well, they leave scars that will always be noticed. But scar tissue is tougher and stronger than skin.

"After the affair, we went through such turmoil. We argued, talked, and grieved. We each questioned whether we'd stay together. We went to counseling and began to look at the differences we had. We got very specific about the kind of partnership we wanted. It was a painful but important process."

We cannot do justice here to describing the complexities of affairs and the ways in which people address and overcome these problems. If you are coping with an ongoing affair or the aftermath of one, we encourage you to seek counseling. You might also read the books on couples communication and intimacy noted in the "Suggested Resources" at the end of the book.

If you have had, or are having, an affair, reflect on the following questions:

- "What was I looking for by going outside of the relationship?"
- "Did I find it, or was it a mirage?"
- "Was I trying to hurt or get even with my partner?"

If your partner has had an affair, you may find answering the following questions helpful:"

- "Did I assume there must be something wrong with me?"
- [If you entered counseling after the affair:] "Was my goal to bash my partner? Myself?"
- [If you chose to stay in the relationship:] "Why did I stay with [him or her]?"
- [If you stayed in the relationship:] "Have I been able to let go of my anger and hurt, or does it continue to cast a shadow on us?"
- [If you and your partner have resumed sexual activity:] "Has our lovemaking been out of a desire to reconnect or out of fear of losing [him or her]?"
- "Have my sexual feelings and responses changed since learning of the affair?"

Ending in Divorce

On the wedding day, no one expects to get divorced, but the truth is that that's how many marriages end. The number of women facing life after the breakup of a relationship is even higher when you include women who have ended civil unions or live-together relationships. Despite jokes about the wild sexual life of single women, being divorced is not the sexiest time in a woman's life. Most newly divorced women admit that they don't like casual sex and are looking for partnerships involving intimacy and mutual caring.

The months after the breakup of your partnership can bring depression, a drop in self-esteem, and a sexual shutdown. These feelings can prompt you to idealize your former partner and fantasize about reconnection. You may periodically have sex with your relocated partner and wonder if the two of you should reunite. You may even find that the sex is better now that you're not in daily conflict.

The more ambiguous and ambivalent you were about the divorce or breakup, the more difficult it will be for you to grieve the loss of the relationship and make sense of your current life. Eventually, however, you will most likely realize that you can't "turn back the clock" and you will move ahead. If you find you can't move on, consider getting counseling and support to make sense of your feelings.

Looking ahead, you may fear that you'll re-create past problems or may not trust your judgment about future partners. It makes sense to take time to know yourself better before rushing into a new relationship. This includes knowing about your own sexuality.

Sex may have been great in your former partnership, or it may have been awful. Now is the time to decide, on your own terms, what sex is going to be like for you in the future. Remember that being single doesn't mean anything negative about your sexuality. You're sexual regardless of your partnership status. Masturbation, fantasy, reading erotica, buying a vibrator, even checking out sexy websites are all safe and friendly ways to continue to be sexual. They don't involve a partner, require a babysitter, or commit you to meeting someone's first cousin from Toledo.

But don't stop here! Think about the ways that physical activity, friendship, and being in charge of your life can work for you. Singleism gets a very bad rap in many cultures. We are saying this: When you go to live life fully, include your sexual health and your identity as a sexual woman.

Ending in Widowhood

Forty-five percent of women 65 or older are widows (Administration on Aging, 2000). In trying to take care of their sexual selves, widows face unique challenges. In most cultures neither they nor older women are viewed as sexual persons. Older women then face a kind of "double indemnity." Young or old, widows often report that they feel no sexual interest immediately following the death of their spouse, but over time interest in sex usually returns. Not only do widows face cultural stereotypes that negate their sexuality, they also may have to contend with strong internal ambivalence.

> "It had been 2 years since James died. I wasn't looking for anyone, but when I met Alec I was very attracted to him. One night we began to get very sexual. Then it hit me that this was the first time in 45 years that someone other than James had touched me this way. I froze. I felt like I was cheating on James."

Grieving the death of a spouse requires considerable time and work. You'll never forget your partner—he or she will always be an important part of your life. But, in time, the grieving process will allow you to reposition your partner to another place in your life, one that is less central, less exclusive, less dominating. The grieving process will eventually free you emotionally to seek new relationships.

This process takes time—2, 4, even 8 years is not an unusual amount of time before someone is ready emotionally to pursue an intimate relationship. And there will still be times of awkwardness or guilt. There is no road map, only your own steady belief that you are going it alone and that you must do what is wisest and healthiest for you. During the interim, while doing the work of grief, it is important to remember that your sexuality didn't expire just because your partner died.

"In my loneliness, sometimes I would try masturbating, but it reminded me I was alone in my empty bed. Instead of being a sexual turn-on, I'd start to cry, and I'd lie there, my hands rubbing my vulva while tears streamed down my face. Then I realized that this was just how my life felt. I'd have good days and still want to weep. I began to allow sex back into my life the same way I did with other things, a little bit at a time—inching ahead. Sex reminded me that I was alive and what I was still capable of. It felt good to orgasm. I began to treasure my sexuality and see it as one of the parts of me that had been there before and was here with me now."

Beginning to Venture Out

Widowed, divorced, or single due to other reasons, you may feel awkward when reentering the dating scene. If you decide to have sex with a new partner, it can be intimidating and downright scary.

"When I was 22, it was hard enough the first time a partner would see me naked. Even though I had a pretty good sex life with my ex-partner, I haven't had sex with someone in a long time and don't know how it will work out."

Beginning a new sexual relationship is even more complex and challenging if you have children living at home.

"Being single with kids meant making a lot of decisions with no road map to follow. I learned to be honest with myself, recognizing my vulnerability about wanting passion and sex in a life full of responsibility and work."

When a single mom decides she's interested in a sexual relationship, she has to consider the effect this will have on her children. She'll have to take into account how old they are, how much time she has to spend with them, and their likely reactions to a new adult on the scene. She'll have to decide whether to bring home the person she's dating to meet the children, whether to have the new partner spend the night with her, and how and when to arrange time to be sexual.

If you are a single mom, many questions specific to your own situation will need to be answered now or in the future. The following questions may help jump-start your thinking about being a single parent and having sex:

- "At what point in a relationship should I introduce a new partner to my kids?"
- "Would I have sex with a friend or only someone I'm in love with? At what point in the relationship would I have sex?"

- "Would I be physically affectionate with my partner in front of the kids? If so, how far would I go?"
- "Would I ever have a new partner spend the night at my home—with or without the children at home?"
- "Would I spend the night at my partner's place?"
- "Would I feel comfortable renting a motel room for 'quickies'?"
- "Am I staying aware of my children's emerging sexuality and their needs for privacy, predictable routine, and my ability to 'go about the business of being a family' without having to deal with a sexually charged environment?"
- "Do I explain to my kids my need to have friends and love, while assuring them of my continued commitment to them as a top priority in my life?"
- "Whether they are young or adults, do my children have the final vote about whether I explore the possibility of a relationship with the person I'm currently seeing?"
- "Parent or not, when the bedroom door closes, how do I feel about my sex life?"
- "And finally, am I practicing safer sex to protect against the transmission of STIs or to prevent pregnancy?"

Remarriage: When One Becomes Two Again

New partner, fresh start. That's the hope you bring to a new partnership. Some women report being surprised that sexual problems experienced before can reemerge in this new relationship. If you've put off addressing a concern, now is the time to tackle it. Review Part V, especially Chapter 15, to gain insight into your sexual difficulties and learn ways to overcome them.

All remarriages or new partnerships begin in loss. If you were widowed, you may experience a normal resurgence of grief when entering a new partnership, even though you're happy to be with this person. If you have been divorced, you are likely to be "sadder but wiser" about partnerships, and it may take several years before you trust that this relationship isn't going to break up.

When it comes to sex in a remarriage, the most important question is: Who else is in the house? If you and your partner are home alone, your sexual activity may be easy to establish, but in many remarriages kids and exes present formidable challenges. If you and your partner have teenagers, they may be uncomfortable with your sexuality and make comments like "You're so gross when you hug each other." This is not going to enliven your relationship. One set of parents coordinating the activities of one set of kids is exhausting enough; imagine the complications when you have up to three sets of parents and two sets of kids requiring coordination and accommodation. You can feel like you're trapped in an endless cycle of figuring out whose kids are staying with which parents on what weekends. This too affects your sex life—big time.

"It was hard to keep my desires in check. After such a long dry spell, I wanted sex when I wanted it, but there were the kids, their activities, our jobs, constant juggling. I wanted this to be simple, but that's not realistic."

Women with children often report that sex in a remarriage can fade quickly if they try to make this new relationship mimic the early days of their first marriage. In a remarriage, you don't have the same control over your freedom, time, or privacy as you probably had when you entered your first marriage. And your children certainly will not go out of their way to make your sex life easier!

Your sexual relationship with your partner will be most successful if you first take care of some basic rules for outside the bedroom. Research indicates that when you remarry, you and your partner need to give up your fantasies about a perfect unified family. You'll need to address conflicts, tolerate stress, and normalize the need for flexibility in the new family structure (Walsh, 1991). You'll need to recognize and combat unrealistic expectations that you may place on yourself. For example, as a mother, you may feel pressure to make the family "successful." If the kids are unhappy in the remarried family, you may feel guilty about taking private time for you and your partner or having any sexual pleasure. Chapter 13 provides helpful suggestions for combating such guilt by identifying and fighting the underlying irrational or self-defeating beliefs and assumptions.

The answers to the following questions will help you build a positive sex life with your new partner while, at the same time, respecting the needs of your family.

- "Have I addressed the emotional baggage from my previous relationship? Should I consider counseling if I haven't?"
- "Have we established a stable household with predictable schedules and clear rules and expectations for everybody?"
- "Have we explained to the children that we sometimes need to be alone in our own bedroom?"
- "Do they know to knock before walking in? Do we have a lock on the door so we won't be accidentally 'surprised' when having sex?"
- "Have we discussed the importance of flexible planning for issues such as custody arrangements?"
- "If our kids are grown, have we discussed how they may find our sexuality uncomfortable when they visit?"
- "Have we discussed how we're going to handle our frustration if sex gets interrupted repeatedly, or if we have to scrap a weekend away, or if we have to go weeks before we're alone?"
- "Have we discussed how it will take time to create this new family and that we're going to have periods of ambivalence and differences of opinion?"
- "Is sex a glue to help us through these times, or do we use sex to avoid discussion?"

- "Do I treat my partner's requests for sex as one more demand on me?"
- "Are we willing to schedule sex so that we are sure to have special time together?"

As you read through these questions, you may recognize problem areas. Chapter 12 provides you with helpful suggestions for enriching your relationship.

Being Single Is Not an Ending

The end of one relationship is not always followed by the beginning of a new relationship. Still, the end of a relationship does not mean the end of your sexuality. Some single women who were previously partnered can honestly predict that there is little likelihood they will find a new sexual partner. Their sexual response to this status is as varied as their circumstances. Some choose not to be sexual at all, others continue to masturbate and explore sensuality, and some even choose to have occasional sexual experiences. These sexual experiences, as we discussed earlier in the chapter, may be driven by passion, neediness, adventure, or desperation.

As singlehood stretches out over the years, a woman redefines herself, including her sexuality, from being partner oriented to being self-oriented. Unlike a woman's young adulthood, later in life her single "sexual self" may not be highly valued by the culture. Women often remark that they have to encourage themselves to stay sexually vibrant. They work to keep sex as part of their life even as they refocus attention and passion on other aspects of life, like family, friends, and meaningful activities.

If you are single, ask yourself these questions.

- "Do I value myself as a sexual person?"
- "Am I willing to continue to explore my sexuality?"
- "Do I regularly allow myself to fantasize, read erotica, masturbate, and enjoy my sexuality in other meaningful ways?"
- "If I'm uncomfortable with my body and with touching myself, am I interested in doing the exercises in this book to help me grow sexually comfortable?" (The exercises in Chapters 13 and 14 will help you.)
- "If I am in a period without physical intimacy, can I get regular massages or facials to treat myself to being touched in nonsexual ways? Do I initiate hugs with my family and friends, ask for and give back rubs, or hold hands when we walk together?"
- "Should I consider some form of body work or exercise by taking a course in Feldenkrais body awareness, martial arts, dance, swimming, or any other kind of movement?"

- "Do I foster my sensuality in the ways that I dress or decorate my home or in the activities I choose?"
- "Do I intentionally think of myself as a sexual person? Do I allow myself to have sex with myself, be curious about sex, and enjoy this deeply important part of me?"

THE 60s AND ON: "THEY SAY THERE'S BEEN A REVOLUTION"

"What amazed me was sex in my 60s. No one told me how much I'd get turned on and how fun it would be. I'm more adventurous than I thought I'd be, trying a vibrator and getting my partner to try one too."

Older adults are breaking the sound barrier of sexuality. We are only at the beginning of understanding what happens to women postmenopause, but what we are learning is both frustrating and reassuring. Frustrating because the cultural "bandwidth" for female attractiveness ignores the beauty of older women and neglects the sensuality of lifelong passion, vitality, and wisdom in women's sexual lives. An older woman may feel she cannot possibly find a partner with such an uneven playing field.

The rules of the game are slowly changing, however, as more older women are dating younger partners. Women are also going online and using their social networks to meet partners. And women are not waiting for a special person to "make them happy." Increasingly, older women are engaging in self-pleasure, purchasing vibrators and masturbating to orgasm. They may acknowledge that sleeping alone or masturbating is not as much fun as partnered sex, but they are also acknowledging that they will not settle for the sexual sidelines in life. Women are orgasmic well into their 90s or 100s. Orgasm and self-pleasuring are part of one's sexual health, and that affects general health.

Where does an interest in sexual health and sexual relating end? Individuals interviewed in palliative-care settings lament the lack of privacy, single beds, staff insensitivity, and general invisibility of their sexuality. Few are asked if they have sexual concerns while they are in terminal care (Lemieux et al., 2004). Age, illness, physical disability, or being single does not stop a person from having sexual health needs. What stops many women is being treated as if they shouldn't have these concerns.

"Sexy grandmother" is *not* an oxymoron. The best-kept secret is sex in one's 60s—that's where the real sexual revolution is embodied. It's a time when the expectation of sexual freedom and comfort is most likely to be a reality. Sex in a woman's 60s is free of time demands. Not only do these women make time for themselves to exercise and pursue personal interests, but they also spend time masturbating and increasing their erotic focus.

Relationships also change. Characteristics of personal strength and assertiveness are valued, and sexual attraction develops from the relationship as well as from appearance. This pattern is in contrast to what younger people experience, where superficial physical attraction is often the initial basis of coupling, and vitality, identity, and depth of personality can be, unfortunately, afterthoughts.

And this sexual revolution isn't confined just to women in their 60s. Used to being ignored as too old or asexual, women in their 70s and 80s have gone about taking charge of their sexuality and proving just how sensual and erotic they can be with themselves and their partners. If they're in long-term partnerships, they find that sex and intimacy can deepen in ways that are possible only for relationships that have been tempered by time, shared trials, and honest communication.

Physical illness, disability, and stress over financial security and retirement can complicate sex during the later years. Widowhood also becomes a significant factor during this stage in life. But healthy or not, partnered or not, women in their later years continue to be sexual people capable of responding to sensual pleasure.

> "What irritates me most in my 70s is the way that people write me off as a sexual has-been. We've always had a good sex life, but we didn't talk about our sex life with anyone else. Then I had a hip replacement, and before I left the hospital the physician suggested that I avoid the missionary position so that I didn't stress my new hip. 'Make love on top,' she said. At first I was embarrassed, but my partner encouraged me to ask questions. The doctor suggested that I go on the web to look at resources and to buy a vibrator. Now we're open to new ideas from anyone! We've been reading erotica out loud to each other, especially on days when my hip or his bad knee is acting up. To be honest, I think you have to be at least 65 to be erotic."

Confusing Aging with Poor Health

A common mistake is to confuse aging and poor health. Being depressed, overly anxious, or irritable isn't part of growing old—it's an offshoot of poor health. Disrupted sleep patterns can also be a sign of depression. Just as cartilage around joints wears away as we age, so does our neurochemical resilience; we just don't bounce back as quickly when we face challenges and stressors. Depression can cause you to withdraw from sexual activities you used to enjoy.

As you age, you may experience chronic medical conditions (like diabetes), mechanical difficulties (like joint or back problems), memory difficulties (like dementia or depression), or fatigue. Remember that your healthcare provider should be part of the solution, not part of the problem, so find medical help that is consistently supportive of you. There may be medications, physical therapy, or a medical procedure that can help you. Use the suggestions for finding a healthcare provider that we give in Chapter 15. Practitioners trained in gerontology will usually be the most knowledgeable.

Accommodate; Don't Capitulate

Sexually active women in their later years observe that issues of physical pain, mobility, and urinary incontinence are the greatest barriers to partnered sex. They find that healthcare providers may not be knowledgeable about their sexual difficulties or are uncomfortable discussing sex with women in their later years. Rather than giving up and going along with the social stereotype that sex is reserved for the young, these women find ways to make accommodations. Chapters 7 and 8 may help you make the physical accommodations you need.

As a sexual woman in your later years, ask yourself these questions:

- "Am I addressing my physical difficulties and willing to consider new ideas for medical care, even if these include medications, physical therapy, learning to use a walker, hearing aid, or other prosthesis?"
- "Am I exercising regularly, including my pelvic floor muscles [Kegels]?"
- "Would I consider an antidepressant medication to improve my mood, sleep, or memory?"
- "Am I avoiding sex because of urinary incontinence?"

Privacy in Assisted-Living Facilities

Some women discover that their interest in partnered sex makes their grown children uncomfortable, and unfortunately many senior housing and care facilities often try to prevent sexual activity between residents and aren't comfortable providing privacy for masturbation either. The lack of freedom and privacy to enjoy sex is a great loss for many residents. Continue to remind your facility managers that older adults have a right to sexual privacy. If senior years are still ahead of you, advocate for the privacy of the seniors in your life who are in assisted-living facilities.

Going the Distance: Your Lifelong Sexuality

Inevitably, all relationships will end, and the majority of married women who live past 80 will be widowed. In youth the possibility of facing this loss seems obscure and unlikely. Most couples who pledge "till death do us part" in their younger years have no concept of what they are promising. Women respond to this loss in different ways. Some may seek a new partner. Other women who are widowed or divorced in older age may choose not to seek new partners but to continue masturbating regularly. They report learning new ways to self-pleasure by using sexual fantasy, vibrators, and dildos. Many cope with loss by learning to refocus their attention and passion on other aspects of their life, like family and social activities.

However they cope, women of age do not appear to meet this challenge by withering and withdrawing. It may seem a paradox, but older single women do not describe their lives as lonely or empty, despite the blatant fact that the majority of them do not have a sexual partner. In fact, they describe less loneliness than at other periods in their life (Friedan, 1994).

Why do women describe less loneliness at an older age? We may be tempted to conclude that sex is not important for women at this stage. That would be erroneous. Sex, intimacy, and touch remain important, but at this stage intimacy has been established in a much broader context.

Women have always been known for their enduring ability to form and nurture meaningful relationships. Whether in the quiet companionship of women quilting together or two friends exchanging voice or text messages in the midst of a hectic day, women tend to weave their lives around relationships.

Women of age have developed a capacity to experience closeness in many deep and abiding forms. This frequently translates into intimacy that does not depend upon, or define itself through, genital sex or intercourse. This does not mean that what is lost or missing is not grieved, but emotionally healthy older women do not seem to waste away or pine for what they do not have. Instead, they draw upon their remarkable abilities of connection to experience intimacy in ways that transcend narrow definitions. Ask yourself:

- "Do I continue to fantasize, masturbate, and enjoy touch?"
- "Do I draw pleasure in remembering positive sexual experiences?" (If memories of sex are traumatic, you may find it helpful to read Chapter 10.)
- "Do I continue to develop myself by being social and nurturing my friendships?"

PART II

Understanding Your Body

Sex research routinely points out how little most women know about their anatomy and sexual function. Our clinical experiences confirm this. In fact, we are constantly surprised by how many of our clients would probably agree with a statement from one client that we've never forgotten: "I really don't know much about sex. I just do it."

Our bodies are central to our sexuality. If sex, in the broadest sense, refers to experiencing pleasure, it is a pleasure we experience in our bodies. If we consider sex in the context of relating to another person, it's through our bodies that we connect and share pleasure. Even love, which we usually consider more emotional than physical, yearns for physical touch and connection. When a woman doesn't know her body, she is less likely to know the pleasure she can feel in her body.

Understanding your body and how it functions is an important way of taking care of your sexual self. This knowledge helps to demystify sex and makes it easier to learn ways to increase your sexual comfort and pleasure. Just as loving someone requires knowing that person, the ability to accept and love our bodies requires us to know and understand them. It's a factor that is critical to healthy sexuality.

In the next three chapters, we offer straight talk about anatomy, hormones, and sexual function. Corresponding exercises to help you become more familiar with your sexual anatomy and more comfortable with your body are in Chapter 13. In this section we hope to answer the questions so often asked in our offices:

- "Is there really a G spot, and if so, how do I find mine?"
- "Why do women have both male and female hormones?"

- "Are all women capable of having multiple orgasms?"
- "Why does it seem so easy for me to orgasm from stimulation of the clitoris but so hard with penetration alone?"
- "Am I more likely to get pregnant when I orgasm?"
- "How do I choose the best birth control method for me?"
- "Is it true that women often get pregnant when they stop trying so hard?"
- "Does intercourse cause premature labor?"
- "Is menopause the beginning of the end of my sex life?"
- "What kind of menstrual changes should I be worried about?"

THREE

Your Body

In their earliest weeks of existence, tiny, developing embryos—biologically destined to be a boy or a girl—are already forming their future reproductive organs. The entire embryo at this point is no larger than a pea, so imagine just how small the tiny genitals and sexual organs must be. At this early stage of fetal development, the egg- and sperm-producing glands are impossible to tell apart. In fact, up until about 7 weeks after conception, developing males and females have virtually the same external genitals. At this point both boys and girls have an "outie," or small bump that's called a *genital tubercle*, and an "innie," which is an opening called the *urogenital slit*.

Despite its early "unisex" appearance, however, the developing embryo already "knows" whether it will be a boy or a girl. This is determined by the chromosomes—XX for girls and XY for boys—that keep development on track. Genes will help the process along by triggering the release of the appropriate hormones at the appropriate times, so that a boy eventually develops a penis and a girl a clitoris. Based on the chromosomal blueprint and influence of hormones, folds of tissue and swellings will develop into a labia or a scrotum. Males will develop testicles, which will produce sperm, and females will develop ovaries, which contain ova, or eggs. As development continues, the clitoris and the tip of the penis (glans) will experience a proliferation of nerve endings, making them highly sensitive to stimulation. The penis and the clitoris, as well as other parts of the vulva, will develop erectile tissue that is capable of becoming engorged with blood when stimulated.

As babies grow into toddlers, parents of sons have it easy when it comes to teaching genital names: *penis*. No confusion about what they are naming—it's right out there and, as for the rest, they can teach about the other parts later. That's why you never hear a toddler running around talking about his *vas deferens*. Parents of daughters have a greater challenge. A girl's genitalia require more names for more parts, and they aren't all that visible. We suspect your parents did what most do—they taught you one name: *vagina*. People readily assume it's the girl's body part analogous to the boy's penis. He has his penis; she has her vagina. But a boy urinates out of his penis, and a girl from her urethra, so there's at least one difference that isn't covered by solely relying on "vagina" as the anatomical name for a girl's genitals. A little girl has a vulva that is immature. It encases her vagina, urethra, and clitoris, but most little girls have no idea what a vulva is or that they even have one.

Why don't girls (and women) know the names of their genital parts? Besides the relatively greater complexity of female genitalia, we suspect it is partly due to parents' apprehension about saying "The clitoris is a part of your genitals that feels good" and anticipating their small daughters' response: "How?" Sticking to the generations-old habit of labeling little girl parts "vagina" may get parents off the hook but is hardly effective sex education. We suggest an alternative: parents can point out that a little girl has a vulva that includes a vagina, a urethra, and a clitoris—one for having babies, one for eliminating urine, and one for pleasure when touched. Women don't have their babies in grocery stores, and girls and women pee and touch for pleasure in private. That's why they're called "private parts."

The terms used to describe female genitals and reproductive organs are either Greek or Latin terms or words made from the names of the male physicians who "discovered" the organ. Popular slang terms for female genitalia do not offer a suitable substitute for the Greek and Latin ones because they aren't consistent or necessarily accurate—they can mean different things to different people. The Latin and Greek words have meanings that are standardized, objectively accurate, and adopted for anatomical description by the World Health Organization. If, at a young age, we were taught what these Latin and Greek terms mean, we would probably have established a better, more knowledgeable relationship with our own bodies. As you are reading this material, if you have any questions about your own physical development or the development of an infant or child that you care for, seek the advice of a medical practitioner. (See Chapter 1 for further discussion about genital names and adult responses to girls' awareness of their sexual parts.)

> "I'm embarrassed to say that, although I am college educated, I didn't know what a vulva was or how to care for my own. It wasn't until I had a daughter, and her pediatrician showed me how to separate the folds of her labia to clean her appropriately—because I hadn't been doing it—that I realized how little I knew. My ignorance hurt her, and I became determined I would teach her what I had never learned."

THE VULVA

Take a mirror and position yourself so you can see your genitals (see Figure 3.1). The visible part of female genitals is called the *vulva*, which means "covering" in Latin. As noted, many people mistakenly refer to a woman's external genitals as her

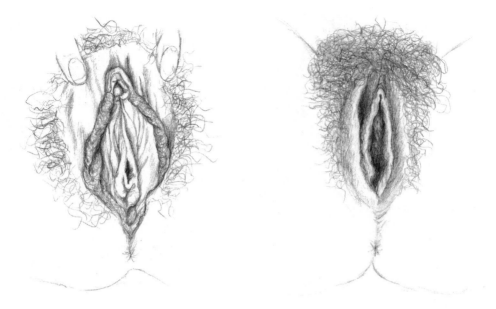

FIGURE 3.1. The vulva. Vulvas differ in appearance woman to woman, as depicted here.

"vagina," but the vagina is actually part of the internal sex organs. Only the vaginal opening is considered part of the vulva, because it's visible from outside the body. The vulva comprises the Venus mound (mons), the labia majora and minora, the vulvar vestibule, the clitoris and clitoral hood, the urinary meatus, and the introitus.

The Venus Mound

The Venus mound is an easier term to relate to than *mons veneris*, its Latin name, which means mount or mountain of Venus, the Roman goddess of love. This is the fatty, cushiony mound directly over the pubic bone. It is an area rich with nerve endings that make it sensitive to touch and pressure. In adults, it is covered with pubic hair. This mound, with the triangle of pubic hair covering it, is the only part of a woman's sexual anatomy that is generally visible when she's nude and upright. Pubic hair has as much variety as hair on women's heads—it can be short or long, wiry or soft, thick or sparse. It may be the same color as the hair on one's head or a contrasting color. Pubic hair thins at menopause, a change that a woman may scarcely notice or that may cause her to experience some feelings of loss.

The Labia Majora

The *labia majora* (Latin: larger lips) are called the outer lips. Referring to the labia majora as "outer lips" is somewhat confusing, because they don't look at all like the inner lips (*labia minora*). The outside of the labia majora consists of fleshy, skin-colored folds, covered with pubic hair. The inside portion of the labia majora, the

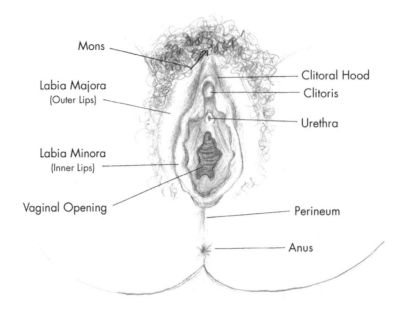

FIGURE 3.2. The visible part of female genitals.

part closest to the inner lips, does not have any pubic hair. The labia majora form a full, rounded oval around the inner lips, the clitoris, the urethra, and the vagina (see Figure 3.2).

The Labia Minora

The *labia minora* (Latin: smaller lips) are the inner lips. The formation of the labia varies from woman to woman, much like penis size and shape vary for men. The shape of the labia tends to be irregular, with less symmetry, say, than eyebrows. Labia vary in thickness, length, and form. The labia have been compared to the petals of a flower. The upper portion of the labia minora forms a hood over the clitoris. The interior skin of the labia minora is pink and often moist. During sexual arousal, blood flows into the labia and the inner lips may more than double in size. The engorgement of the labia during sexual excitement contributes to a woman's sexual pleasure. The labia are rich in nerve endings, making them most sensitive to stimulation. The labia protect the opening, also known as the *introitus*, of the vagina. They are also useful for helping to direct a stream of urine.

The Vulvar Vestibule

The vulvar *vestibule* (Latin: entrance court) is a small area of the vulva protectively enfolded by the labia minora. The pink skin of the vestibule remains moist; otherwise just walking around would be irritating to the labia minora. Perhaps not easily visible to you as you are separating the folds of your labia to explore your vulva is the "Hart's line." This line, sort of like a partial outline of the vestibule, delineates the vestibule from the labia. This may seem like a lot of detail, but if you have pain with sex (see Chapter 8), this anatomical area might well be the site of that pain.

The Clitoris

The term *clitoris* comes from the Greek word *kleitoris*. How the name originated and what it means is uncertain. The best guess is that it means to titillate, to seek pleasure (Angier, 1999). The clitoris has only one purpose and function: pleasure and sexual excitement. It is covered and protected by the labia minora. The clitoris is a small, rounded organ composed of erectile tissue. Similar to a man's penis, this spongy erectile tissue can become engorged with blood and increase in size during sexual arousal. The *glans*, or visible part of the clitoris, has thickly clustered nerve endings, even more than the head of a penis, making it an organ often described as "exquisitely sensitive." The root of the clitoris runs below the surface and is also extremely sensitive. The shaft of the clitoris separates into two parts, wishbone fashion, where the shaft is anchored to the pelvic bone. The clitoris, including the parts that can't be seen, becomes engorged with blood during sexual stimulation and is important in sexual arousal and orgasm. The clitoris is protected by a clitoral hood, or *prepuce* (Latin: foreskin), which is part of the labia minora. This hood of protective tissue can be manipulated to expose more of the clitoris. Women can masturbate by rubbing the exposed portion of their clitoris or by stroking the shaft of the clitoris below the clitoral hood. Thrusting during penetration may cause a tugging on the clitoral hood, which can affect clitoral stimulation and thus become one of the major sources of pleasurable sensation.

The Urethra and Urinary Meatus

The *urethra* (Latin and Greek: to urinate) is a duct or tube that carries urine out of the body from the bladder. Its opening, called the *meatus* (Latin for opening or passageway), is located in the vulvar vestibule, above the vaginal opening and below the clitoris.

The Introitus

Introitus (Latin: going inside) is the name of the vaginal opening. You cannot see the introitus unless the lips of the labia are spread open. This would be a little like stretching the tissues of your cheek to get a look at the inside of your mouth. A ring of muscles, called the *bulbocavernosus* and *ischiocavernosus muscles*, surrounds the introitus. These powerful muscles can contract, and if orgasm occurs during penetration, they actually "hug" the penis, finger, or vibrator inside the vagina. The introitus has many nerve endings, making it very sensitive to stimulation. Technically, the introitus belongs to the group of external sexual parts, the vulva, because it can be seen from the outside.

INTERNAL REPRODUCTIVE SEXUAL ORGANS

The Vagina

The *vagina* (Latin: sheath) is the organ that gets all the publicity as a female genital part. Perhaps that is because of the vagina's function. The vagina envelops and contains the penis during heterosexual intercourse, and it becomes the birth pathway to the world for the newborn. The vagina also is a passageway and connection from the uterus to the outside of the body (see Figure 3.3). Menstrual blood leaves the body through this passageway. The vagina is a closed muscular tube, 3 to 5 inches in length, but expandable. It's a little bit like the inside of an empty mouth. A penis, tampon, finger, or newborn inside the vagina will cause it to expand.

The vagina is a closed passageway; objects inside the vagina can't wander to other areas of the body. The only connection to the rest of the body is through a very small opening of the cervix called the *os* (Latin: mouth, opening). The os opens enough to allow menstrual blood to exit and semen to enter. If a woman has surgery in which her cervix and uterus are removed, the top of the vagina is stitched so that there is no opening from the vagina to any other internal body part.

The vagina remains moist in large part due to mucus discharged by the cervix. These secretions serve as a self-cleansing mechanism to flush away dead cells and

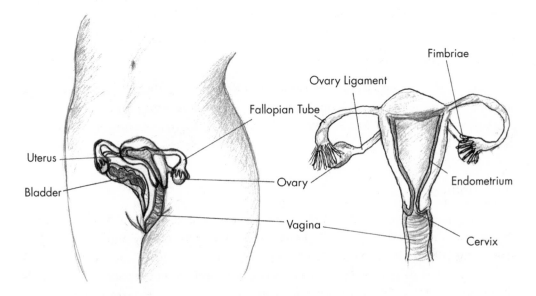

FIGURE 3.3. Internal reproductive sexual organs of a woman.

bacteria and keep the walls of the vagina healthy and moist. The amount, color, scent, and consistency of cervical secretions can change throughout a woman's monthly menstrual cycle, and can be affected by medications, infection, pregnancy, or menopause.

Sexual arousal can dramatically increase vaginal wetness. One source of lubrication is a clear, slippery discharge from two glands (Bartholin's glands) positioned near the introitus. The bulk of vaginal lubrication during sex, however, is the result of a process called *transudation*. When a woman is sexually excited, the spongy tissue that lines the walls of the vagina engorges with blood. As the tissue swells, it pushes these tiny beads of clear, slippery fluid through the walls of the vagina. The fluid consists of the water derived from the plasma engorging the surrounding tissue and small amounts of electrolytes and protein. The upper portion of the vagina is lined with more spongy tissue, so that most of the lubrication is produced closest to the cervix. Hormonal changes or medication side effects can reduce lubrication secretions, causing vaginal dryness during sex.

The vagina is pinkish in color and has a rippled texture that you can feel if you explore with your fingers. The portion of the vagina closest to the opening, or introitus, is sensitive to touch and sexual stimulation, but the upper portion of the vagina, closest to the uterus, has fewer nerve endings. During sexual arousal, this upper portion of the vagina either lengthens and balloons out or compresses, depending on the type of stimulation. We describe this and other physiological reactions of the genitals in Chapter 4.

The Hymen

Most baby girls are born with a membrane called the *hymen* (Latin: membrane; also Greek: god of marriage), which partially covers the opening to the vagina. We aren't sure why the hymen exists; it's just there. The hymen can be tough and thick in some women and practically transparent in others. The absence of a hymen is not proof that a woman or girl has had sexual intercourse. As you can see from the definition, the term refers not only to the membrane but also to marriage. In fact, in many cultures the intact state of the hymen is important evidence that a bride is virginal, and penetrating the hymen on the wedding night is necessary to secure the dowry, the price of the bride, and the woman's reputation (Brumberg, 1997). In some countries, engaged women seek operations to replace their hymens so they won't bring shame on themselves or their families.

After puberty, the hymenal tissue is usually elastic and easily stretched to accommodate penetration of a tampon, finger, or penis. Prior to puberty the vaginal and hymenal tissues can be easily hurt or torn. Some girls will have no evidence of a hymen by the time they reach adolescence. Participation in sports or other vigorous activity as well as even minor accidents, such as falling on the crossbar of a bicycle, can injure or break the hymen. Some girls lose their hymens by inserting fingers into their vaginas while experimenting with masturbation. Others lose their hymens due to the intrusion of sexual abuse.

A hymen may have one, two, several, or no openings. An *annular* hymen has one opening in the membrane. A *septate* hymen has two distinct openings. A *cribriform* hymen has numerous openings, almost honeycomb in appearance. An *imperforate* hymen means no opening is evident. If a hymen is both imperforate and thick, a minor surgical procedure may be needed to open the hymen later on. This is rare.

The Gräfenberg Spot

Ernst Gräfenberg was a German gynecologist who described an area within the vagina on the anterior (upper) wall, between the opening (introitus) and the cervix, that is particularly sensitive to stimulation. In the 1970s and 1980s Drs. Beverly Whipple and John Perry collaborated on research studying the patterns of orgasmic response in women by focusing on what they called the Gräfenberg spot, or G spot, after Gräfenberg (Ladas et al., 2005; Perry & Whipple, 1981). They reported what many women and couples already knew from experience—the G spot responds and swells when stimulated, often resulting in orgasm for many women. The spot is described as a small area of tissue, possibly erectile tissue similar to the nipples or the clitoris, that appears to enlarge in size during sexual arousal. This spot isn't typically detected during a pelvic examination because the tissue isn't in an aroused state during such an exam.

During orgasm, stimulation of the G spot may cause some women to expel a clear or milky white fluid from the urethra, an ejaculation, which is a different composition from urine (although some women may also expel a small amount of urine). This "female ejaculation" is not confined to an orgasmic response from stimulation of the G spot, although that is how it came to the attention of the researchers. On the basis of the research of Dr. Whipple and others, it appears that the expulsion of fluid during a state of high sexual arousal is an absolutely normal phenomenon, though it doesn't happen for all, or perhaps most, women. For those women who have this experience, the amount of fluid they expel and the circumstances under which this happens can vary dramatically.

There continues to be debate over whether a G spot exists, and if so, what it is and whether every woman has one. A slowly growing consensus in the medical community is that a gland or glands along the urethra (perhaps paraurethral, periurethral, or Skene's glands—experts can't seem to agree) are the remnants of the embryonic prostate gland that would have developed had there been a Y chromosome present to trigger masculine development. In some textbooks, these glands are now referred to as the "female prostate gland." These glands secrete fluid into the urethra and likely account for ejaculation when it occurs. Research suggests that some women do not have these glands, and if they do, the size and density of the glands can vary dramatically. This would account for why some women ejaculate and others do not and why some women can experience intense arousal from vaginal stimulation while others cannot.

The Uterus

The *uterus* (Latin: belly, paunch, womb) is about the size and shape of an upside-down pear. The walls of the uterus are very powerful muscles, about half an inch thick, which cover and surround a central area. Every month the uterus prepares for the possibility of nurturing a developing fetus. The lining of the uterus is called the *endometrium* (Greek: within the womb). Each month the lining becomes soft and thick. During menstruation the endometrium is sloughed away, then renewed again the next month unless implantation of a fertilized ovum (egg) occurs. Numerous strong, stringy tissue ligaments support the uterus and tie it to the bony structures of the pelvis—which is a good thing, since a 40-week-pregnant uterus expands to about watermelon size. There is also a rich blood supply to the uterus. Women often experience a pleasurable contraction of the uterus as part of their orgasmic response.

The Cervix

The *cervix* (Latin: neck) is located at the bottom of the uterus. The narrowed neck of the bottom of the cervix protrudes into the vagina and can be seen easily during a pelvic exam. You can probably locate your own cervix by probing with your fingers; it feels something like the rounded part of your ear or the tip of your nose, at times a bit softer. The opening of the cervix, the os, is the only passage into the uterus. The cervix functions as a protective barrier to the uterus, constantly producing mucus to keep out unwanted bacteria. This self-cleansing operation works so well that health-care providers have concluded that douching should not be recommended for routine vaginal care.

The opening of the cervix changes very little after a woman has a baby. Although labor contractions lead to a complete dilation of the cervix at the time of birth, afterward the body adjusts and the cervical opening contracts.

Some women report that they experience a pleasurable sensation from thrusting during sexual intercourse derived from stimulation of, or pressure against, the cervix. Other women may experience this sensation as unpleasant or even painful.

The Fallopian Tubes

Droopy and delicate, the *fallopian tubes* (named for Gabriele Fallopio, an Italian anatomist) extend from either side of the uterus. The *infundibula* (Latin: funnel), the flared ends of the fallopian tubes, are fringed with microscopic strands called *fimbriae* (Latin: fringe). The tubes, infundibula, and fimbriae are constantly in motion, swaying back and forth, ready to capture the egg released from one of the ovaries and draw it into the adjacent fallopian tube. The tiny passageway of the tube is about the size of a daisy stem.

Eggs aren't mobile by themselves, so they are propelled along the fallopian tubes toward the uterus by muscle contractions. If pregnancy is going to occur in any given cycle, fertilization of the egg by sperm happens when the egg in the fallopian tube is about a third of the way to the uterus. Within a few days the fertilized egg reaches the uterus, where it implants in the endometrium. The fallopian tubes also sweep the sperm toward the egg.

The Ovaries

The *ovaries* (Latin: *ovum*, egg) have two jobs. One is to produce the powerful message-senders—hormones—that regulate the menstrual cycle as well as serve other functions (discussed in Chapter 5). The ovaries also produce eggs (*ova*) for reproduction. A girl baby starts out with a million or more follicles that could develop into ova, but by the time she is prepubescent the number has dropped to about 300,000, the rest having been reabsorbed into the body (Strong & DeVault, 1988). Despite this dramatic drop in the number of egg follicles, she will have more than enough for the years ahead. She will actually cycle only a few hundred eggs in her reproductive lifetime. Although ovaries are the size of a small nut, they can hold eggs numbering in the millions, and each egg is no bigger than a fine pencil dot. The ovaries do not float free in the abdomen—they are anchored by ligaments to the abdominal wall.

PELVIC FLOOR MUSCLES

When people began to stand on two feet, evolution, as always, adapted to this change. A powerful structure, sort of like a sling, developed to help support the internal organs. The pelvic floor muscles make up the largest muscle group in the body. Located around the vagina and the anus, the pelvic muscles are responsible for urinary control, assistance in maintaining posture, and keeping the internal organs in place (see Figure 3.4). They are also very important in sexual response. The opening of the vagina is ringed by strong muscles that create the physical tension that sheaths and stimulates a penis during intercourse. The nerve source for the pelvic floor muscles is the same as for the clitoris, vagina, and vulva, so contraction of the muscles can produce sexual pleasure. These muscles also contract during orgasm—at least during the orgasms that are triggered by the clitoris.

Like other muscle groups, the pelvic floor muscles can lose their tone. If the muscles are weak or overly tense, or if a woman has no sense of voluntary control over these muscles, the quality of her sexual response—including orgasm—can be greatly diminished. The tone of the pelvic floor muscles affects whether or not there

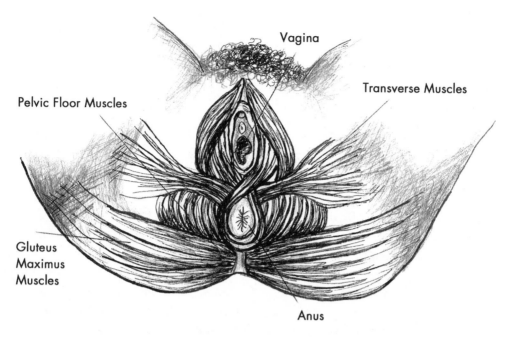

FIGURE 3.4. The pelvic floor muscles.

is "stress incontinence" (an involuntary dribbling of urine that can occur, for example, when a woman sneezes).

Pelvic floor muscle exercises—tightening and then relaxing the pelvic muscles—can improve a woman's voluntary control over these muscles, intensify her sexual pleasure (especially during orgasm), improve urinary control, and help tone the vaginal opening after childbirth. A description of these exercises, called Kegels, can be found in Chapter 8. (You may be aware of sexually pleasurable feelings in your pelvis when you practice these exercises.)

Some women experience painful muscle spasms in the pelvic muscles. These spasms, or cramps, can feel like a charley horse and make penetration painful or impossible. The large pelvic muscles are the only muscles in the body to have muscular tone when they're at rest. Even physically fit women who are very aware of the presence or absence of muscle tone may be unaware of muscle tension in the pelvis, which can contribute to muscle fatigue and chronic pelvic tension. Muscle spasms are involuntary, much like blinking is reflexive if there is a threat of something hitting the eye. Sometimes the pelvic muscle spasms occur for unknown reasons that may be psychological in origin. We think that some women carry psychological stress in their pelvic region, similar to the neck and back muscle tension that other people experience.

Women who have had uncomfortable sexual experiences—for whatever reason (vaginal irritation, infection, sexual abuse, or other causes)—may involuntarily tense their pelvic muscles, as a learned defense against pain or discomfort, when intercourse is attempted. The cycle of attempted penetration and muscle pain can be frustrating for a woman and her partner. The good news is that treatment is effective. We encourage any woman who is experiencing vaginal, vulvar, or pelvic muscle pain to seek help. Chapter 8 offers many suggestions for dealing with pain and maintaining your sexual relationship in a positive way.

THE NERVES OF SEXUAL RESPONSE

Neurons, Neurotransmitters, and Neuropeptides

Neurons are excitable cells that receive and transmit signals up and down the nervous system. Can you imagine your central nervous system containing billions and billions of *neurons*–and that every one of them knows what its particular job happens to be? When you feel the sting of a mosquito bite, certain neurons are doing their job. When you startle at the boom of a thunderclap, neurons are at work. The neurons are clustered in specific "neighborhoods" in the brain to carry out their functions. (Actually, they reside in something more like gated communities since they communicate only with others within the neighborhood.)

If you could see a neuron, it might look to you like a tree with little branch-like projections called *dendrites* (bringing information in) and *axons* (sending information out). A synapse, part of the neuron system, includes a tiny but essential gap. Across this gap an electrical "push" connects and makes it possible for communication to occur between neurons in their "neighborhoods."

Neurons secrete *neurotransmitters* and *neuropeptides*, chemicals that communicate between neurons to initiate a specific physical or emotional reaction. These chemicals cross the gap between neurons, moving a signal farther down the line, often resulting in a message registering in the brain or a command for a body response to occur. This communication process happens far more quickly than the blink of an eye.

Neurotransmitters and neuropeptides both serve as messengers, but they differ in how they are manufactured and how long they remain active. Neurotransmitters are smaller molecules and are fast acting—they do their thing quickly and then are often reabsorbed into the neuron, to be used again. Neuropeptides are larger molecules that can travel farther and have longer-lasting effects when they activate nerve endings. Unlike neurotransmitters, they aren't recycled when they've finished their job; they simply degrade. The neurons "hold" various types of neurotransmitters and neuropeptides within until certain stimuli alert the neurons to release them. The messengers we're concerned with in this book are the neurotransmitters dopamine, norepinephrine, and serotonin and the neuropeptides oxytocin and vasopressin— the messengers that affect sexual interest, attraction, arousal, affection, attachment, and orgasm. We will describe their function in later chapters.

Nerves

Neurons are individual cells; when they come together they form a nerve. A number of nerves play a critical role in sexual response. The *pudendal nerve* is the primary nerve group responsible for a woman's experience of sexual response. Originating in the spinal cord, the pudendal nerve carries much of the sensory information—the physical feelings—of the clitoris and other areas of the genitals and is responsible for the pelvic muscle contractions of orgasm. The same nerve activates the vaginal secretions during the excitement phase and signals the tissues to engorge with blood. Other nerve pathways important in sexual responsiveness are the *hypogastric, pelvic,* and *vagus nerves.* The physical sensation that results from stimulation of the vagina, cervix, and some of the pelvic floor muscles is due to the response of these nerves. In fact, there apparently is no direct neural pathway linking the pudendal nerve and the uterus, so the sensations and contractions of the uterus during orgasm come from another neural pathway. The same is true for the G spot.

BREASTS

A woman's breasts have two primary functions: sexual pleasure and nourishment for infants. Breasts are considered an "erogenous zone," or area of the body that can be extremely responsive to sexual stimulation. They consist of fatty tissue that protects their many milk-producing glands. A system of ducts funnels the milk to the nipple, where it is let down by a hormonal signal triggered by a sucking infant. As glandular organs, breasts are a part of a woman's genital and reproductive system. Breasts are sensitive to hormonal changes. For example, during sexual stimulation, breasts of women who have not yet been pregnant may enlarge. Breasts can also undergo changes in size during certain times of the menstrual cycle and become enlarged and feel tender just prior to a menstrual period. During pregnancy, breasts typically become larger, and the nipple and areola may darken in color.

Nipples are made of erectile tissue that is responsive to stimulation. Nipple stimulation causes the release of hormones—the same hormones that cause uterine contractions during orgasm or during nursing. With sexual arousal and orgasm, nipples are typically erect. As all women know, being cold can also stimulate nipple erection, as can other tactile sensations.

Numerous medical conditions can cause breast problems or changes. Evaluation of breasts and nipples should be a normal part of health maintenance. Your healthcare provider can teach you how to perform breast exams, which should be done monthly. Some women pick a specific day of the month, such as the first, or the date corresponding with their birthday, to remember to perform breast exams regularly. Breast examination is a routine part of good gynecological care; self-care exams should not take the place of regular medical exams.

If the media is an accurate barometer of our culture's attitude toward women's breasts, then clearly they exist primarily for display purposes. Carefully selected models, provocatively airbrushed; enhanced photography and filming; and clothing designed to reveal breasts are hallmarks of American graphics, be they print, film, or live. No wonder women often express dissatisfaction with their breast size and shape and breast alteration is a frequent medical request. In fact, normal breasts—breasts on real women—don't typically look like Barbie-doll breasts. Normal size includes large and small, droopy and firm.

Typically, one breast is larger than the other, or a different shape. Nipples and areolas (the darker-colored area around the nipple) vary just as much in size and shape from one woman to another. Depending on the pattern of a woman's hair distribution, she may have hairs growing at the outer edge of the areola. We believe that so much media attention is focused on an exaggerated idea of beautiful breasts that many women are needlessly self-conscious about their breast or nipple size or shape and therefore are unable to experience their breasts as a full sexual part of themselves. In Chapters 6 and 13 we take a closer look at the importance of body acceptance and suggest ways to make peace with our bodies and to hold them in greater esteem.

FOUR

Sexual Response

Annalise is a 5-year-old with a wispy ponytail poking through her cap. She's the star player on her soccer team, but not because she's proficient at making goals. Her coaches and the spectators cheer her because she kicks the ball *toward* the appropriate goal. Annalise is at an age when the most common coaching call heard on the field, as the peewee players run wherever the group seems to be going, is "Wrong way! Wrong way!"

Although Annalise is a long way from needing personal guidance about sexual responsiveness, throughout history the interpretation of female sexual response has too often mirrored Annalise's fledgling soccer team. Despite some wise "coaching" from researchers and clinicians over the years, a lot of confusion and chaos has surrounded women's sexual response. Unfortunately, no one has been hollering, *"Wrong way! Wrong way!"*

For example, if we could capture and distill some moments from thousands of years of history regarding how women's sexuality has been viewed, in our dominant Judeo/Christian culture we might start with Eve and that apple. How biting an apple had anything to do with sexual awareness is left to biblical scholars, but the pervasive conclusion is that it represented female sexuality as so explosively dangerous that it had to be controlled externally. *Wrong way! Wrong way!*

The mythological danger of women's sexuality has pervaded across cultures for millennia, but in 19th-century Europe and America a shift in perception occurred from woman as temptress to a more genteel stereotype. Women were viewed as sexually bored and passive, while their male counterparts possessed and displayed sexual prowess and lust. Women were to be well bred, while sex was about breeding—the two were not supposed to overlap. Again, *wrong way! Wrong way!*

Even during the past 50 years, when women were again perceived as just maybe being capable of lust and sexual enjoyment, until recently, how they responded to sex was assumed to follow a male script of becoming horny, wet, and orgasmic—in that order. Anything that departed from that 1-2-3 linear progression was automatically viewed as dysfunctional. Once again, *wrong way! Wrong way!*

In Chapter 3 we discussed sexual anatomy—the parts of the body involved in reproduction and sexual enjoyment. In this chapter, we want to take this discussion one step further, to make clear how these parts come together and function in sexual situations. We want not only to dispel the "wrong way" that sexual response has been described in the past but, also, to provide an understanding of sexual response that is more accurate and useful.

FIRST, SOME BACKGROUND

Sex wasn't studied in people until after the United States had the hydrogen bomb, television, the Salk polio vaccine, and space travel. It wasn't that clinicians were not interested in how women and men worked sexually but that study required observation in a clinical setting—which was simply deemed inappropriate. Instead, scientists made extrapolations about people based on the information they amassed by studying animal sexual behavior. In the 1950s Alfred Kinsey provided the medical community with access to the first comprehensive scientific data on human sexual behavior—not through observation but through a large survey that revealed what people said they did sexually.

During the same decade William Masters was curious and bold enough to undertake studies with human subjects in a controlled setting, observing their sexual activity and charting and filming their responses. The studies that he and Virginia Johnson conducted in the late 1950s and early 1960s provided the most information ever gained, to that point, about sex and people. Sexual activity was finally being acknowledged as a fundamental part of the human experience, not just a by-product of reproduction. As a result of their observations of more than 10,000 episodes of sexual behavior, they mapped out four stages of sexual response. They suggested that when men and women engage in sexual behavior, they first experience *excitement*—the penis becomes erect and the vagina becomes wet. Dramatic body changes occur very quickly during the excitement phase, but then things seem to settle down to a slower pace as the excitement intensifies during the second phase—the *plateau* phase. Once the excitement reaches a heightened threshold, *orgasm*, the third phase, occurs. Orgasm can be a single or a multiple event, but once it occurs, the body goes through a process—the *resolution* phase—of returning to its normal, nonaroused state.

During the late 1970s and early 1980s, critics of the Masters and Johnson model insisted something was missing. Harold Lief (1981), Helen Singer Kaplan (1979), and others suggested that before the body shows signs of excitement there has to be a desire for sex. Kaplan proposed a three-phase model for sexual response that added a *desire* phase to the front end of Masters and Johnson's model and combined the excitement and plateau phases into a second phase, the *arousal* phase, and the orgasm and resolution phases into a third phase, the *orgasm* phase. Her model, often referred to as the "triphasic model of sexual response," has been widely adopted over the past 30 years by medical and mental health experts. It has influenced what we have considered to be a normal as opposed to a dysfunctional sexual response.

This triphasic model of desire, arousal, and orgasm implies that each phase leads to the next, with orgasm being the anticipated end-point of sexual activity. Following this line of thinking, a person could easily, and incorrectly, conclude that anything less than passion, physical arousal, and orgasm is an inferior sexual experience. In recent years we have become increasingly aware of shortcomings in this model. First of all, the model more often reflects the sexual experience described by men than by women. Most men, for example, will insist that they didn't have a sexual experience unless they ejaculated. Many women, on the other hand, report that lovemaking and self-pleasuring can be fulfilling and satisfying without an orgasm. Another shortcoming of the triphasic model is that many men and women report having hot, satisfying sexual experiences despite the lack of any apparent signs of sexual desire outside of the bedroom. Discussing sexual experience as a series of physical reactions has the additional shortcoming of overemphasizing the importance of biological factors for a satisfying sexual response. As we point out throughout this book, sex is not just biology, but also an intimate relationship that a woman has with her own body. This relationship is not dependent on hormones, blood flow, or the G spot but on a woman's history, self-concept, and comfort with her body.

For the reasons described above, in recent years scholars and clinicians have been moving away from the triphasic model. New ways of conceptualizing how men and women respond sexually have been proposed (Whipple & Brash-McGreer, 1997; Basson, 2005). For example, for decades it has been assumed that one's libido drives sexual behavior—that is, sexual hunger seeks sexual gratification. Rosemary Basson proposed a nonlinear model for female sexual response that suggests that sexual hunger is not the sole motivation for sex and that orgasm is not always the sought-after outcome. Her model suggests that a woman may engage in sex because of sexual desire or because of a desire for emotional intimacy. Further, sexual desire may not trigger sexual activity, but might become evident only *after* the woman is sexually excited. The outcome of sex could be an orgasm or a sense of satisfaction arising from pleasurable sensations and emotional closeness to her partner or all of the above. According to this model, satisfaction, with or without orgasm, is a valued outcome of any sexual encounter.

Now that we have attempted to discredit the triphasic model, we're going to turn around and use the three phases of the model in our discussion about how the body responds in sexual situations. We're going to talk about desire, arousal, and orgasm not as stages, but as a useful way for highlighting the distinction between wanting sex, physically and emotionally responding to sexual stimulation, and having an orgasm. Any of these experiences can occur alone or in combination with one or more of the other experiences. Understanding how each of these experiences is influenced by physical and psychological factors puts us in a better position to understand how we respond sexually and how we can enhance that sexual response. It is also helpful in deciphering problems that can occur in each of these three areas. In Chapter 15 we discuss strategies for overcoming problems of low desire, lack of arousal, and inability to orgasm.

SEXUAL DESIRE

Sexual desire is referred to in the academic literature as *libido, drive, passion, sexual instinct*, and *sexual motivation*. In less scholarly arenas, words like *turned on, horny, hot, frisky*, and *randy* are popular labels for this innate biological drive. When we talk about sexual desire, we're referring to being interested in or receptive to sexual activity. What does that mean? Put simply, when a person either hungers for sex and seeks it out or responds to sexual stimulation with a hunger to enjoy the stimulation fully, she is displaying sexual desire. On the other hand, a person who not only has no interest in initiating or engaging in sex but also fails to enjoy sexual activity when it occurs lacks sexual desire.

As we discussed earlier in this chapter, for many years we assumed that sexual desire was a primary motivator for sexual activity and a prerequisite for becoming sexually aroused. We assumed further that in the absence of factors that can thwart this normal drive, people will regularly act on opportunities for sexual expression, including sex with a partner or masturbation. Actually, a woman's motivation for engaging in sex is extremely varied and frequently *not* motivated by spontaneous desire. The motivation for engaging in sexual behavior is often relational—to express love, to experience an emotional connection, to avoid conflict, to fulfill a sense of obligation, or to meet the partner's sexual needs. In recent years researchers, healthcare practitioners, and therapists have come to acknowledge what women have always known (even if their insight was never previously validated): powerful desire and arousal often arise *from* consensual sexual activity, even if the "ignition" was not sexual.

Behind the Scenes

Sexual desire is the product of a complex interaction of powerful social, psychological, and biological factors. Recall a sexy scene in a movie. Chances are that the scene depicted two people who hungered to be intimate with each other. The scene probably made their sexual desire appear simple and straightforward—their behavior a natural consequence of attraction and passion. To create a sexy scene like this, however, was anything but simple and straightforward. What you didn't see in the scene, and thus were not aware of, was what went into creating the ambiance that made the scene memorable. If the scene was warm and romantic, the lighting may have been deliberately muted and softened to create this mood. If the scene was intense and pulsing, it may have been accompanied by the sound of rhythmic crashing and receding waves, replicating the thrusts and withdrawal of sexual intercourse. You didn't see the director orchestrating the actors and crew; the cameramen zooming in and controlling the scope and focus of the lens; technicians capturing, enhancing, and muting myriad sounds; stage crew working the lighting and props; and all of the other behind-the-scenes activities that came together to create a memorable sensual scene.

In the process of producing sexual desire, your body has every bit as much going on behind the scenes as you will find in any movie. Let's look at the cast, crew, stage, and props that lead to sexual desire.

The Biology of Sexual Desire

Brain Activity

We have always known that the brain plays a critical role in sexual desire, but in recent years advances in technology have made it possible for us to begin to map out how specific parts of the brain contribute to and manage sexual desire. For example, with the fMRI (functional magnetic resonance imaging) we are able to get an "inside view" of what's going on in the brain when a person views a sexy picture or video. Preliminary research suggests that parts of the brain that manage intense emotions (amygdala and insular cortices), manage memories (hippocampus), maintain awareness of what our bodies are experiencing (anterior insula), and tune in to the thoughts and intentions of others "light up" when a person is exposed to a sexual stimulus. It appears that as the brain becomes aware of a sexual stimulus, a complex process occurs at lightning speed that judges the stimulus, compares it to memories, judges whether it is potentially pleasurable, assesses how the body is reacting to the stimulus, estimates whether the stimulus is safe or threatening, and so on. Receiving and evaluating sexual stimuli, the brain subsequently cues the body to respond in certain ways.

As with other body functions, the brain and central nervous system must work as a director coordinating all the other responding parts if sexual desire is to be experienced in any meaningful way. If not, basic external cues like an attractive person showing sexual interest or internal cues like engorgement of a woman's clitoral tissue would not be experienced as a sexual feeling or opportunity. Returning to our movie scene for a moment, it would be like one of the actors having a script and reading his or her part alone. Without the other parts—not to mention the camera, set, background music, and so on—the words would be a monologue without much meaning.

Hormones

Hormones are essential to the rhythms and cycles of female sexuality. Hormones are chemicals secreted by endocrine glands that signal the start-up and shut-down of activities in all parts of the body. The discussion of hormones in this chapter is confined to those connected with sexual responsiveness. How the menstrual cycle and reproductive hormones work is covered in Chapter 5.

Androgens are the hormones associated with sexual desire for both sexes. They're produced in the ovaries and the adrenal glands (about 50% of the androgens in the bloodstream come from adrenal glands). The androgen we are most familiar with is testosterone, generally known as a male hormone. Testosterone is as important to male sexual development and maturity as estrogen is for women. Men have many more times the testosterone than women, but this does not mean that men have a correspondingly higher sex drive. A higher level of androgen is required for male sexual desire than for female desire, so "normal" is different for men and women.

Women are more sensitive to androgens than are men. An intricate hormonal system protects women from overexposure to androgens, because if women have too much androgen the hormone can have masculinizing effects on their distribution of body fat, muscular development, and hair growth—and, even more serious, the potential for the development of ovarian cancer.

Although sexual responsiveness can be influenced by the dramatic hormonal fluctuations that occur during the menstrual cycle, it is not regulated or controlled by the menstrual cycle. In most animal species sexual activity is directly connected to the reproductive/hormonal cycle, so that sex occurs only during the fertile time of the female. Humans are different from other animals. Researchers have concluded that our sexual functioning and responsiveness does not follow a pattern that can be tracked readily by cyclical hormonal changes. Unlike animals, we can desire sex and be highly responsive regardless of where the woman is in her menstrual cycle.

In terms of sexual function, *estrogen* enhances sensitivity to sexual activity and creates a physical climate conducive to sexual behavior. It helps the vaginal tissue remain elastic and contributes to lubrication. Despite all of the research that has been done on the hormone estrogen, its role in sexual desire remains unclear other than its contribution to increased sexual comfort, which understandably will influence a woman to be more receptive to future sexual encounters, and its role as a mood elevator.

Pheromones

There is another set of chemicals, called *pheromones*, that are linked to sexual attraction for both men and women. You are attracted to others and they are attracted to you partially due to the pheromones you and they secrete. Although there is scientific evidence that pheromones exist, little is known about them. A major difference between pheromones and hormones (about which much more is known) is that hormones are secreted and circulated inside the body through the bloodstream, and pheromones are secreted outside the body through the sweat glands, skin, and urine. Interestingly, although we do not consciously detect pheromones by the sense of smell, the olfactory function must be working for pheromones to be effective; no sense of smell, no pheromone-related attraction. We don't have to be aware of pheromones for them to have an effect. We do know that odors are one of the most powerful triggers of memory and interpersonal connection.

Neurotransmitters and Neuropeptides

In Chapter 3 we described chemicals that communicate between neurons to trigger a specific physical or emotional reaction. Evidence suggests that there is an important balance in the brain of neurotransmitters that stimulate sexual interest (dopamine and norepinephrine) and ones that inhibit sexual desire (prolactin and serotonin).

Anthropologist Helen Fisher (2004) has speculated on three systems in the brain that have evolved for mating and reproduction, all three of which are influenced by neurotransmitters or neuropeptides. She refers to one brain system as *lust*, which she describes as essentially sexual desire. Lust doesn't discriminate; it doesn't restrict its focus to one person but instead targets any sexually desirable target. Lust, according to Fisher, is driven by testosterone, but elevations of the neurotransmitter dopamine can drive up testosterone levels and increase the overall sex drive.

Fisher refers to the second brain system as *romantic love*. She describes romantic love as a drive, not a feeling, and suggests that it is stronger than the maternal instinct, the sex drive, and even the will to live. This drive, an evolutionary imperative to keep mates together beyond copulation, prompts people to take risks they wouldn't otherwise take and to focus on the loved one to the point of obsession. In the throes of romantic love, even the sense of pain is modified. The anxiety associated with this attraction is indescribable: Will the phone ring? Will I lose him? Why isn't she answering my calls? This drive is propelled by the neurotransmitters *dopamine* and *norepinephrine* and a significant reduction in *serotonin*. If a person "gets dumped" while at the height of romantic love, dopamine remains high while the person fervently searches for a way to regain the person who has been lost. If romantic love ends badly, the suffering can be intense. Eventually, however, after neurotransmitters return to a more balanced state, most jilted lovers go on to pair-bond with someone else.

Even in the most successful instances of romantic love, this highly intense state is not permanent, and for good reason. From an evolutionary point of view, being initially obsessed with one's partner may facilitate pair-bonding, but if it goes on too long it can distract from and interfere with the "hunting and gathering" that's required for long-term survival. Romantic love at most lasts a year or two before giving way to a third brain system—*attachment*. Lust and the craving for emotional union and obsessive behavior characteristic of romantic love give way to a sense of calm, security, and social comfort between the partners. Orgasm, childbirth, eye-gazing, touching and holding, sex, and domestic experiences like holding an infant trigger the release of the neuropeptides *vasopressin* and *oxytocin*, which help sustain a bond that was initially forged out of lust, romantic love, or both. The evolutionary value of this third brain system is that it helps sustain a relationship for the long haul, helping to ensure that offspring are provided for until maturity. In a letter to her husband John Adams in 1793, Abigail Adams captures wonderfully the essence of attachment—"Years subdue the ardor of passion, but in lieu thereof friendship and affection deep-rooted subsists, which defies the ravages of time, and whilst the vital flame exists" (McCullough, 2001).

Fisher's work on these three brain systems provides valuable insight into three common questions about sexual desire and attraction that often come up during sex therapy. One question is how a partner could show such enthusiasm for sex during the courtship phase of the relationship and then become practically asexual once the marriage has occurred. An embittered partner might accuse the spouse of pulling a "bait and switch," intentionally providing sex just long enough to manipulate the partner into a marriage. In the vast majority of these cases we find no evidence of a bait and switch, but rather, a person who long experienced sexual inhibitions that were temporarily overridden by the biological intensity of romantic love. In such cases, it makes sense that, after the dominance of dopamine and norepinephrine and the suppression of serotonin subside, the partner's sex drive will return to its original baseline, even if a strong loving attachment has developed.

The second common question is "When I truly love my partner, how can I feel attracted to another person?" A common variation of this question is "If he really loves me and finds me attractive, why would he want to look at other women?" Remember, as Fisher points out, lust doesn't discriminate; it just responds. You could be sitting at an outdoor café with your loved one when an extremely attractive person strolls by. Your attention is momentarily, almost involuntarily diverted to the attractive person. It doesn't mean you are going to run off with the stranger; rather, more than one of your brain systems are working. One system, your sex drive, is reacting to the attractive person, but the third system—attachment love—reasserts itself and you remain comfortably with your loved person at the café.

The third common question in sex therapy is often raised by couples who have been together for 5, 10, 15, or more years. They will come to therapy lamenting not only that things aren't like they used to be but also that the old feelings just aren't there. Although we maintain that couples can enjoy passionate, hot, loving sex throughout their lifespan, a return to the blissful state of intense romantic love is neither realistic nor desirable. As exciting as biologically driven romantic love can be in the short run, we suggest to our couples that in the long run it cannot compete with the stable connection that rests on history and trust rather than hopes and promises. We then work with the couple to discover the richness of sexual intimacy that can occur only in the context of a deep, healthy attachment.

That's Not All, Folks

The central nervous system, hormones, neurotransmitters, and neuropeptides all play an important role in producing sexual desire, but in the end, sexual desire is the product of so much more. Upbringing, religious values and beliefs, previous sexual experiences, body image, relationship satisfaction, current life circumstances, expectations, attitudes about sex, and general health play an equally important role in facilitating or interfering with sexual desire. See Chapter 15 for a discussion of nonphysical causes for low sexual desire.

SEXUAL AROUSAL

Sexual arousal involves the narrowing of concentration so that other things are tuned out as sexual responsiveness is tuned in. There are intricate body responses and intense emotional responses as well. All of the changes we describe certainly happen with masturbation, but if sexual activity is with a partner, then the interaction with that partner, including his or her pleasure, the scope of the relationship, the context of the sexual activity, and the feelings behind the sexual activity will all contribute to the experience. If, for example, your partner is breathing heavily and nibbling, nuzzling, and stroking your earlobe, you may respond with a welcoming arching of your body and an intense excitement that matches your partner's. This section will explore what is happening in your body as sex becomes increasingly exciting. Although each woman's response will differ and may even vary widely from one sexual experience to another, sexual arousal includes some specific physiological changes common to most women. See Chapter 15 for advice on dealing with sexual arousal difficulties.

Blood Flow Changes

Physical arousal can last minutes or much longer. During this time your blood pressure rises, breathing becomes more rapid, and pulse rate increases. As sexual excitement intensifies, blood flow to the vagina and vulva increases, resulting in vasocongestion, the process by which vaginal tissue becomes plump and swollen with an increased volume of blood. Blood flows in, and the hydraulics of sexual arousal temporarily keep the blood from flowing back out. If you squeeze the base of one of your fingers, you can cause congestion of blood into that finger. You can even see it change color. The most receptive parts of the vulva, particularly the labia minora, may also change color, to a deep pink or burgundy. The primary source of blood for vasocongestion during sexual arousal is the pudendal artery.

Vasocongestion also contributes significantly to sexual sensitivity. The labia majora become engorged and retract, similar to how the petals of a flower open. In most women the clitoris will become erect, but this does not happen for everyone. Some women develop a skin mottling, resembling a rosy skin rash, that begins on the trunk of the body around the upper abdomen and can spread to the breasts, buttocks, back, and even the arms, legs, and face. This is called a "sex flush." Blood engorges the nipples as well, causing them to become erect.

Lubrication

The presence of lubrication is an important feature of sexual excitement for women. Lubrication is the product of a process that happens within the tissues of the vagina: *transudation*. Facilitated by estrogen, the vaginal walls "sweat" with lubrication, which is a clear, slick fluid we've heard described as "an engineer's dream" because it's a nonoily lubricant. During arousal, blood flows to the genital region and the spongy tissue of the walls of the vagina engorge with blood. This swelling pushes tiny beads of this intercellular lubrication through the walls of the vagina. The composition, odor, and amount of this vaginal secretion vary from woman to woman, as they can vary for you as an individual at different times of your life.

Internal Evidence of Sexual Arousal

During sexual arousal, you will generally not be aware of the physiological changes going on inside of your body. This is partly because there are fewer nerve endings in the inner parts of the vagina. Also, the external organs, especially the clitoris, become acutely sensitive during arousal and their responses can easily overshadow the more subtle sensations coming from farther inside your body. There are exceptions. Changes near the vaginal opening are more noticeable than those in the inner vagina because of the rich supply of nerve endings near the entrance. In addition, sexual play and direct stimulation are often concentrated in the area around the clitoris and the opening to the vagina, which will draw your attention there. Another exception is the G spot. When stimulation is focused on this portion of the sexual anatomy, the spongy tissue swells and becomes quite distinct. The focused stimulation of the G spot can lead to intense sensations inside the body.

When the primary sexual stimulation is focused on the clitoris, the innermost portion of the vagina, nearest to the uterus, begins to expand. Think of a strawberry. As the pale fruit ripens, it becomes plump and red. During sexual excitement, as blood engorges the vagina, it too becomes plump and "ripe." As the strawberry rounds out in its ripeness, its flesh pulls away from the center, creating a space. The sexually aroused vagina also rounds, and its expansion creates a space. In contrast to the deepest part of the vaginal ballooning, the opening of the vagina swells, giving it the capacity to grip a finger or penis.

During arousal, the uterus also changes size due to blood engorgement. As the inner part of the vagina expands, the uterus is elevated and pulled forward, which changes the position of the cervix. As noted, some women enjoy the physical sensation of feeling their partner's penis or a dildo push against the cervix, a sensation that is enhanced by the body's arousal.

When sexual stimulation is focused more internally, on stimulation of the G spot, the physical changes are different. Even though there is blood engorgement and considerable swelling of the tissue, the muscles around the entrance of the vagina tend to open rather than grip. The innermost part of the vagina expands less than it does during intense clitoral stimulation. The uterus and cervix press against the upper portion of the vagina, actually compressing it a bit. During the height of arousal coming from G spot stimulation, you may experience a bearing-down pressure, as if you were pushing against or expelling the stimulating hand, penis, or vibrator. It is unlikely that your partner will notice these subtle physical differences in how you respond to clitoral and G spot stimulation.

Other Physiological Changes during Female Sexual Arousal

Along with rapid breathing, increased heart rate, vasocongestion of the internal and external genitals, and heightened concentration tuning other stimuli out, you will likely experience a generalized tension throughout your body. This makes sense. For a few moments, try to breathe rapidly, and you will find that at least your upper body muscles meet this "stress" almost automatically, by tensing and focusing. (When sex therapists work with women who are tense during sexual activity due to fear, first they help these women distinguish the physical responses of fear from the normal physical tension of sexual arousal.)

Changes also occur in the clitoris. As noted, a fold of skin called the "prepuce," or "clitoral hood," covers the clitoris. The skin of the clitoral hood is normally loose, not taut like the skin that covers your fingers, for example. It is connected to the labia minora, as explained in Chapter 3. During intense sexual arousal, the clitoris is retracted up against the pubic bone. Ironically, it becomes much less visible and prominent when excitement is highest and the labia the most swollen. The clitoris is thus protected against direct stimulation, which may feel far too intense to be pleasurable.

Breasts also change during intense sexual arousal. Women's breasts may swell as much as 25%, especially in women who have never breast-fed. The nipples typically become erect during arousal, and as arousal increases, the areola—the darkened circle around the nipple—begins to swell. Indeed, the areola can swell so much during arousal that it can look like the nipple has retracted. These breast changes recede as soon as sexual arousal diminishes.

"Plateau" of High Sexual Arousal

Sexual arousal often reaches a plateau that is a highly erotic, focused period of intense sexual tension. This phase lasts moments or many minutes, depending on the individual woman, the circumstances, her health status, and how relaxed or anxious she is. Masters and Johnson (1966) delineated and named this phase of sexual response and described it as being the sustained height of sexual tension. A state of protracted, intense sexual pleasure can be supremely gratifying and complete in itself.

ORGASM

Orgasm is the briefest phase of sexual response, lasting only seconds. Often called "climaxing," "coming," or "getting off," orgasm is the rhythmic pulsing that occurs as your body releases sexual tension. Orgasm is often depicted in the media by thrashing, moaning, gasping, writhing, and fascinating gyrating behavior. Such portrayal may be entertaining but is woefully noninstructive or worse. We believe it perpetuates the myth that a woman's orgasm is a spontaneously occurring event, happening as she is swept away in a consuming tidal wave of unbridled passion. Instead, we have come to know that a woman's orgasmic response is learned through experience, experimentation, and self-awareness. And we certainly don't expect to see an intense, spontaneous orgasm "just happening" for a woman who is sexually inexperienced and unaware of her body's responses, no matter how skilled her lover may be. Let's look at this more closely.

When boys hit adolescence, there is a direct connection between pubertal development and ejaculation. For girls, however, there is no connection between the beginning of puberty—such as the appearance of pubic hair—and orgasm. In studies of boys the findings are consistent and clear: hormonal factors much more than social factors determine sexual response, including orgasm. For girls, social factors appear to be a much stronger determinant than sex hormones for becoming orgasmic. "Social factors" were not consistently defined in these studies. Our own clinical work and the work of other sex therapists support our view that orgasm for women is more learned than spontaneous. It is important to note, however, that for many girls orgasm can precede pubertal development or sexual activity with any partner.

This learning process is most likely ongoing, perhaps beginning during childhood, when a girl might explore her vulva, vagina, and clitoris, and continuing on through her adult life as she communicates with her partner about her body's sense of pleasure and sensitivity. In other words, a woman's orgasmic response, including the overly acclaimed multiple orgasm, depends first upon a woman's curiosity about, knowledge of, and experimentation with her body and how it responds. One abiding myth is that if a woman masturbates, she "uses up" sexual energy that could go to her partner and therefore should give up masturbation once she's in a partnership.

There is no research to support this myth, and in fact we find that self-pleasure enhances sexual pleasure in a partnership.

The Clitoris and Orgasm

The clitoris exists for sexual pleasure alone. Its only function is to trigger a common form of orgasm—a clitoral orgasm. This doesn't mean that orgasm happens in the clitoris. The clitoris is the source of some orgasms, just as the G spot is the source of other orgasms. Either way, the orgasms are felt not only in the clitoris but also in the pelvis and entire genital region. The pleasure of the orgasmic pulses isn't confined to these body areas: most women describe orgasm as an intense, entire-body experience.

The G Spot and Orgasm

As explained in Chapter 3, the G spot is a small area of erectile tissue felt through the front wall of the vagina that becomes engorged during sexual arousal and is especially sensitive to stimulation. The sensations of an orgasm generated through stimulation of the G spot are described by women as being different from the orgasms generated primarily through the clitoris. They say that the G spot orgasms feel like they occur deeper inside the body with fewer pelvic floor muscle contractions. When orgasms are evaluated in laboratories by technical measurements, this is borne out. The G-spot-stimulated orgasms result in less activity in the pelvic floor muscles and more activity in the uterus and cervix. It should be kept in mind that because more than one nerve group can be stimulated at the same time, simultaneous G spot stimulation and clitoral stimulation are mutually enhancing.

Pelvic Floor Muscles

As we discussed in Chapter 3, the pelvic floor muscles are very important to a woman's sexual pleasure. During orgasm, these strong muscles contract, involuntarily, in intervals of 0.8 second. Sometimes they are felt very strongly and at other times more like a gentle ripple. A woman may experience 3 to 10 of these contractions during an orgasm. It's interesting to note that men too have 0.8-second rhythmic contractions of similar pelvic floor muscles, so both sexes probably feel similar sensations during orgasm.

The muscles have different names and locations. Some of them form a figure-eight shape around the anus and vaginal opening (see Figure 3.4 in Chapter 3). Others actually circle the vagina in a way similar to how two hands wrap around a can of soda. As the muscles contract during orgasm, so do the vagina, urethra, and anus, together producing a highly pleasurable sensation. A woman can enhance her sexual pleasure by gaining more voluntary control over her pelvic muscles—getting them in shape by exercising them just as she does with other muscles in her body. Research has shown that women who have stronger pelvic muscles (measured by how tightly they can voluntarily contract those muscles and how long they can hold the contraction) are more arousable and have stronger and more predictable orgasms (Lowenstein et al., 2010). So exercise those muscles! Kegel exercises—to strengthen pelvic muscles—are described in Chapter 8.

Uterine Contractions

The uterus also contracts during orgasm. Some women describe this sensation as intensely pleasurable and satisfying. Other women are barely aware of when it happens. If a woman has consistently experienced pleasurable uterine and deep vaginal contractions, having her uterus and cervix (a total hysterectomy) removed for medical reasons can represent a great loss for her. Removing the cervix and uterus does not involve removal of the G spot, so the pleasure a woman can feel from stimulation of the G spot can continue to be very intense even following a hysterectomy.

Uterine contractions are not always pleasurable. Very low or widely fluctuating estrogen levels may make the uterine contractions painful. This could be associated with childbirth, menopause, or the blocked ovarian production of estrogen and should be discussed with your healthcare provider.

Chemical Reactions in the Brain

While parts of the body go through involuntary albeit pleasurable contractions upon orgasm, an important chemical reaction takes place at the same moment in the brain. Research is ongoing, but it appears that when we experience an orgasm the reward center of the brain (the *nucleus accumbens* in the forebrain) is bathed with a flood of dopamine, which causes an intense, momentary sense of pleasure. As wonderful as this pleasure might be, out of necessity it has to be very brief, lest we become victims of an incapacitating stupor. The pleasurable flood of dopamine is immediately followed by a spike in prolactin, a hormone that acts as an antidote for dopamine.

As discussed above, orgasm triggers the release of the neuropeptide oxytocin, which reinforces bonding with the sexual partner. Partly tongue in cheek, and partly not, Helen Fisher warns: Be careful with whom you share an orgasm—you could end up falling in love.

Multiple Orgasms

Women have the physical capacity to have more than one orgasm during the same session of sexual activity, whether through masturbation or with a partner. Men usually require a "cool-down" period after an orgasm; women usually do not. In fact, for some women, orgasm may not completely resolve sexual tension.

Multiple orgasms have been given a lot of sensational attention in the media, but they are not achievable for all women and certainly not essential for sexual pleasure and satisfaction. Some women find they are so physically sensitive after an orgasm that further stimulation can be uncomfortable rather than pleasurable. We have found that women and their partners may feel pressured to experience multiple orgasms, as if this were a superior accomplishment. Some couples strive to experience multiple orgasms with a "We'll get this or die" approach, which is not particularly conducive to increased pleasure or satisfaction. We realize that we are debunking the glamour of multiple orgasms. Think about it. Human beings also have the physical capacity to eat four doughnuts instead of one, but proving or exercising that capacity is certainly not essential for enjoyable dining, and pushing oneself to do so could actually detract from the experience.

Keeping Orgasm in Perspective

All sexologists agree that many women—perhaps most women—do not experience orgasm regularly from sexual intercourse alone. We can't give you the exact percentage, because the research on women and orgasm does not always include information about how a woman is having her orgasm—whether by intercourse alone or by intercourse combined with additional stimulation. What we want to stress is that not experiencing an orgasm with sexual intercourse alone is not a sexual dysfunction. It is normal.

Equally important is the fact that most women do not orgasm every time they make love, and they are quite satisfied. It's not that they are trying to talk themselves into being satisfied with a less-than-optimal experience. On the contrary, for many women *satisfaction*, which can be physical such as orgasm, or emotional such as closeness and connection, or both, is the ultimate objective of a sexual encounter—not solely or necessarily orgasm.

Finally, the question has long been debated whether an orgasm increases the chances of conception. Elizabeth Lloyd (2005), a philosopher of biology, reviewed and rejected 20 different theories suggesting that female orgasm has an evolutionary purpose. After examining the theories and the presence or absence of research support, she concluded that orgasm offered no advantage for natural selection and is a "happy accident" in evolution. Komisaruk, Beyer-Flores, and Whipple (2006), in their review of the scientific literature, disagreed with Lloyd's conclusion. They cited studies they believe suggest that orgasm may influence the probability of a woman becoming pregnant. Although there is no clear answer to this question, focusing on orgasm as a solution for infertility is of questionable value. Given that a majority of women do not orgasm regularly as a result of intercourse yet conceive successfully, if orgasm does indeed influence conception, that influence, at best, is a very subtle one.

For more information about orgasm concerns, refer to Chapter 15.

SEXUAL RESPONSE AT MENOPAUSE AND LATER

Sexually, a woman's body "works" fine during menopause and the later years. She remains robustly capable of functioning in all aspects of sexual response. Yes, a woman might say that she would prefer to have her body of younger years, but the preference is usually qualified: "I want my body then but my mind now." Because it doesn't work that way, we need to deal with menopause and changes in our bodies—including sexual changes—adaptively. We'll say it again: one of the most pernicious myths about female sexuality is that sex is for the young. Not so; *sex and sensuality are natural, valued experiences throughout a woman's entire life.*

Desire

Does menopause mark the beginning of the end for a woman's sexual interest? With the dramatic hormonal changes associated with menopause, one might certainly think so. In actuality, however, this is not at all the case, and some women actually report an increase in sexual interest and activity in later years. In a 2006 study of more than 2,000 women between the ages of 20 and 70, 24% of premenopausal women reported low sexual desire, compared to 29% of the naturally postmenopausal women. (The same study found surgically induced menopause—the effect of a total hysterectomy—has a greater impact than natural menopause on sexual desire, especially for younger women. This finding is not surprising since the change is usually abrupt, surrounded by stressful circumstances, and may include grief over premature loss of the capacity to reproduce.) More telling was when the researchers factored in whether the decrease in sexual desire was a source of distress. Fourteen percent of the premenopausal women reported being distressed over their lack of sexual interest, compared to only 9% of the naturally postmenopausal women (Leiblum et al., 2006).

Other national studies of naturally postmenopausal women have shown that emotional well-being and quality of the relationship had a greater impact on sexuality than aging itself (Bancroft et al., 2003; Pfeiffer et al., 1972). Perhaps most interesting was the result of a survey of 1,328 women over the age of 40, in which 53% of the women in their 50s reported finding sex more satisfying than when they were in their 20s (Frankel, 2005).

Nevertheless, medications and medical treatment can affect all aspects of sexual response, and as you age, chances naturally increase that you will undergo medical treatment for some illness or condition. See Chapter 15 for an overview of medically induced sexual difficulties and possible interventions.

Arousal

Arousal appears to be the most affected aspect of a woman's sexuality following menopause. The mucous membrane tissue of the vagina and part of the vulva may have become thin and prone to irritation and minor injury. Lubrication diminishes during and after menopause, so these sensitive tissues are more susceptible to damage from vigorous sexual activity, especially heterosexual intercourse and other penetrating sexual activities involving the use of fingers, dildos, or vibrators. The cushiony thickness of the vaginal walls and the Venus mound has decreased, so some of the insulation against active sexual play is diminished, particularly sex involving penetration or lengthy periods of direct stimulation.

Some studies suggest that, with aging, the clitoris becomes less sensitive because of decreased blood flow and engorgement during sexual arousal. Other studies report that the clitoris becomes more sensitive because of the changes in the clitoral hood and supporting tissues around the clitoris, which diminish and leave the clitoris more exposed. If you notice a change in sensitivity, adjust the intensity of clitoral stimulation during sex to a level that is pleasurable to you. Decreased sensation in the clitoris, vagina, or labia may indicate damage to the blood vessels or nerves, which can occur with diabetes and some neurological diseases. Many physicians have been trained only to recognize the possibility of neurological or vascular disease in their male patients with erectile dysfunction and may not be sensitive to women's concerns. As with all aspects of your health, be persistent in getting the medical attention for your symptoms that you deserve.

Orgasm

We know that regular sexual activity and orgasm help maintain a woman's sexual health. Women who masturbate or have regular sex with a partner actually continue to lubricate more rapidly and have more estrogen circulating in the body, even if they show signs of vaginal atrophy (thinning of the lining of the vagina). In fact, "use it or lose it" may be truer for women than for men. Because vaginal tissue tends to atrophy and lose elasticity due not only to lowered estrogen levels but also to lack of stimulation and stretching, we also recommend masturbation with a penetrating, dildo-shaped vibrator. Using lubrication, a deep penetrating vibrator can create a satisfying sense of fullness and can help maintain healthy tissue, promote lubrication, and minimize shrinking of the vagina. The same results can be obtained through regular sexual intercourse (approximately once a week), but this latter method is not always an option or an interest for some women as they grow older.

Pelvic muscles are integral to orgasm for women and men. We also know that throughout life if your pelvic muscles are strong, your orgasms and sensations will be increased. As noted, Kegel exercises—squeezing and relaxing the pelvic muscles—can promote strength in these muscles, which are prone to lose elasticity. See Chapter 8 for specific instructions regarding Kegel exercises.

Uterine contractions that occur as part of orgasm can change in intensity and sensation as a result of menopause. Some women find that the contractions, which they may have previously felt as pleasurable, now become uncomfortable or even painful. In some cases hormone therapy also referred to as hormone replacement may help. Your healthcare provider may recommend an antispasmodic medication. It is important that uterine pain be evaluated because pain can be a signal of a medical problem. Any bleeding that you can't account for should be reported promptly to your healthcare provider.

Maintaining Sexual Health

When you are sexually aroused and enjoying penetrative sex, vaginal pain can be a big sexual downer. The vagina in menopause needs some assistance to stay healthy and user friendly. To maintain sexual health in menopause and beyond, we recommend that you lubricate, moisturize, and stretch your vagina on a regular basis.

Lubricate and Moisturize

The hormonal changes of menopause can dampen desire because of the discomfort of dealing with the symptoms and because of reduced estrogen and androgen. In some cases hormone therapy can promote healthy vaginal tissue and adequate lubrication, but this is a decision that should be made with the guidance of your healthcare professional. Using a non-petroleum-based lubricant can be very helpful to protect against irritation and dryness. Also consider using moisturizers like Replens or KY Liquibeads. Both are available over the counter and are inserted in the vagina twice a week to maintain moisture and decrease feelings of dryness and pain. See Chapter 15 for further discussion of lubricants and moisturizers.

Stretch

Besides using lubricants during sexual activity and keeping the vagina moist with local estrogen or nonestrogen vaginal products, stretching the vagina regularly can help prevent pain. If you are having regular, pain-free penetrative sexual activity, you do not need to stretch your vagina. But if you feel pain or are not as active with penetration as in the past, we suggest stretching.

The vagina is surrounded by muscles. These muscles can either tighten or become too lax during the perimenopausal and postmenopausal periods. A woman keeps her vagina and supporting muscles in great shape and increases her overall comfort through regular stretching exercises for the vagina (Foley, 2005).

Even if you think you will not be engaging in any penetrative sexual activity, the vagina remains an important part of your body and in need of attention as part of your general physical health. For instance, you will continue to have regular gynecological exams or may have a yeast infection and need to insert a suppository. There are many reasons to continue to make sure the vagina is comfortably accommodating penetration.

Try stretching every day. There are two types of stretching exercises that have proven to be helpful. The first are Kegel exercises, described in Chapter 8. The second type of stretching keeps the vagina comfortable during penetration. This exercise can be done during your regular shower or bath. With wet fingers, gently insert one or two fingers into the vagina and push slowly up into the interior space. Then make a small circular motion with your fingers, assuring that all the walls of the vagina are comfortable being touched. Next, using your index finger or thumb, gently press all the way around the opening of the vagina (the introitus) in clock-like fashion. Try to pull the introitus open as you move your finger around the circle. If you're having trouble picturing this, imagine opening your mouth and then taking your finger and pressing gently out in a circle against your lips, as if stretching your mouth wider. The introitus will respond to this stretching and, as a result, you should have greater vaginal comfort when being penetrated. To remind herself to do the stretches every day, one woman wrote in waterproof magic marker on her shampoo bottle: "STRETCH."

STAY TUNED

We are only beginning to understand the rich complexity of a woman's sexual response. We know that it spans a lifetime and that women who live in cultures that honor older women are less likely to become sexually inactive. Their continued sexual activity points to a fundamental truth: *sexual response is one of the most enduring and pleasurable parts of our humanity.*

FIVE

Reproduction and Beyond

From the first period of menarche to the last period of menopause, from puberty to sexual activity in your 90s, your sexuality evolves with the cycles of your body. Although sexuality in our modern world is viewed broadly, exceeding reproductive concerns, from a rudimentary standpoint reproduction remains a primary purpose of sexual behavior. While it's possible to write a book about male sexuality and spend very little—if any—time on reproductive function, that's not so for female sexuality. Your sexuality is experienced through the lens of your reproductive potential. For example, if your body is functioning normally, you will have menstrual periods every month for a very long time, and your sexual choices will be made, in part, around those cycles. Your decisions and experiences regarding pregnancy will have an impact not only on your sexual activity but also on your sexual self-image. For these reasons, women bring us questions like the following:

- "I want to have sex during my period. Is this weird?"
- "Is PMS all in my head? My sister says she never has it."
- "Now that I'm pregnant, I'm more interested in sex than ever, but for the first time in our relationship, my husband doesn't want it. What can I do?"
- "How do I know what birth control method to pick? And when do I start?"
- "My doctor says we can have sex again now that the baby is 2 months old, but I just don't want to. Why not?"
- "We've been trying for almost 2 years without a pregnancy. My friends keep telling me stories about women who got pregnant the minute they gave up. Does stress have something to do with conceiving?"
- "Infertility has taken all the fun and romance out of our sex life. It's all sex-on-demand and failure. Will sex ever be what it used to be?"
- "Is there any way to prevent our sex life from changing when I reach menopause?"

In this chapter we discuss the physiological cycles of women's bodies and how these cycles impact sex, beginning with a discussion of hormones and their powerful impact on women's cycles and continuing with menstruation, pregnancy, infertility, menopause, and beyond. Because Chapter 4 introduced the sex hormones that are most prominent in sexual pleasure, we'll touch on them only briefly in this chapter.

HORMONES: THE AMAZING MESSENGERS

Even when viewed in this age of technological marvels, our bodies contain a communication system that is astonishingly complex. Along with the central nervous system, invisible chemicals called *hormones* communicate with every part of the body—every cell, in fact—providing operating instructions. Hormones are produced by glands: in women, the adrenal glands, the thyroid gland, and the ovaries. When the hormones have a job to do, they are released into the bloodstream. Every process the body goes through, like menstruation, gets its start-up and shut-down instructions from hormones, often in combination with signals from the central nervous system.

Sometimes even a tiny amount of a hormone can have a big effect, depending on how sensitive the receiver is to that particular chemical. Some receiving organs have very alert receptors and respond strongly. Think about the sensitivity of your fingertips. Nerve endings in fingers are distributed in such a way as to be very sensitive to texture. If we want to experience the smooth feel of satin, for example, we use our fingers rather than our elbows to examine the cloth. In the same way, organs and cells vary in their degree of sensitivity to certain hormones, as can each individual woman.

Hormones operate by changing the chemical process within a cell: the cell or organ reacts when the hormone enters it. If we add baking soda to vinegar, we see an instant foaming action that happens only when the ingredients are combined. (Of course, the endocrine system that regulates hormonal action is much more complex than this culinary analogy.)

Neurotransmitters, described in Chapter 3, interact with hormones in intricate ways to signal body functions and responses to occur in working order. How and where hormones and neurotransmitters are released in the body so as to carry out their functions differs. Suppose you live and work in Washington, D.C. It's a gorgeous day; you generally take the Metro, but today defines itself as a walk-to-work day. Well, neurotransmitters are like the Metro—they are released from nerve cells and "transport" quickly (instantaneously). Hormones pace along differently: released from glands, they move through the body carried by fluids, so their impact isn't as instantaneous. Neurotransmitters and their receptors affect hormones, and, in turn, hormones affect neurotransmitters. The effects are especially sensitive around reproductive health and sexual response.

Hormones that regulate the changes of the menstrual cycle are part of a governmental system that is headed by the hypothalamus, an organ found deep in the skull at the base of the brain. We can think of the hypothalamus as having an office in the basement of the Pentagon. In this office, the hypothalamus is bombarded with information from the outside world, while at the same time it has the job of keeping things running smoothly within its domain: the body. The hypothalamus keeps track of reproductive status by monitoring different body signals, including the levels of hormones (estrogen and progesterone) being released by the ovaries. Hormone output from the ovaries can vary greatly during the menstrual cycle. To regulate the menstrual cycle, the hypothalamus communicates with the nearby pituitary gland by producing a chemical called *gonadotropin-releasing hormone*, or *GnRH* for short. The hypothalamus releases GnRH a little at a time to signal the pituitary gland when and by how much to respond. Think of it as e-mail instructions, sent every hour or so. Based on instructions received from the hypothalamus, the pituitary gland releases one of two regulating hormones: FSH or LH. *FSH* (follicle stimulating hormone) stimulates the growth of ovarian follicles for the production of a mature egg, and *LH* (luteinizing hormone) stimulates the release of that mature egg from the ovary. Later in this chapter, we discuss how these hormones regulate the menstrual cycle.

Hormones are difficult to pin down in medical parameters. A blood test can show the healthcare provider the level of different hormones at a certain time on a certain day, but these levels change continuously, so that the same test several days later would probably produce very different results. Each active hormone is changing at a different rate as well. It's like an orchestra production of a symphony: the trumpet players may sit with their instruments in their laps for most of the piece, but when it comes time for their part in the musical production, they will be heard and appreciated. Because of this complexity, it's not surprising that precisely how some of these hormones function is not yet fully known or appreciated.

Estrogen

Estrogen signals an embryo to develop as a female and then stimulates her body at puberty to develop breasts and fully mature her vulva, vagina, clitoris, and internal reproductive organs. Somewhere between the ages of 8 and 12 or 13, hormonal changes cause a girl's nipple area to swell and small breast buds to develop, a process that will take years. At times this will be uncomfortable for her. Estrogen will also determine the way in which her body shape and body fat distribution will differ from a boy's. Estrogen will provide the vagina and vaginal opening with strength and elasticity. The pelvic girdle bones will widen an inch or two at puberty, preparing her body for the future possibility of giving birth.

Estrogen affects a young woman's skin and complexion and helps determine when the growth of her long bones, like arms and legs, will stop. In concert with genetic factors, it will determine the distribution of her body hair. Of particular importance, estrogen is active in almost every cell in the body. For example, it will protect against the loss of bone density as a woman ages, and it can be a preventive factor for some cardiovascular diseases as well. The longer lifespan of women, relative to men, may well be due to their hormonal makeup.

Estrogen (as well as a number of other hormones) is the Internet provider of the body. Just as a long-distance carrier allows you to make phone contact with a distant friend or relative, estrogen levels help communicate to the hypothalamus where you are in your menstrual cycle. This information influences what instructions are sent from the hypothalamus to the pituitary gland and, ultimately, to the ovaries.

Estrogen comes mostly from the ovaries, but fatty tissue in the body also produces estrogen. When a woman reaches menopause and her ovaries no longer produce very much estrogen, fatty tissue will continue to make estrogen by converting other hormones present in the body.

Androgens

Androgens are produced in small amounts by the ovaries and the adrenal glands. This hormone is incorrectly referred to as the male hormone. Although a form of androgen called testosterone is extremely important in the fetal and pubertal development of boys' sexual characteristics, androgens are important for women's health and sexuality as well. The role of androgens in a woman's sexual response is discussed in Chapter 4.

Progesterone

Progesterone means "pro" (for) "pregnancy" (gestation), reflecting the fact that pregnant women have very high levels of progesterone. This hormone is produced by the ovaries and, in small amounts, by the adrenal glands. It is barely present in the first part of a woman's menstrual cycle but is made by the ovaries after ovulation each month. Man-made or synthetic progesterones are called "progestins" and are a primary ingredient in birth control pills. Progesterone is a very important hormone for the menstrual cycle and pregnancy. It helps create a mature uterine lining, keeps the uterus from contracting too much, and helps the body allow a fetus to attach and grow.

Pheromones

Pheromones, as explained in Chapter 4, are chemicals that we may secrete for the purpose of attracting others. Interestingly, pheromones may also be involved in "menstrual synchrony," which is a tendency for women who live together to have menstrual cycles at the same time or very close together.

THE MENSTRUAL CYCLE

The menstrual cycle for a woman has been compared with the moon's cycle because the typical menstrual cycle mimics the lunar cycle of 28 days. Although it is termed *menstrual* cycle, the cycle refers to the entire, and repeated, reproductive cycle a woman experiences during the fertile years. It is important to note that variations are normal. Some women have very predictable menstrual cycles of 28 days, while other women have shorter or longer cycles. Cycles of 24 to 38 days are considered within the normal range. Deviations from this "normal" pattern, such as having a period at a predictable interval for 3 months in a row and then having a cycle that goes 32 days instead of 28 days, sometimes occur.

Phases of the Menstrual Cycle

On the first day of your period, lowered estrogen and progesterone levels have signaled your body to let the blood and tissue from the lining of the uterus (endometrium) slough off and leave the body through the cervix and vagina in the form of menstrual blood. Over the next 3 to 7 days you will shed about four tablespoons of menstrual discharge.

Follicular Phase

The follicular phase is the first half of the monthly cycle, and it includes the days of menstruation. It also is the time for an egg to begin maturing. For this to happen, the hypothalamus "notices" the low levels of estrogen and progesterone and communicates to the pituitary about what will be needed for an egg to mature properly so that it is prepared for the important phase of ovulation (see Figure 5.1). The pituitary sends FSH for this part of the job. Actually, the pituitary is zealous about its job and stimulates many follicles. Follicles are extremely tiny sacs inside the ovary, and each follicle holds one ovum (egg). All these follicles become revved up by their own production of estrogen, which causes the endometrium to thicken. Soon the follicles unite, sending the hypothalamus, via the messenger estrogen, the message to stop the pituitary gland from sending additional FSH and to start sending LH. The pituitary complies and sends LH back to the follicles, where things now become selective. LH suppresses the activity of all of the follicles but one, which is groomed for complete maturity. As the follicle matures, it swells a bit and can resemble a tiny blister as the egg it contains ripens. This phase takes about 2 weeks.

Ovulation

Ovulation is the shortest part of the menstrual cycle, lasting only a day or so. The ripened egg (ovum) bursts through the sac (follicle) that contains it. Sometimes a woman will notice a little cramping at the time of ovulation on one side in her

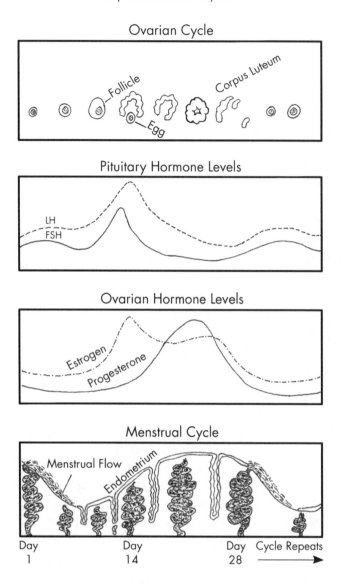

FIGURE 5.1. Phases of the menstrual cycle.

lower abdomen. This cramping is called *mittelschmerz*, a German word for pain in the middle of a cycle. The fallopian tubes become active at this point. The fimbria, or graceful, fringe-like ends of the tubes, curl and close around the transient egg, encouraging it into the fallopian tube. As soon as the egg is released, the menstrual cycle enters its last phase.

Luteal Phase

Let's go back to our empty follicle, which has been abandoned by its adventuresome ripened egg. Now the follicle undergoes a dramatic transformation. It doesn't remain an empty sac for very long. LH changes activities inside the follicle. Where there had been fluid, the cells change in composition and color, becoming the *corpus luteum* (Latin: yellowish body). Under new management, the follicle—now called the corpus luteum—again produces estrogen. The corpus luteum plans for the future and starts producing the "pro-pregnancy" hormone, progesterone. The estrogen and progesterone stimulate an increased blood supply in the lining of the uterus, just in case a fertilized ovum implants itself during the next week or so. Meanwhile the prodigal egg, conveyed by muscular contractions in the fallopian tube, stays for a few days before moving along to the uterus.

Of course, big things could happen to the little egg. If the egg becomes fertilized by sperm and attaches to the uterine lining, the corpus luteum keeps up the campaign for progesterone, which takes on the regulating function of maintaining a pregnancy. Progesterone aids in the development of the fetus and prevents contractions from beginning too early. If fertilization does not occur, after a few days the pituitary gets the message that all the progesterone that is needed has been produced, and it stops sending LH. On about day 24 of the cycle, without a pregnancy, the corpus luteum collapses and begins to deteriorate. The drop in progesterone and estrogen output signals the body to begin the menstrual period. Very soon, however, the low levels of hormones alert the hypothalamus to remedy the situation, and the cycle begins again.

MENSTRUATION

Menarche, or the first menstrual period, is often a developmentally defining moment for young girls. You will likely remember when and where you started your first period and the emotions and experiences you had around this event. A girl can expect to begin her period between the ages of 9 and 15, usually anywhere from a few months to a few years after she has begun breast development. Prior to her first period, she may have some months in which she notices a nonirritating clear or whitish vaginal discharge on her underpants.

Across cultures, menstruation has been misunderstood and mythologized, sometimes leading to the isolation of women during menstrual periods, with the isolation associated with shame and degradation (Northrup, 2010). Through the course of history it has been difficult for people to understand a biological imperative to bleed monthly, and because of this, the forefathers of medicine (such as Aristotle) posed several theories based on their rudimentary understanding of the woman's body—all of them noxious—such as that menstrual blood is fermented with impurities men are able to eliminate through sweat but women are not (Angier, 1999).

We've come a long way, with most cultures accepting menstruation as a very natural process.

Sex during Menstruation

It is important to know that having sexual intercourse, including ejaculation, is quite normal during menstruation. You can also use a vibrator or have oral sex if you choose. Whether or not to have sex during a menstrual period is a personal choice to be made by you and your partner.

Sex during menstruation is, however, a bit more complicated than choice. All aspects of sexual response "work" during your period, except, perhaps, attitude. One study compared menstrual shame with sexual decision making. A woman who experiences shame about menstruation is less likely to engage in sex during menstruation. And it may go further than that. Her attitudes may influence her sexual choices: "Once in sexual situations, a woman who fears negative evaluation may focus more on her partner's judgments of her than on her own desires, safety and pleasure" (Schooler et al., 2005, p. 326). Other research shows that experiencing negative feelings about menstruation is associated with lower sexual frequency (aside from menstruation) *and*, significantly, riskier sexual behavior (Allen & Goldberg, 2009). A study of young women's perceptions about sex during menstruation showed that their attitudes ranged from "gross" to "messy" (Allen & Goldberg, 2009). We want to stress here that avoiding sexual contact during active menstruation would involve approximately one-quarter of a woman's fertile life. As is repeated over and over in this book, relationships and time in a relationship make a difference in the decision about sex during menstruation.

> "I love having sex when I'm on my period. I already have a 'full' feeling in my pelvic area, and I get really turned on. It's a bit embarrassing, but we both even enjoy the mess of it. We take a shower afterwards, so, so what!"

> "I was absolutely certain you couldn't get pregnant during your period, so I felt 'safe' then. But my nurse practitioner told me to be sure to use condoms, because some women ovulate near the beginning of their period or might even spike ovulation during their period."

> "The only partner I'm interested in during my period is my heating pad."

Menstrual Blood Flow Abnormalities

> "I'd never had any problems with my periods, but one month, days after my period had stopped, there was blood when I went to the bathroom. I was pretty nervous—seeing blood when you aren't supposed to is scary! My doc was really good. She checked things out and decided that I just had some bleeding with ovulation that month."

We find that women who experience changes in their menstruation patterns tend to experience this as more worrisome than temporary changes in other bodily functions. Perhaps this is because blood, aside from menstruation or giving birth, is normally a cue that something is wrong. Many times there are innocuous causes for irregularities in cycles, but nothing can replace the security of being "in charge" of your sense of well-being—so call your healthcare provider if you're concerned.

Amenorrhea (No Menstrual Periods)

If you are sexually active and miss a period, the first thing you and your healthcare provider think of is pregnancy. There are, however, other reasons for menstrual periods not occurring, ranging from minor to serious problems. If you are in your 40s, you may be in perimenopause—the period when the body undergoes changes leading up to menopause.

Hypermenorrhea (Heavy Periods)

Heavy bleeding can have many causes. This is not a time for self-diagnosis: call your healthcare provider. If you have twice the volume of bleeding than is normal for you during your period, or if you bleed for more than a week, call. If you are coping with a chronic medical problem that has heavy bleeding as a symptom, check Chapter 7.

Spotting

Spotty bleeding in between periods also demands medical evaluation or attention. Causes may range from a normal response to ovulation to a serious medical problem. Some women have spotting following sexual intercourse. This should be discussed with your healthcare provider. A physical injury, such as a minor abrasion, can also cause spotting. Be persistent in seeking a cause for your spotting.

Cramps

Cramps with menstrual periods were once thought to be "in a woman's head." In the late 1970s, however, the presence of too much of a hormone called *prostaglandin* was discovered to be the main reason that women have cramps during their periods. The accumulation of prostaglandins during the second 2 weeks of the menstrual cycle can cause a strong cramping of the muscles of the uterus, similar to the aches that occur when one engages in exercise and has sore muscles the next day. This cramp, or spasm, can reduce blood flow to the uterine muscles. When there isn't enough blood, there isn't enough oxygen, which can cause pain. Cramps are also caused by pelvic congestion of fluids (creating the bloating sensation many women experience).

The good news is that many women can find ways to relieve menstrual cramps. Eighty percent of women can find relief from their cramps by taking antiprostaglandin medications. These medications include aspirin, ibuprofen, fenoprofen calcium, mefenamic acid, naproxen sodium, and naproxen. Cramps can certainly "cramp" your interest in sex, but clinicians actually recommend orgasm as a remedy for cramps! Masturbation or partner activity leading to orgasm (if you are up to it) can help. As discussed in Chapter 4, sexual arousal involves the congestion of blood in the pelvic region, and orgasm dissipates this congestion.

Premenstrual Syndrome

PMS became a popular term in the 1980s for premenstrual syndrome when an article appeared in the widely read *Family Circle* magazine. The article described PMS as a cyclical cluster of symptoms affecting numerous women (Northrup, 2010). To diagnose PMS properly, two factors must be present. First, PMS can occur only in a woman who is menstruating and ovulating regularly; the term relates to the *cycle* rather than the symptoms. This means that women who are pregnant, are taking birth control pills, haven't started periods yet, don't ovulate for some reason, or are postmenopausal do not experience PMS, even though they may experience some of the same symptoms. Second, for the diagnosis of PMS to be accurate, a woman must have several consecutive days when the symptoms are absent.

Up to 100 physical symptoms have been associated with PMS. The more distressing physical symptoms women complain of include weight gain of several pounds, bloating and fluid retention, cramps, change in appetite (food cravings or nausea), backaches, joint/muscle pain, sleep problems, fatigue, and headaches.

Emotional symptoms include crying, irritability, anxiety, depression, impatience, mood swings, difficulty concentrating, and feeling emotionally withdrawn. We want to stress that PMS is characterized by several symptom-free days, so if you are experiencing these physical or emotional symptoms *without relief*, you could have an undiagnosed depression or other medical illness and should talk with your healthcare provider.

PMS can cause havoc in a woman's sex life. Because the symptoms include emotional fluctuations as well as physical discomfort, neither the woman nor her partner knows what to expect. Some women find that their energy goes into symptom management, and they become self-absorbed. They tune in to their bodies but tune out their sexual feelings and, many times, their partners too.

> "My husband joked that he wanted me to put a sign on the refrigerator telling him whether it was okay for him to touch me. I realized I was being unfair to him. He's a really good guy, and he couldn't predict what kind of response he would get from me! When I realized this, I went online and found some really helpful advice."

> "We never had sex. I mean never. I was getting so preoccupied with either my symptoms of PMS or my period that I shut Terry out completely. She finally got fed up. She said either I fix this or she would be out of here!"

If you have PMS, there are a number of things you can do to get help and to help yourself. The following suggestions have been beneficial to many women.

Medical Evaluation

An evaluation should take into account other medical conditions that may be present. For example, we know that although PMS is not depression, women who already have depression or anxiety will be more likely to experience PMS. A medical evaluation can determine whether the use of antidepressant medication may be helpful or whether hormonal treatment, diuretics, or over-the-counter medications may be indicated.

Relaxation Techniques and Stress Management

The most current treatments for PMS all include a combination of mind and body approaches. They encourage the woman to seek medical help and to manage the challenges of daily life through relaxation and stress management techniques. Yoga, guided imagery, progressive muscle relaxing techniques, relaxation tapes, meditation, and other techniques have proven to be useful in managing PMS.

Nutrition

Keeping blood sugar fairly even throughout the day is one way to use diet to help control PMS symptoms. Reducing salt and drinking plenty of water can help reduce bloating and water retention. Eliminating or reducing caffeine and alcohol is recommended because both can trigger irritability, anxiety, and other problems associated with PMS.

Exercise

A regular, moderate regimen of exercise is a reliable way to help manage PMS. Exercise promotes cardiovascular health, an overall sense of well-being, regulation of fluid retention, brain production of endorphins (chemicals that make you feel good), weight management, elimination of toxins in the body, and a natural alleviation of depression.

Planning for Sex

Sex and PMS aren't mutually exclusive. When you are taking care of the physical symptoms of PMS, you may feel that you are doing all the planning you can tolerate. But, as we say throughout this book, sex is a quality-of-life issue. You have a right to its pleasures. Because stress can increase the symptoms of PMS, relaxing, enjoyable sex can be quite therapeutic. Pick a time when you can dedicate an hour to sexual activity, time when you won't be exhausted. Make a plan that is reasonable—don't try to create the sexual atmosphere of a lifetime with expectations that are far too grand. Assess your bedroom plan: it should be an opportunity for pleasure without adding so many extra pressures that it undoes what you are striving to create.

Premenstrual Dysphoric Disorder

The symptoms of premenstrual dysphoric disorder (PMDD) may be very similar to those of PMS, but they are more severe. PMDD is *not* PMS. If PMDD is suspected, your healthcare provider can review a symptom list. There are no medical tests that reveal PMDD, but there are factors that influence the syndrome, such as history of anxiety, depression, substance abuse, and lifestyle. Keeping a symptom diary and working with a healthcare provider are important. Many of the suggestions for PMS discussed here apply to the treatment/relief of PMDD.

CONTRACEPTION

In the early decades of the 21st century, we enjoy a sexual freedom (if there is such a thing as sexual freedom) that was not reliably available to our foremothers. That freedom was due to birth control. A woman's ability to choose the timing of pregnancy has had a tremendous impact.

This book, which stresses self-responsibility and awareness in regard to female sexuality, would not be complete without a discussion of birth control. Being heterosexually active is inextricably connected with biological reproduction and the potential for pregnancy. No matter what your religious convictions or cultural mores are about pregnancy and sex, the consequences of regular heterosexual activity, including not only pregnancy but also STIs, need to be considered carefully, in consultation with your healthcare provider, before you choose to be sexually active. Consider the following in making your choice:

1. Make your decision about which birth control method is right for you before you have sexual activity that involves—or may lead to—contact of a penis with (in or near) your vagina.
2. When reviewing the birth control methods, consider their potential effectiveness not just for birth control but also for protection from exposure to STIs. Read the section in Chapter 9 titled "One More Time: Safer Sex."
3. Determine whether any of the methods are unacceptable to you for cultural or religious reasons.
4. Decide whether you want exclusive or shared control over, and responsibility for, the birth control method. For example, an IUD would provide you

with a high protection against pregnancy (although no protection against STIs) and would be entirely within your control, whereas using condoms is a shared responsibility (and provides the most protection, other than abstinence, against STIs).

5. If you are in a committed relationship, include your partner in the decision-making process, incorporating his values and preferences.

6. Factor in any medical limitations. For example, if you are a smoker, you may not be able to use an oral contraceptive method.

7. Consider when you may want to become pregnant in the future and include this concern in your discussion with your healthcare provider.

8. When you have made an informed choice of a birth control method, seriously assess whether there are any reasons you would not consistently use this method; then address these concerns.

With the exception of abstinence and the use of a condom with spermicide, the birth control methods discussed here do not prevent STIs, although diaphragms and hormonal methods may reduce the risk of pelvic inflammatory disease. All effective methods of birth control reduce anxiety about unwanted (or "prewanted") pregnancy and at least in this dimension have a beneficial impact on sexual activity.

50 Candles for the "Pill": Enough to Light a Fire?

We don't have to explain what we mean when we say "the Pill." Perhaps people don't know the history, but almost everyone knows that the Pill is an oral contraceptive, highly effective in preventing unwanted pregnancy, that it has been around for decades, and that it became an icon because of the reproductive freedom it offered to women. Sadly, the Pill, with its freedoms (which, as part of the broader social revolutions of the 1960s, extended far beyond sexual freedom), can come with a cost, and research is showing that that cost can be sexual interest and pleasure, a very serious consideration for some women and couples.

Here's how the Pill works. The hormonal parts of the menstrual cycle that prompt ovulation are suppressed by a combination of manufactured estrogen and progesterone, swallowed every day by 100 million women worldwide in the form of a pill. Ovulation is prevented by the ingested pills mimicking pregnancy. But it is also well documented that women taking the Pill produce less testosterone, so the body's sexual response can be affected as well. Testosterone is the hormone most intensely associated with women and sexual interest. Too little, and sexuality is measurably diminished. Women who take the Pill not only produce less testosterone, but also have much higher levels of SHBG, sex-hormone-binding globulin, a glycoprotein that binds, or attaches to, testosterone. By binding testosterone, SHBG keeps testosterone from its receptors and renders the bound testosterone ineffective. SHBG emits from several sources and is activated for many reasons. Sometimes it is way overactive. The testosterone that isn't bound by SHBG is called "free" or "bio-available," meaning it circulates in the body and does the jobs it is intended to do. In women, the major job is to enhance sexuality in various ways, especially igniting sexual desire and contributing to pleasure. In ordinary circumstances, very little of a woman's testosterone is "free," but, as explained in Chapter 4, women are much more sensitive to testosterone than men.

The upshot? The amount of free testosterone retained by women who take the Pill is fractional compared with women who have never used the Pill (Wallwiener et al., 2010; Schaffir, 2006; Panzer et al., 2006; Caruso et al., 2004; Bancroft et al., 1991; Northrup, 2010). There may be evidence that SHBG levels remain higher even when women discontinue taking the Pill (Panzer et al., 2006).

Does this indicate that the Pill may be a bad choice for some women, aside from the usual health concern warnings? Yes—and there is little evidence to predict for which ones. Studies have shown that a "significant" number of women experience distressing sexual problems. The most prevalent is low sexual desire, but sexual arousal and interest are also implicated. Pain with sex is reported more frequently with women who take the Pill, as is discomfort with penetration related to decreased arousal (Panzer et al., 2006; Caruso et al., 2004). There isn't, however, enough information to discuss whether supplemental testosterone would be helpful, and testosterone is not FDA approved in any form for women in the treatment of sexual problems.

Some studies and reviews did not conclude that the lower available testosterone levels in women taking the Pill resulted in significant sexual difficulties (Bancroft et al., 1991; Schaffir, 2006). One reviewer reflected that women's sexual response is simply too complex to deduce that sexual problems could be due to oral contraceptives.

It's possible that enthusiasm about the Pill freeing couples from the worry of an unintended pregnancy increases sexual interest and activity and overcomes whatever difficulties may have been caused by less free testosterone. Women in strong relationships also report less distress.

It also may be difficult to rely on self-reports of low sexual desire. Sex therapists and healthcare providers are, at times, confounded by what a woman means when she reports low sexual interest. Women are acutely sensitive to their partners' sexual desire. Could they mean that they perceive their desire as low only because they are comparing it with that of their partners? Early analyses of sexual response (beginning with Masters and Johnson) may also have created an unrealistic standard comparable to the perfect body standard (Masters & Johnson, 1966).

In light of the possible problems with sexual response, we recommend that any decision to start taking the Pill be made very carefully. Your healthcare provider may not be familiar with the issues raised here, focusing, responsibly, on whether you have health counterindications for even taking the Pill. You may need to be persistent and thorough in your research about the Pill and its potential effects on your sexual responsivity. Many professionals in organizations like the International Society for the Study of Women's Sexual Health (*www.isswsh.org*) and researchers publishing in journals like the *Journal of Sexual Medicine* or *Archives of Sexual Behavior* are studying these concerns.

Avoiding Sexual Intercourse

Avoiding intercourse is a reliable way of avoiding pregnancy. For abstinence to be effective, it must include preventing ejaculate from coming into contact with the vaginal introitus. Sperm are motile (they swim), so couples should be cautious even if their sexual activity does not include intercourse.

Natural Family Planning

In natural family planning—sometimes referred to as the "rhythm method"—you abstain from sexual intercourse during fertile periods of your menstrual cycle. Generally this is determined by charting basal body temperature, which is the lowest body temperature reached during waking hours. Your body temperature rises during the phase of your cycle after ovulation, when progesterone is higher. You can also chart your cervical mucus and vaginal discharge, because there are changes in the consistency of the mucus near ovulation.

Natural family planning is the most effective if sexual intercourse is avoided during the first half of the cycle. The accidental pregnancy rate is high, but this method can be fairly reliable for women who have a regular menstrual cycle and follow the procedure carefully and consistently. It is important to note that women with irregular menstrual cycles are often unable to use natural family planning.

The disadvantages of this method include the fear of accidental conception, which may impact sexual responsiveness, and a feeling of pressure, in one or both partners, to have intercourse during the "safe" times because the number of these days is limited. The advantages are that both partners participate in this decision and assume mutual responsibility.

Preventing the Egg from Maturing

Hormonal control—using synthetic hormones in various combinations—works to suppress ovulation. The hormonal effects vary according to the composition of the medication used. Some hormonal contraceptives, like birth control pills, are a combination of synthetic estrogen and synthetic progesterone (progestin). The effect of estrogen is to stop ovulation by inhibiting the FSH. The effect of progestin is to reduce fertility by preventing the secretion of LH and altering the cervical mucus so that sperm can't penetrate.

The primary advantage to hormonal control is its effectiveness and simplicity. A woman using this method doesn't have to think about birth control during lovemaking or chart body changes during her menstrual cycle; she only needs to remember to take pills or get the injections or the hormonal implant. (The disadvantages of birth control pills are described above.)

Implanon

Implanon is an effective progestin contraceptive implant. During an office visit a healthcare provider inserts a thin rod, about the size of a matchstick, in the upper arm. It is permanent, effective for up to 3 years (although it can be removed at any time), and its effects are fairly quickly reversible. You don't have to worry about remembering to take pills or to be concerned about the "safe" days of your cycle. Issues discussed under oral contraceptives apply to both Implanon and Depo-Provera (discused below). Although Implanon is a progestin-only compound, the sexual side effects remain a consideration for any hormonal birth control method. One study on the progestin-only method showed no sexual side effects (Graham et al., 1995) but this study was too limited to be conclusive.

Mini-Pills (Synthetic Progesterone)

The mini-pills are very effective and can be used in some cases where the Pill is not medically indicated. Breast-feeding mothers are able to use this contraceptive. Of course you and your healthcare provider would need to review your specific circumstances and health status. One reason women toss this away as an option is that the pill *must* be taken at the same time *every day*.

Depo-Provera

With this method, ovulation is prevented by an injection of progestin, which is effective for about 3 months. (Actually, ovulation sometimes occurs with progestin-only methods, but the other effects of progestin prevent pregnancy.) Most women have irregular spotting at first with Depo-Provera, and about 50% experience the complete cessation of their periods if they use this method of birth control for a year or so. Depo-Provera is used worldwide. Progestin can also be administered in pill form.

Keeping Sperm from Doing Its Job

Spermicides

Spermicides are topical creams or gels, foams, and suppositories that are designed to kill sperm. Most condoms contain a spermicide, but you should check the packet to make sure; otherwise a separate spermicide should be obtained. Furthermore, spermicidally lubricated condoms do not provide as much protection as a condom plus spermicide. To be effective, spermicides should be used with condoms or other barrier methods such as a diaphragm. The disadvantage is that sexual activity will be interrupted briefly to apply the spermicide. With creativity, however, this disruption can be minimized by making the application of the spermicide part of the lovemaking, as opposed to treating it as a time-out.

Intrauterine Device

There are currently only two intrauterine devices (IUDs) available in the United States: a nonhormonal copper-wrapped device and a progestin-releasing device. An IUD is inserted into the uterus by a healthcare provider under careful conditions and only after a thorough evaluation of the appropriateness of this contraceptive for the woman requesting the device. There are important considerations for choosing this method, which your healthcare provider will review with you.

The uterus responds to the insertion of an IUD by producing inflammatory cells and white blood cells in the uterine lining, preventing sperm from surviving in the uterus or reaching the fallopian tubes. The hormonal IUD alters the cervical mucus so that sperm cannot penetrate easily. The hormonal IUD has recently been approved to treat heavy menstrual bleeding; women who had excessive periods prior to using the hormonal IUD experienced a notable difference in menstrual blood loss after implantation. It was once believed that IUDs allowed fertilization to take place but prevented the fertilized egg from implanting in the uterus. Recent studies indicate, however, that modern IUDs prevent pregnancy by preconception mechanisms, especially by thickening the cervical mucus so that it is impenetrable to the sperm. Even though IUDs have been used effectively for decades, the precise reasons they work is not fully understood or defined. The progesterone IUD has many of the same effects as Implanon or Depo-Provera.

Contrary to popular belief, IUDs do not cause infections. However, they can enable sexually transmitted organisms to more easily enter the fallopian tubes. Only women who are in permanent, stable, and monogamous relationships should use IUDs. Multiple sex partners increase the risk of pelvic inflammatory disease. This and other risks and side effects should be discussed thoroughly with your healthcare provider. A hormonal IUD may be an effective alternative to the Pill.

Keeping Egg and Sperm Apart

Withdrawal Method

Some couples rely on the male withdrawing his penis from the vagina when he experiences ejaculatory inevitability—the feeling that ejaculation is about to happen at any moment. This method has serious drawbacks, including a high rate of undesired pregnancy and the interruption of sexual activity at a moment when both partners are at a heightened point of arousal. We do not endorse this as an effective birth control method.

Condoms

Condoms can be very effective—but not if they are sitting in a jacket pocket or on a bedside table. Aside from abstinence, condoms with a spermicide are the only effective (although not perfect) protection against sexually transmitted infections. Condoms are thin latex "rubbers" that, ideally, are rolled onto the erect penis before there is any contact between penis and vagina.

For condoms to be most effective, proper use is essential. Condoms should be used only once and then discarded. Room should be left at the tip of the condom for the semen to collect following ejaculation. Using a "retain" double-latex ring in addition to the condom can prevent slippage of the condom. These rings are available at most condom shops or sex paraphernalia shops and at some pharmacies. They can also be purchased at several of the "sex store" websites we list in the "Suggested Resources" section. Condoms should not be lubricated with petroleum jelly or any other oil-based substance, because these can break down the thin latex coating. If additional lubrication is needed, a water-based lubricant can be used.

A large study of college students revealed several interesting facts. It appears to be assumed that (1) women are responsible for birth control and (2) men don't want to use condoms (Edwards & Barber, 2010). Women are hesitant to initiate condom use and far too frequently avoid the issue altogether by just leaving the condoms in the drawer. Here's where a little dialogue would go a long way: both men and women *underperceived* their sexual partners' desire to use condoms. So TALK!

A drawback to using condoms is that sexual activity can be interrupted when the time comes to put on the condom. With imagination and creativity, however, putting on a condom can be quite erotic and happily incorporated into the lovemaking.

Vasectomy

A vasectomy surgically alters the *vas deferens* (the tube that connects the testicle to the penis) so that sperm cannot unite with the fluid expelled during ejaculation. This procedure is permanent and has the advantage that birth control does not have to be considered during sexual activity. Although a vasectomy can sometimes be reversed, there are no guarantees that the surgical repair will be effective.

Diaphragm or Cervical Cap

Both the diaphragm and cervical cap are made of flexible latex and are fitted specifically to a woman's body by a healthcare practitioner. It is important that you have the opportunity to insert the diaphragm/cap and check its position while you are in your clinician's office. The purpose of the diaphragm/cap is to prevent semen from entering the cervix. A spermicide must be used in conjunction with these methods. Interrupting sexual activity to put in a diaphragm/cap is a drawback to its use. It is difficult to eroticize the insertion of a diaphragm/cap because it has to be placed correctly, but this drawback can be avoided by inserting it up to 2 hours before sexual intercourse is anticipated. Normally a diaphragm/cap won't be dislodged by urination, a bowel movement, or other normal activity, but the position of the cap or diaphragm should be checked prior to intercourse.

Female Condoms

The female condom offers some protection against STIs. These condoms are made of polyurethane—prelubricated plastic about twice the thickness of the latex condoms but still very thin. They are one size, soft, and have a flexible ring at each end. The condom is closed at one end, like a male condom. The flexible ring that inserts into the vagina is positioned over the cervix, much like a diaphragm. The condom acts as a barrier between the penis and the vaginal wall. The condom extends outside from the vaginal opening and is visible. At first it may seem disconcerting and cumbersome to users who are not accustomed to seeing a vaginal/vulva contraceptive, but once a woman gets more comfortable using it, she often remarks that she likes being in charge of contraception and the protection of some of her vulva as well as her vagina. Additionally, women with latex allergies appreciate this nonlatex alternative.

Interrupting the Journey of the Egg by Tubal Ligation

A surgical procedure altering the fallopian tubes so that a mature egg cannot travel through the tubes is an effective, permanent form of birth control. As with vasectomy, before choosing this method women should carefully consider whether a pregnancy might be desired in the future. *This method is not reversible.*

The procedure is commonly done through a laparoscope, which is a unique telescopic instrument inserted into the abdomen. As with any medical procedure, complications can occur. Research shows that about 2% of these procedures have some type of medical complication. Other than the need for a brief period of sexual abstinence immediately following surgery, this procedure does not impact sexual function.

Preventing Implantation of a Fertilized Egg

The "morning after" pill, a high-dose estrogen or combination estrogen-progestin pill, can be administered under medical supervision within 72 hours after intercourse; its effectiveness is most potent within 12 to 24 hours. This hormonal intervention alters the lining of the uterus so that a fertilized egg does not implant, and it alters the corpus luteum so that fertilization cannot occur. It is a legal form of contraception. It also changes the character of the cervical mucus, alters tubal motility, prevents ovulation, and may cause nausea and vomiting, depending on the hormonal composition of the pill used. It has a 75% rate of effectiveness—which means that one out of four women using this method gets pregnant.

What Could Be Coming

Male contraceptive pills have been "gestating" for many years but have yet to come to full term. That this has been so difficult to achieve makes sense, actually. With women, only one egg per cycle needs to be managed in some way. Sperm is in never-ending supply, replenishing itself and numbering in the millions. These barriers aside, this form of contraceptive is aggressively being pursued. A very promising compound in development is a form of application that will knock out not only sperm but also STI germs or viruses.

PREGNANCY

"When the results of the pregnancy test were positive, my feelings came in a flood. I felt scared and happy and anxious all at the same time."

The significance of pregnancy for our discussion about female sexuality is that girls and women generally associate their sexuality with reproduction and often view their bodies in the context of having the capacity to bear children. This capacity is inextricably linked with being a woman, and each woman has to manage this complex awareness in her own way.

The ever-present issues surrounding conception—as much a part of being a woman as are breasts, ovaries, and a vagina—have tremendous significance in the course of a woman's life. Think of the challenges a 24-year-old single woman faces if she decides to have a tubal ligation because she does not want to be a parent. Think of the grief of a couple coping with invasive and expensive technology in the hopes of conceiving or a 14-year-old girl who ignores obvious signs of pregnancy because she can't bear to consider the consequences. Consider the 38-year-old single woman who is considering donor insemination because her "biological clock" is ticking and she is not in a relationship. Reflect for a moment on the agonizing choices many women have to make between career and motherhood. Imagine the challenge confronting the lesbian couple who may face multiple layers of "coming out" to employers, coworkers, and family members because of their choice to become pregnant or a gay couple standing up to discrimination and disapproval as they process an adoption. There are as many personal and poignant stories about reproduction as there are individual women in the world.

Prenatal care cannot begin too early to help assure a healthy outcome for woman and child. Books on pregnancy focus on all possible aspects of pregnancy, labor, delivery, and the postpartum period and are an excellent and easily obtained resource. Your midwife or physician can guide you to the resources most relevant to your needs.

Our goal here is to provide an overview of possible sexual activity during pregnancy and the postpartum period. In addition, we address the possible impact of infertility treatments on sexuality. We are not at all suggesting that the areas we have selected to discuss are the most important issues regarding pregnancy—only the most pertinent for our consideration of sexuality.

Sexual Activity during Pregnancy

Sexual activity during pregnancy refers to masturbation or activity with a partner resulting in high sexual arousal, including lubrication, blood engorgement of the genitals, and often orgasm. Pregnancy, of course, brings enormous physical, emotional, and hormonal changes, as well as the anticipated presence of the new baby. Each stage of pregnancy—and, in some cases, special circumstances related to pregnancy—tends to create different challenges and raise questions about sexual activity.

> "When I was pregnant, I got worried that sexual activity or my exercise class might hurt the baby."

A developing fetus is well protected against physical sensations from the outside. The cervix has a mucus plug that blocks any direct passage of foreign material into the uterus—the baby's growing place. The fetus is enclosed in a protective amniotic sac of fluid, so jarring movements are experienced by the developing baby as a rocking or bobbing. Sexual activity should definitely be suspended, however, if there is any bleeding, loss of amniotic fluid, or contractions or on the advice of your healthcare provider.

Pregnancy, Previous Miscarriage, and Sex

In her book *Men, Women and Infertility*, Aline Zoldbrod (1993) describes the distress of a woman who suffered a miscarriage: "[She] was frightened of having sex while she was pregnant and said that she pictured the 'fetus attached to my body by only the thinnest of threads.' This woman saw her husband's penis as a 'giant intruder that will destroy the baby'" (p. 55). Women in a similar circumstance may find that they entertain fearful scenarios about sexual activity during pregnancy. The dangers may not be in line with reality, but women who are apprehensive because of previous loss will not find simple reassurance adequate. We recommend talking—early and often—with your prenatal health practitioner if you identify with these concerns. The practitioner can talk with you about your specific fears and help you prevent those fears from escalating. Any sexually stimulating activity, including masturbation, should be cleared with your healthcare provider as well.

Sex in the First Trimester of Pregnancy

Breast tenderness is common during early pregnancy. Most women experience some breast growth along with increased breast sensitivity. Touch that once was fun, playful, and arousing may become uncomfortable. The additional rush of blood to sore breast tissue during sexual arousal may make breasts exquisitely tender for a time. Couples can compensate for this by experimenting with controlled touch and nipple stimulation, being careful to avoid anything the woman finds uncomfortable, and maintaining a special awareness of the need for gentleness.

Early pregnancy often includes two other physical experiences that are incompatible with feelings of sexiness: nausea and extreme fatigue. It is helpful to remember that these early symptoms tend to diminish after the first 3 months, although feeling tired and needing more rest are normal for the duration of pregnancy.

One liberating factor for women who have just become pregnant and their partners is that they don't have to put energy into *not* getting pregnant. Some women who were constantly anxious about getting pregnant discover that, once pregnant, they can relax and enjoy sex.

Even in the first trimester of pregnancy the genitals and vagina swell and engorge with blood, contributing to a feeling of pelvic and genital fullness. This, in turn, can lead to enhanced sensitivity and arousal during sexual stimulation. Vaginal secretions are also increased.

Sex in the Second Trimester of Pregnancy

Pregnancy is a time for you to learn about your body in ways you never have before. Typically, you will ask questions about your body, its changes, and the baby's development. You can take this opportunity to learn about, and practice control of, your pelvic floor muscles—muscles involved not only in labor and delivery but also in the pleasurable contractions of orgasm.

The second trimester is generally physically more comfortable than the first. Vaginal tissues have engorged with blood, making them similar in appearance to tissue engorged during sexual arousal. The extra blood supply often changes the color of the tissue to a more vivid or darker color. When these factors combine—increased blood engorgement making genitals more sensitive, alleviation of some of the uncomfortable symptoms of earliest pregnancy, more self-awareness about your body, and increased confidence in the pregnancy's viability—you may find yourself more sexually aroused, interested, and responsive than ever before. In fact, some women experience their first multiple orgasms during this phase of pregnancy. In some cases, pregnancy creates an increased blood supply to the pelvic area, which can also contribute to increased arousal and orgasmic response *after* pregnancy. There is a "however," and that is that the SHBG discussed earlier in this chapter doubles during pregnancy, and free testosterone is comparably reduced. This may be—and often is—compensated for by the vascular changes we've described.

Even if you are highly sexually responsive and desire sex, know that your partner may not share your enthusiasm. The partner who is overly anxious because of fears of hurting the fetus should find the time to talk openly, ask questions, and explore these concerns with his or her healthcare practitioner. This anxiety can occur whether you are in a heterosexual or lesbian relationship.

Sex in Late Pregnancy

Adjusting to body changes during later pregnancy becomes a unique part of a woman's sex life. If motivated to overcome the challenge of making love with a bulging, pregnant abdomen, couples can continue to have sexual contact throughout pregnancy, and you can continue to masturbate, unless medically advised not to.

Adapting sexual positions to accommodate pregnancy can give you an expanded sexual repertoire. Intercourse is far from the only sexual experience you can have, but if you desire penile penetration, you may find that rear-entry positions are both comfortable and erotic. Face-to-face sexual intercourse may work best in a side-by-side or sitting position. Sexual intercourse with you lying on your back and your partner on top will work best if he props himself up on his hands to avoid too much direct pressure on your abdomen. This isn't a precaution due to danger to the baby but because it might be uncomfortable due to pressure on your bladder and diaphragm. If you are in a lesbian relationship and accustomed to using vibrators or dildos for penetration and arousal, you will likely need to discuss your sexual preferences and comforts (for both of you).

Concerns about Sex Starting Labor

Orgasm causes uterine contractions, and nipple stimulation with hands or mouth frequently causes strong uterine contractions as well. However, it is important to note that uterine contractions are present throughout pregnancy. In fact, as pregnancy proceeds, a woman will be aware of Braxton Hicks contractions, which aren't labor contractions but more of a rehearsal. Real labor is not going to start because of an orgasm unless the body is ready to go into labor anyway.

There are hormones associated with both sexual activity and labor. Oxytocin is a hormone associated with the beginnings of labor and one of the hormones released during sexual arousal. The uterus becomes more sensitive to oxytocin as pregnancy comes to its last few weeks. The increasing sensitivity to oxytocin builds up and culminates in the spontaneous initiation of labor.

Prostaglandins may also be associated with the onset of labor. Because semen carries a higher concentration of prostaglandins than any other substance in the body, semen coming into contact with the cervix may sometimes help induce labor. In fact, engaging in sexual intercourse and allowing the deepest penetration possible, with the penis actually touching the cervix, is a method of using sex to start labor in a full-term pregnancy, as described by Sheila Kitzinger (1985) in her book *The Complete Book of Pregnancy and Childbirth* (p. 151). To ensure the effectiveness of this method, make sure your partner's penis remains inside of you for a few minutes after ejaculation, so that the cervix is in direct contact with the semen.

This natural method of inducing labor seems to work for some women, although discomfort due to the physical state of being at the end of pregnancy may be a barrier to trying. Also, it is very important to caution against trying this method if the mucus plug has loosened (there may be some bloody "show"), if there is any leaking of amniotic fluid, or if there is any other medical contraindication. It is best to discuss this option with your healthcare provider before attempting it.

Sexual Activity after Pregnancy

Pregnancy and childbirth involve the chemical release of the hormones oxytocin and vasopressin. When a woman has a baby, she is positively flooded with these hormones—the hormones of attachment and security (Fisher, 2004). Much of what we've learned in recent years comes from neuroimaging. Neuroimaging shows vividly which part of the brain "lights up" according to the stimulus. The three processes identified with all types of love, categorized by Helen Fisher (2004) as romantic love, attachment, and sexual drive, are ignited by separate hormonal systems. Like siblings vying for attention, these three systems can compete with each other. With attachment as a "biological imperative" it makes sense that the newcomer (romantic love or sexual drive) will actually *biologically* "trump" attachment. Or at least it might cause conflict in a new mother in circumstances where intimacy with her partner would seem like a logical progression. Christine Northrup calls the postpartum period *The Fourth Trimester* (Northrup, 2010). The first few months are a bit like extended pregnancy, only with the baby on the *outside*, and very vocally, too.

Hormonal and other physical changes postpregnancy can be profound. Some women experience postpartum depression and feel completely overwhelmed for a time. Mood changes, crying jags, and feelings of being overwhelmed are normal responses soon after childbirth. Nevertheless, these should be addressed with practitioners if you haven't rebounded by the time of your first postpartum visit. Estrogen and progesterone levels are low soon after childbirth, and this may cause vaginal dryness. Nursing mothers may also experience some thinning of vaginal tissue due to low estrogen. You may be able to compensate for this condition by using supplemental lubrication or an estrogen cream, but before trying one of these, discuss the possibility with your healthcare provider.

Physical discomfort can be anticipated to some degree after childbirth. Some women have to heal from an episiotomy (an incision in the perineum to prevent tearing of tissue during childbirth) or a Cesarean section. The episiotomy site may remain tender for weeks or months after childbirth, making the pressure and stretching of vaginal penetration uncomfortable for a time. For a few weeks after childbirth you may have heavy bleeding, like an extended menstrual period, and your breasts may be sore from milk engorgement.

Just after pregnancy you may wonder whose body it is, anyway! You seem to have more body secretions than you ever imagined would be possible. If nursing, your breasts may leak and sometimes even squirt breast milk when stimulated. Some women love and regret nursing all at the same time; they cherish the bonding and closeness with their infant and, at the same time, sigh and wonder if they will *ever* have claim to their bodies.

Body Changes

After childbirth, the vagina, cervix, and muscles in the pelvic floor may be changed. Although some changes are normal, you may experience them as *abnormal* for you. Just as your household (pets too) goes through a process of adjustment with a new baby, you will go through a process of adjustment to your body as its "new normal." The differences themselves may be very minor, but coupled with all the other recent life changes, they may lead to some distress that you did not anticipate. Talk with other moms, friends, or family members about their adjustment and remember that you *will* feel like yourself again.

Postpartum time is a time for tenderness, sensuality, and connection and not a calendar counting down the weeks until you can resume sexual activity. Realizing this sounds easier than it is, but you are in this experience with a partner who can feel extraneous and confounded about what to do and when as far as closeness to you is concerned. Connection with your partner doesn't have to be one more thing on your list to do. Touching, holding, kissing, and caressing can be comforting, reaffirming, and a gentle way to connect. It doesn't have to take inordinate amounts of time. Even a few moments for a hug, kiss, and smile looking into your partner's eyes can remind both of you that you are in this together. Communicate openly about this "fourth trimester" and don't be afraid to address negative thoughts and responses. If you can keep talking and touching (and not talking in anger), you will negotiate this transition time.

When you do resume sexual activity, respect yourself and your timing. Don't expect that some sort of switch will be turned on and you'll necessarily feel powerful sexual feelings. Let go a bit and tune in to your partner. Humor is always good. Talk so that you know what each other's expectations are. At some point if you suspect you are using your status to avoid sex, seek help. This manner of dealing with ambivalence or conflicts about being sexual with your partner will compound itself if it is not addressed.

Some couples like the wetness and earthiness of sex after pregnancy. They report that they feel freer than ever before because it is impossible to hold on to some high-gloss and/or pristine notion of sex. They enjoy the stickiness and fun of milky breasts that can squirt a stream of milk several feet, vaginal secretions that are more copious, and even the occasional leakage of urine during orgasm because of the temporary relaxation of pelvic floor muscles.

Cesarean Section

If a woman has given birth by C-section, she is recovering from major abdominal surgery as well as childbirth. For a while, it may seem to her that it is all she can do to pull herself to a sitting position or get out of bed. Her healthcare team should give her information on C-section recovery, including care of her incision, abdominal exercises, and what she can expect in the healing process. In addition to the physical discomfort, there may be feelings of not having had her baby the "right way." It can be very helpful for a woman to talk about these feelings with her nurse, midwife, physician, and other women who have had C-sections.

> "A few weeks after my C-section, Tashi and I tried to have intercourse. My vagina wasn't sore, and I wasn't bleeding much. But it hurt at my C-section incision. Thank goodness Tashi is very easy-going. He said we would take it easy—and we did. We kept asking each other how we were doing. In a way, it was like birth: Tashi coached me through my entire experience, and now I was coaching him through this one."

After a C-section, you will need to pace lovemaking and intercourse in concert with your returning strength and flexibility. Because you are recovering from major abdominal surgery, you may feel protective of the surgical incision and perhaps self-conscious about your shaven pubic hair. If the C-section was unexpected, you may also be recovering from the exhaustion of labor and the disappointment that things didn't go "naturally."

When a woman has a C-section, she becomes the teacher for herself and her partner. She will need to think about what feels good to her, where she would like to be touched. For some women, the incision scar remains extremely sensitive; for others it is a nonissue. If a woman has fear about the incision splitting open with the strain of lovemaking, she will need to talk with her healthcare provider to reassure herself. This may be true for her partner as well. (In reality, surgical incisions are closed in multiple layers and do not burst open.)

INFERTILITY

> "When the pregnancy test after our latest procedure turned out to be negative, after all we'd gone through, I was devastated and felt dead inside. We'd already long given up on some romantic notion of conceiving, and now I felt like giving up on the whole business."

Infertility is often a profound personal experience. Medically, infertility is defined as a year of being sexually active without using birth control during intercourse and not getting pregnant. The term is also used for women who are able to get pregnant but have a pattern of repeated pregnancy loss. As many as one in seven women experience infertility, and about half of that number go on to successfully complete a pregnancy. Most infertility is traceable to a medically defined cause, but about 3% of the time no cause can be determined—everything looks just fine, but pregnancy doesn't occur. Even for those infertility cases where a cause is evident, treatment and intervention are not always successful.

Often treatment becomes a gamble with very high stakes. You may begin infertility treatment with very firm ideas about how far you will go, but the seemingly endless array of treatment options holds out the tantalizing possibility that the outcome will be a baby. For many couples, taking another chance seems worth yet another risk and investment of hope.

Sexual Difficulties Related to Infertility

Infertility and Postovulation Sex

If you are in active treatment for infertility, you probably have experienced sex as a means to an end: pregnancy. The timing of intercourse around ovulation is prescribed and planned and therefore may have little or nothing to do with pleasure or sexual desire. In addition, you may experience tremendous frustration because so little of your reproductive life or sexual life is in your control during the period of active treatment.

What we have observed is that a woman in this situation will often have perfunctory sex around the prescribed time for intercourse, will prop up her pelvis afterward to get the ejaculate fluid moving in the right direction, and will thereafter do anything possible not to disturb any potentially fertilized egg. For many couples, the days following ovulation and active attempts to get pregnant are days of self-imposed abstinence. What they don't realize is that the uterine contractions caused by orgasm, the thrusting from sexual intercourse, and the fluid from semen will not keep a fertilized egg from implanting in the uterus or dislodge a newly implanted embryo.

Sexual Problems in Response to Infertility Treatment

It would be more common than uncommon for you to complain of temporary sexual difficulties at some point during infertility treatment. Having sexual intercourse not motivated by desire can be a daunting experience for anyone. Sometimes couples are successfully able to separate out their "functional" sex from what they consider to be the real essence of their sexuality together. This can be challenging, however, and it is common for one or both partners to find themselves avoiding sex at times.

This happens because sexual contact can be such a vivid reminder of what they are longing for (pregnancy); instead of being a source of relief and pleasure, sex in these circumstances is a reminder of pain and loss.

Sexual Problems Caused by Infertility Treatment

Sexual problems actually caused by infertility treatment are much less common. If this happens to you, you need to talk with your healthcare provider to determine whether the problem is occurring as a result of the infertility treatment or as part of a preexisting problem.

> Mavis was in her bed on her back with her knees flexed and her eyes tightly closed. She didn't want to disappoint Sherm, but she certainly wasn't into sex this time. Mavis hadn't noticed that Sherm reached for lubricant. His hands touched her body for several moments. When he inserted two lubricated fingers into her vagina, Mavis felt her stomach muscles go rigid. Her entire body became stiff with hyperawareness. Sherm's fingers felt like a speculum to her, and she flinched away from his hand. She began to cry with the intensity of her reaction.

Mavis was already tense due to a recent medical procedure related to her infertility evaluation. Afterward, her reactions during sex with her partner were tense, anxious, and avoidant. In circumstances like the ones faced by Mavis and Sherm, it is likely such an emotional response would be disarming to both the woman and her partner. If this has happened to you, we would advise you to resume sexual activity gradually, paying particular attention to your responses and avoiding any circumstances, at least for a brief time, that can re-create the problem. This may mean that you will refrain from sexual intercourse temporarily. It may mean changing the time/place/initiation/position to see if that will alleviate the stress, or at least decrease it. Although couples who are in the midst of infertility treatment don't want to miss even one month of opportunity, we believe that ignoring sexual problems only compounds the stressful situation.

Body and Self-Image Problems

How can the hidden stresses of infertility impact your body image, self-esteem, and sense of sexuality? We can count the ways!

First, reproductive and sexual organs are pathologized or at least scrutinized for possible pathology; it's difficult to maintain a positive sense of self and body in the midst of infinitesimal medical assessments of what is going wrong. Second, you have connected your personal identity with being able to conceive a baby—a natural enough connection, given the circumstances. Third, sex becomes inadvertently paired with a sense of failure and loss; each menstrual cycle brings a reminder that the wished-for baby is yet out of your reach. Fourth, medical and hormonal treatments (if you are in such treatment) have their own impact on emotions and feelings. Fifth, infertility is socially isolating: you may be out of synch with your own goals to start a family, while your friends and family members may be proceeding quite nicely with the same goals. To make matters worse, friends and relatives can be everything from clueless to sympathetic regarding your plight and often inadvertently cause you and your partner to feel even more isolated due to their lack of support and understanding.

What to Do about Sexual Problems Associated with Infertility

Just relax. What couple experiencing infertility doesn't cringe to hear those words? Still, there is something to be said for taking a break from infertility treatment for a few months if this is feasible. Some couples find it helpful to step away briefly from the stress of trying to conceive and to find comfort in being relaxed and enjoying lovemaking that isn't on demand.

Change the routine. As therapists, we are always stressing that sexual activity is much more than intercourse. Couples can experiment with nondemand (not focused on penetration or orgasm/ejaculation) sexual activities and be pleasantly gratified.

Don't focus on the success stories of others. This a conundrum—the more you focus on the success of others, the more negative you feel about yourself. Along the same lines, be critical of much of the advice offered by others. For example, the exhortation "Don't get discouraged; think about the positive things you already have" sounds good, but it's much easier said than felt. If you take such exhortations to heart, you may find yourself on a slippery slope to more social isolation. Your feelings of failure will only increase when you realize (probably quickly) that you can't live up to the well-intentioned but often naïve advice of others.

Our recommendation is to be sure that you have interests and activities that are compelling and important to you, preferably physical ones. One woman found something healing in tending her flower garden. If this seems peripherally related to sex and intimacy, consider it more carefully: if you identify and practice focusing on activities other than basal temperature and ovulatory cycle, you will have an experiential foundation for pleasure, sensuality, and other positive responses. You will be able to build on that success to explore enjoyable, not just functional, sex and intimacy.

THE SECOND PART OF ADULT LIFE: MENOPAUSE AND BEYOND

As life expectancy continues to increase, you can look forward to having as many adult years postmenopause as you have during adult reproductive years. Menopause indeed brings challenges—not since adolescence has your body gone through such developmental changes.

Menopause Terminology

Menopause has long been misunderstood, so it's not surprising that the terms used to describe phases around menopause are confusing. If a woman has hot flashes and irregular periods for a few months and consults her healthcare provider, she may be told she is menopausal, premenopausal, perimenopausal, in the climacteric, or in a "situation that will just bear watching for a few months."

Physical Changes Associated with Menopause

A number of physical changes are associated with menopause. We will briefly discuss them here and also refer you to the "Suggested Resources" list at the end of this book. In Chapter 4 we discussed the impact of menopause on sexual response.

Ovarian Estrogen Production

During the perimenopause, estrogen production by the ovaries declines to about 10% of the level of the estrogen produced prior to perimenopause. At menopause, the ovaries disregard the signals to produce estrogen. It's the body's way of indicating that the woman's reproductive time is coming to an end. Ovarian-produced estrogen is called *estradiol;* only this form of estrogen decreases dramatically at menopause. *Estrone* estrogen, manufactured by and stored in the body's fat cells and other tissue, continues to be present in the bloodstream because its production isn't controlled by ovarian function.

Changes in the Vulva and Vagina

The vulva and vagina are very responsive to estrogen levels. Elasticity, lubrication, and thickness of the vaginal walls are affected by declining estrogen, and the tissues of the labia majora and minora become less engorged during sexual arousal. The mucous membrane lining of the vagina is particularly susceptible to irritation, minor injury, and infection as the capacity to produce lubrication decreases. Normally thick and cushiony, the vaginal walls can thin during and after menopause. The actual size of the vagina shrinks, as does the uterus. The cervix may atrophy (shrivel) and flatten out to the wall of the vagina. The Venus mound, or mons (described in Chapter 3), loses plumpness and definition, and the inner labia may shrink and in some women, whose estrogen supply has been completely suppressed, disappear altogether.

Changes in the lining of the urethra and bladder can cause irritation as well, leading to an annoying need to urinate frequently. Supporting muscles to the internal organs lose elasticity because of reduced blood flow to the pelvis. This is especially distressing if it leads to involuntary urine loss (urinary incontinence) when coughing, laughing, exercising, or having sex. Some women experience thinning of their hair, including pubic hair. This can be as distressing for a woman as it is for a man.

Taking Care of Your Vaginal Health

Maintaining physical health requires vigilance and commitment. For many women, vulvar and vaginal health care is relegated to personal hygiene and an (at least) annual gynecology appointment. In fact many women still refer to "down there" when talking about their genitals, as if "down there" was a vague destination, disembodied from them. But, whether or not a woman is sexually active, her genitals are a part of her body and, like any part of one's body, need some attention and care. Taking care of both the vulva and the vagina is part of a woman's good physical health and is simple and easy.

First, find a healthcare provider who is interested in answering your questions. Make sure you check out any of the following suggestions with your healthcare provider before beginning.

Vaginal lubrication is a normally occurring moisturizer inside of the vagina. Since the vagina and the inner labia of the vulva are mucous membranes, like the inside of the mouth, the vagina and inner labia need to have regular moisture. Just as saliva lubricates the inside of the mouth, vaginal mucus is produced in the upper walls of the vagina and bathes the vagina and inner labia with a continuous film of lubrication. This process goes on from before a woman is born until she is menopausal. The process of lubrication is stimulated in part by the presence of estrogen in the body. Lubrication not only helps during sexual activity; it protects the vulva and vagina from getting too dry, itchy, feeling painful, or experiencing tiny cracks from all the dryness. This can contribute to a woman feeling a burning sensation after urination or sexual activity as well.

Vaginal dryness is a normally occurring reaction to any of the following:

- Taking antihistamine medications, like hayfever medicines. These are medicines that dry up your sinuses, and they can dry up other parts of your body too.
- Taking some antidepressants or other psychopharmacologic agents.
- Many treatments for illnesses, like radiation, chemotherapy, or other medications, can cause dryness.

Lubricants can be purchased at *www.drugstore.com* or at any drugstore. They are usually located in the same area where condoms are sold or may be in the section for women's health with menopausal products.

Many women are also able to take localized estrogen in the form of a small suppository in the vagina (Vagifem), a ring placed over the opening of the cervix (Estring), or a cream applied directly to the vulva and vagina (like an estradiol cream). The doses are small, and the estrogen stimulates normal lubricating activity in the vagina, providing a steady source of natural moisture for the walls of the vagina and maintaining vaginal health. Many women report that they experience positive side effects in increased urethral comfort and decreased urinary leakage with the use of this localized estrogen.

Some women cannot take estrogen in any form due to a medical condition, but in some cases, after treatment ends and they are released by their physician to do so, they are able to use topical estrogen. The local estrogen, available by prescription, must be approved by a woman's healthcare provider. It is worth checking with your doctor or nurse practitioner about this if the symptoms we described apply to you.

In addition to moisture, a woman can practice simple techniques of vaginal stretching. These are described in Chapter 4.

Hot Flashes

Hot flashes, or flushes, have sometimes been called "power surges." A hot flash may not seem so empowering to a woman overcome by a sudden flush of heat radiating to all parts of her body. She is more likely to feel claustrophobic than powerful. Hot flashes happen to most perimenopausal women as their bodies react to dramatic fluctuations in estrogen. Though not entirely understood, hot flashes often are triggered by a stimulus, such as sitting in an uncomfortably warm room or experiencing stress and pressure. Most women on hormone therapy experience significant relief from hot flashes. Vitamin E and herbal remedies are also reported to be effective, though you should check with your healthcare provider to make sure they are safe for you to take.

Secondary Health Concerns

Cardiovascular Concerns

Heart disease is the number-one cause of death in postmenopausal women. Although men tend to have heart attacks during their 40s, women seldom do because of the protective effect of their estrogen prior to menopause. Estrogen and progesterone both influence a woman's cardiovascular system. As estrogen production declines, "bad cholesterol" (LDL) tends to increase because blood lipid patterns have changed. Once they lose the protection of estrogen, women are more prone to heart attacks and stroke. Whether hormone therapy may help postmenopausal women regain some cardiovascular protection remains unclear.

Osteoporosis

Osteoporosis means porous bones. As women age, their bones lose density. This is a gradual process of aging, but it's noticed most dramatically at menopause, when estrogen levels drop. Bones can become significantly more brittle and, at the same time, take on a honeycomb quality, making them much more susceptible to break-age. Hormone therapy and supplemental vitamin D with calcium can substantially help this serious health problem.

Mood Swings and Decreased Concentration

Menopause has been blamed for a number of emotional problems. If menopause caused such problems as depression, anxiety, and memory loss, it would stand to reason that estrogen therapy or homeopathic treatments would then undo these symptoms. In fact, estrogen and other therapies do not cure clinical depression. The bottom line is that menopause may bring some temporary emotional disequilib-rium, but it is a normal, not debilitating, condition. If you find you have lost interest in activities you used to enjoy; if disturbed sleep is not responsive to estrogen or homeopathic treatment; if you feel consistently sad or hopeless or unable to concen-trate effectively; and/or if someone close to you expresses concern about your mood, get an evaluation for clinical depression. Don't delay or let a medical practitioner minimize or rationalize these concerns Menopause is a natural function and transi-tion, just as puberty is. Although symptoms occur that may need medical interven-tion, menopause is not a disease.

Hormone Therapy

Hormone therapy, or HT for short, most commonly involves estrogen, or estrogen combined with progestin, a synthetic form of progesterone. If you are one of the women who cannot take estrogen, there are now effective treatment alternatives that you can discuss with your healthcare provider.

HT can greatly relieve the symptoms of menopause, but no decision about hor-mone therapy should be made without careful, individual evaluation and discussion with your healthcare provider. Fewer than half of women who are postmenopausal are on hormone therapy, despite the obvious, even life-prolonging benefits many women could receive from this treatment. However, hormone therapy is not for every woman. Women are complex individuals; personalities and preferences differ, and so do reactions to hormonal intervention. Tailoring the hormonal replacement to one's individual needs is most important.

We recommend that you discuss hormone therapy with your healthcare pro-vider before you need it. If you're not satisfied with your healthcare provider's knowl-edge and interest in menopausal women, get another opinion. Pay attention to new information about hormone therapy as it becomes available, but be discriminating. Go with the "preponderance of evidence," not with the latest news flash. Some news-media stories about medications include incomplete information or initial findings that are later contradicted by further scientific investigation. Hormone therapy is no substitute for self-care. You've heard it before, but the essentials for managing your health are still good nutrition and exercise.

The Good News Along with the Bad

Social factors strongly affect life satisfaction, and in a social and relational context sexual desire for women is profoundly impacted. If you are in a relationship where you feel positive and secure, you are much more likely to experience satisfaction with your sexual relationship, even if there are some self-described sexual difficulties with you or for your partner. The same goes for hormonal changes: they are trumped by a positive relationship (Dennerstein et al., 2005). We are aware that partner loss for a variety of reasons occurs as age progresses (and, of course, for younger women too). But older women with outside interests are not inclined to curl up with the cat and just stay put. Older single women are known to have decreased sexual desire, but this does not always correlate with dissatisfaction. One study showed that 90% of doctors believed that menopausal women felt loss with menopause. Only 30% of women expressed that response. Half the women in the study reported relief instead, a fact the doctors didn't believe (Lindh-Astrand et al., 2007). And if a woman does experience loss, perhaps it is more associated with societal ageism and the loss of social status women notice as they age.

Your Brain Postmenopause

We have always assumed that as our bodies wrinkle, creak, and gray, our brains are going through equal—and irreversible—degrading. Barbara Strauch, the health and medical science editor for the *New York Times*, has drawn upon the work of researchers to bring surprising information to light that refutes this assumption in *The Secret Life of the Grown-Up Brain* (Strauch, 2010). First, amusingly, no one will step a toe over the line to define what *age* middle age is. The variance Strauch found was 28 years—a whole generation in real time! Second, you may wonder what relevance information about our brains has for menopause and sex. This will become evident.

There are some brain changes with growing older that fit hand in glove with the prevailing concept that every year our brain cells are dying, never to revive. One is the pretty universal problem with name recall. Another is what Strauch refers to as our increasing distractibility: we walk 25 steps into another room and forget why we're there. But there are gains as well.

Here's just a sample of what is newly discovered, from impeccable research and neuroimaging:

- Brain cells (specifically the myelin coating of neurons) continue to grow with age.
- We grow happier, calmer, more adaptable, and better able to see the big picture. This capacity appears to be a function of aging itself.
- In tests involving conclusions about a situation, older people are more positive and more likely to see several sides rather than making one assumption, like their younger counterparts.

- Although negative experiences and images are much more potent than positive or neutral ones, older individuals "sort things out" much more positively, and this is *not* a kind of disembodied haze. It is highly adaptive.
- There is no scientific evidence for empty-nest syndrome or midlife crises. Conversely, people should not retire too young.
- When confronted with brand-new technology or information, older people process more slowly and utilize the information more ineffectively. *BUT—and this is big*—if confronted with something new that relates, even minimally, to what they already know, Strauch says, "The middle-aged brain works quicker and smarter, discerning patterns and jumping to the logical endpoint" (Strauch, 2010, p. 48).
- Robust older brains change. Younger people use one side of their brain for one type of task and the other side for another. Their elders use *both sides simultaneously*. This boosts brain power and literally widens the scope of problem solving.

Your brain is your most important sexual organ. As described in Chapter 3, the brain receives stimuli, sends signals, and allows you to interpret those signals. Do you want to keep advancing your brain and assist your body to its maximum capacity? You may yawn when you hear this, because it is so often repeated, but exercise regularly and with commitment. *Regular exercise increases the neurons in the brain* (Strauch, 2010). Review your diet, supplements, and medications. *Concentrate* when you are hearing about new material. Many people just tune out, which contributes to brain stagnation. Choose some tasks or play requiring physical dexterity. Be socially interactive and involved (don't shrug and say "I feel self-conscious in groups"). It will help your cognition. Be altruistic: it is one of the fundamentals of wisdom and well-being to reduce self-centeredness. It also lights up the reward center of your brain. Laugh, relax, and have fun. Your older brain is preparing you to do just that.

PART III

Making Peace
with Your Body

If you're alienated from your own body, you're shut off from an important source of pleasure and deprived of a vital means of connecting with special people in your life. In many parts of the globe, media incessantly remind women that their bodies are woefully imperfect and that the quest for happiness is a quest for youth and beauty. For many women, to engage in sex is to focus on their perceived inadequacies rather than on pleasure and intimacy.

Feelings of alienation from your body can be intensified even further if you have been sexually abused, have contracted an STI, have been diagnosed with a serious illness, find sex physically painful, or live with a disability. In the face of any of these challenges, you may even feel betrayed by your body. As a defense, you may try to distance yourself from all physical feeling and sensation. You may try to retreat to a world of thoughts and words, devoid of any pleasure that can come from touch, caressing, or the mingling of bodies.

In Part III, we examine the challenges that can alienate women from their bodies and explore how they can take care of their sexual selves by making peace with their physical selves. In this section you can learn to have a positive sexual identity that includes your physical appearance. You can come to terms with your uniqueness as a female and learn to feel comfortable in your body. The following chapters provide specific self-help strategies to help you move from fear to knowledge and from victimhood to empowerment. Exercises for those who want to take this work further are in Chapter 13.

Chapters 6–10 address the questions our clients frequently bring us:

- "I haven't been able to rise above the media's portrayal of women and feel good about the way I look, so how can I teach my daughter to do it?"
- "I'd love to love my body the way my partner claims to love it, but how can I deny what I see in the mirror?"
- "Where can I get information about having a good sex life in spite of my cancer?"
- "Does disability have to mean asexuality for me?"
- "How do I deal with my developmentally disabled daughter's sexual maturation?"
- "Having sex hurts, and the more I try to 'get over it,' the tenser I get, and the tenser I get, the more it hurts—what can I do besides stop having sex?"
- "What kind of sex is safe for me if my partner has an STI?"
- "How do I tell someone I'm about to have sex with for the first time that I have an STI?"
- "I thought I had put that awful abusive experience behind me years ago—why is my sex life suffering now?"
- "When sex is supposed to be experienced with abandon, how can I keep enough control over it to feel comfortable when just kissing makes me freeze up?"

SIX

Body Image

ARE OUR BODIES OURSELVES?

From the first flood of breath into our lungs to the last flutter of our final exhalation, we make our sexual journey in our bodies. For too many women, much of the journey is spent yearning to be elsewhere: any place but in their own body. Our bodies are ourselves, to quote a well-known book title, but far too many of us ask, "Does it have to be this body?" What drives this all-too-common body dissatisfaction?

In Part I, we discussed the emphasis placed on female desirability early in childhood. All people rely on cultural values for individual guidance about what is typical and expected behavior for that society, and, accordingly, women are vulnerable to cultural "suggestions" about what constitutes female desirability. Cultures that are considered "market driven" often pressure women with idealized images that create personal dissatisfaction and prompt women to strive for body perfection. By encouraging women to seek unobtainable perfection, a strong market is sustained for industries peddling fashion, cosmetics, plastic surgery, fitness, weight reduction, and so on. Cultures that are considered "values driven," on the other hand, often pressure women with idealized expectations, with the outcome being control and submission. In this way the prevalent values and beliefs within these cultures often restrict a woman's choices or freedom of movement.

Regardless of whether they are products of a market-driven or values-driven culture, women throughout the world struggle with unattainable expectations. Varying from place to place, these expectations are diverse and include being perfectly thin or perfectly round, physically fit or fragile, beautiful, fertile, chaste, or adventurous. *All* women, not some women, are subjected to the impossible dilemma of not meeting fictionalized standards. Some women may "make the cut" for a period of

145

time, only to face the inevitable fall from perfection. Even those who are temporarily elevated for their beauty or their virtue find it is a precarious perch.

> Rosa, 15, shivered in the chill of the stark room, curling her toes against the cold tile floor. She was nude except for a light cotton gown, and she waited nervously for what would happen next. She twisted a plait of her black silky hair nervously when two women, also wearing cotton gowns, entered the room. The women smiled briefly at her, but with no real connection. Rosa needed connection.
>
> "This is my, um, first time. My first shoot. Who decides, like, about hair and stuff?"
>
> One woman flicked momentary eye contact with Rosa and said, "We'll get to that."
>
> The gown was slid to Rosa's waist. A huge brush, soft as down, dipped in an earthy-colored powder, was dappled on Rosa's shoulders and breasts. One of the women rouged her nipples, causing Rosa to blush vividly. No one but she had ever touched these youthful breasts before.
>
> Weeks later Rosa stared at the glossy magazine picture of herself propped on the machine where she was working out. In the picture Rosa was wearing a creamy silk shift, and her rouged nipples were apparent under the soft material. The wind machine had pressed the material against her skin, creating an allure in the picture Rosa had never seen in herself. She took stock of the magnificent girl in the magazine ad who was supposed to be her. She had been buffed and tinted and curled and posed and lit and dressed.
>
> *How is this me?* Rosa wondered, as she climbed into her third hour on the Stairmaster, going nowhere.

There are women who rise above this socialization and deserve our admiration, but most women struggle with this issue for most of their lives. Most women are familiar with the statements we've just made about body image and probably agree with them, but this doesn't mean that their behavior or self-esteem is free from being influenced by what is defined as desirable. These messages can become so distracting that a woman loses track of herself.

We all know—or are—women who vehemently denounce buying into *The Beauty Myth*, as outlined by Naomi Wolf in her 2002 book that exposed our dominant culture's selling (with major market success) *dis*satisfaction, yet who will turn around and reject their own bodies for their societal shortcomings. We have heard countless statements by women despairing over their inherited traits:

> "I feel like a frog. All of the women in my family seem to have inherited these skinny legs and barrel belly."

> "My hair is impossible: seaweed-on-a-rock."

> "Is every girl in our family doomed to be 5 feet tall?"

Or acquired ones:

"I will never look 18 again."

"I avoid mirrors—my belly is so round since I've had kids."

An unfortunate reality is that body dissatisfaction and sexual dissatisfaction are in bed together. Many women who avoid sexual activity hold out for the perfect body, imagining that such a body will create perfect sexuality.

Exercise: The Journey from Corsets to Ab Crunches

As girls stepped into the 20th century 100 years ago, they did so by throwing off the corset and other cumbersome clothing and by the 1920s had adopted the loose-fitting flapper dress. This physical freedom was accompanied, however, by a new tyranny. When women were no longer laced from the outside through corsets, they began in earnest to establish internalized control of their bodies through both diet and exercise.

From the mid-20th century onward we girls and guys have been wearing the same pants and shirts. Why hasn't this change brought freedom? Because Victoria's secret is that there is an alter-image to the woman who jumps into her casual khakis. The elastic that used to encase a woman's abdomen and bottom in a girdle now comes in a spandex form that passes for a dress, skirt, or top. The purpose isn't to modulate her form but to provide a new way to emphasize and focus on the rigidly developed and defined muscles and fat-free body that she has achieved through rigorous exercise. Brumberg (1997) observes that "the pressure to control the body has been ratcheted upward by an even more demanding cultural ideal: a lean, taut, female body with visible musculature" (p. 123). The goal of exercise is not so much being healthy, but being a perfectly delineated "10" in spandex.

Body Control Measures

The Surgical Solutions

Plastic surgeries, breast augmentation, and liposuction—procedures that go the extra mile toward body perfection—are now considered acceptable. But they don't come without real physical risk, including at times serious surgical complications. In the market-driven culture of body perfection, the American Society of Plastic Surgeons (ASPS) reports that cosmetic surgery reflects the national economy: when the economy is strong, cosmetic surgeries (which when elective are paid for by the consumer) increase (ASPS, 2007).

There was a time in history when women's feet were mutilated by means of a practice called "foot binding," which attempted to shape what was then considered the perfect foot: a tiny one. Nowadays the mutilation of foot binding to achieve this goal would rightfully be considered abusive, and efforts to curb the trend undoubtedly would be swift. This is in sharp contrast to our benign acceptance of surgical intervention as a method of beauty enhancement. A study comparing women who had cosmetic surgery with those who did not (von Soest et al., 2009) looked at satisfaction, self-esteem, and psychological problems. Notably, women who had cosmetic surgery were more focused on their appearance than the control (no surgery) group. The 6-month follow-up showed that women were satisfied with their surgery from an appearance standpoint. Consumers and researchers correlate positive body image with self-esteem, but the self-esteem improvement attained through cosmetic surgery was quite modest and was no different from that of the control group. Elective cosmetic surgery appears to have no effect on psychological problems. Each woman must decide for herself whether the breast augmentation or face lift or tummy tuck will give her the reassurance and confidence that she associates with "being pretty."

Labiaplasty—the process of surgically altering a woman's genitals to make them smaller or tighter—and hymenorraphy (sometimes called *revirginization*), the process of piecing together the remnants of hymenal tissue in the vagina to make the hymen look intact and to convince a future sexual partner of a woman's virginity, have gained popularity in different cultures. Ironic that these very cultures may also condemn the practice of female genital cutting (FGM) that takes place in other cultures. All of these genital surgeries to shape the labia, deny prior sexual penetration, or prevent penetration or pleasure are of grave concern to most healthcare professionals. These procedures can sometimes reduce genital sensation and pleasure. Although the practices may seem vastly different from one culture to another, they are all ways of creating the "perfect female" and represent attempts to increase a woman's desirability and potential for mating. These practices are not necessarily foisted on women by men; ironically in all cultures the woman herself or her mother or her other female family members, far from preventing or discouraging the practices, often support them—desiring the anticipated benefit that these young women will be marriageable and conform to socially accepted standards for female gender and identity. Education and greater understanding about the risks and problems associated with genital cutting will reduce these practices, but long-standing traditions take time to change. It's important to remember that these customs derive from male-dominated societies in which women were not treated equally.

The greater cross-cultural phenomenon of female genital surgeries elected by women will not be reduced by education alone. Many women seeking these surgeries have high levels of education. It will require a cultural redefining of who owns a woman's body. We vote for each of you—no matter your age—to take back your body, your sensations, and your shape, no matter what shape you are in. This will have a profound impact on your sexuality.

Are Lesbian Women Immune?

How's this? Lesbian women aren't generally included in research about body image—just because they aren't attracted to men. Despite Ellen DeGeneres being Cover Girl cosmetics' "cover girl," our dominant culture has stereotyped and often perpetuates negative views about what is *presumed* to be "lesbian appearance." If a woman is judged to be less attractive than average, or presents as more androgynous in dress or action, she is likely to be quickly assigned the label of "lesbian" whether that fits her personal identification or not.

Easier—and Harder

Laura Kelly, an associate professor at Monmouth University (Kelly, 2007), sums it up: the multiple dilemmas a lesbian woman experiences can lead to what she calls "body silence." Many lesbian women consciously choose to dress in nongenderized clothing and low-maintenance hairstyles. This likely contributes to the dominant culture's misattribution—that lesbian women possess more "masculine traits." There are, of course, women who do choose to appear "butch," where they deliberately take on a more masculine appearance. The women who may have the most dilemmas, however, may be the "femme" lesbians. These women—as so many women—identify with the dominant cultural norms of appearance and may strive to be thin and attractive. For lesbian couples in general, though, the cultural ideal of thinness as attractiveness holds less sway than for either gay couples or straight couples.

> "Body silence" is not the same thing as body acceptance. Each woman must think through what appearance means to her and to a relationship.

Anorexia and Bulimia

No argument is persuasive enough to alter the perception of a woman who has been convinced by magazines, the mirror, the mall, or her peers (and sometimes even her parents) that she is fat. How far can this distorted thinking go? It can go to starvation and death. Anorexia is purposely restricting the intake of food, and bulimia is purposely restricting the body's retention of food. With bulimia, eating is not restricted, but the body disgorges the food it has taken in, through induced vomiting or laxatives or both. Even if this is only an occasional behavior, it is too much. We want to stress that marketing and media do not cause anorexic or bulimic behavior, but they do contribute to its prevalence as a disease.

Behavior close to starvation comes with hidden costs. The body and brain don't care if the behavior is intentional. Energy will be conserved toward survival, so creativity, production, involvement with others, normal alertness, and judgment are all impaired. The body systems compensate for the starvation as long as possible, but eventually life-sustaining processes will break down.

Women who deliberately starve themselves become obsessed with food, almost or entirely to the exclusion of other interests. This isn't voluntary. It is the brain's mechanism against life-threatening peril. Furthermore, it appears that engaging in anorexic/bulimic behaviors creates a cycle wherein the distorted thinking connected with these behaviors becomes reinforced, making it even more difficult to stop.

Anorexia and bulimia are devastating to sexuality. The closer a woman comes to paring off all of her body fat, the lower her sex hormone production drops. In fact, her reproductive system shuts down: menses cease, and getting pregnant becomes difficult or impossible without medical intervention. Sexual desire is dampened or nonexistent. Body hatred or extreme body self-consciousness tends to quench the flickers of sexual interest that might remain.

If you have binged and purged even once or twice, we advise you to have a consultation with a social worker, psychologist, clinical nurse, or physician who has expertise in eating disorders. If you are severely restricting your food intake and find that you are fearful about continuing (or stopping) this behavior, the same advice applies. If you are the parent, relative, or friend of a person whose eating behaviors worry you, you may not know where to turn or what to do. Many communities have support groups for concerned "others" at local medical centers. You can join an online support group such as *www.something-fishy.org* or find out more about eating disorders on websites such as *www.healthlinkusa.com*.

Fat: The World on My Plate

Fat: What Is It?

Fat isn't easily defined. One woman with the tiniest, normal, visible indent that her bra makes in her back under a tank top will declare herself "gross" and cover up with an oversize T-shirt; she feels ashamed if her body has any curve or contour. A woman of ample body size may comfortably wear a garment that doesn't seem suitable to the observer because it reveals too much fat. These women have distinctly different responses to their body size.

When the Pounds Add Up: Overweight

Few personal stories have been as candid and inspiring and powerful as Oprah Winfrey's detailed account of her struggle with excess weight. This gifted woman—one of the most influential entertainers of our time—allows us access to her most private thoughts and feelings as she was about to accept her Emmy (Greene & Winfrey, 1996):

"And the winner is Oprah Winfrey." I was stunned. Stedman and my staff were cheering. I wanted to cry. Not because I won, but because I would have to stand before this audience of beautiful people and be judged. And not for being a winner.

I felt so much like a loser, like I'd lost control of my life. And the weight was symbolic of how out-of-control I was. I was the fattest woman in the room. (p. 2)

Sometimes weight becomes a real problem physically, medically, emotionally, and/or psychologically. A woman who carries around many extra pounds has a bigger burden than the literal weight. She will be prone to measure herself first, before any personal accomplishment, by what she considers a primary personal failure. Weight is certainly no gauge of capability, talent, humor, skill, moral strength, intelligence, or success in relations with others, sexual or otherwise. But being overweight obscures these assets, as if it were a shield beyond which little else can be seen or appreciated (Esposito et al., 2008).

How many times have we heard statements from women to the effect of "When my weight is down, I feel sexy and interested, but the more I weigh, the less I desire"? Genitals, brains, hormones, and nerve endings do not become dormant as a result of additional weight. In many cases, however, the internal looping dialogue about weight is so complete, body weight so distracting, that a woman cannot focus on her sexual feelings.

In North America, there is an increasing emphasis on thinness as the ideal for body attractiveness in both genders and across ethnicities. Being male or female, young or old, African American, Asian American, or Latina American does not afford protection. In one study, a greater dissatisfaction with her body contributed to a woman's increased reluctance to insist on condom use and safer-sex strategies. Women feared that their lack of body attractiveness would cause them to be rejected, and their fear of abandonment led to higher risk taking during sexual activity (Wingood et al., 2002; Molloy & Herzberger, 1998; Kelly, 2007; Legenbauer et al., 2009; Hormes et al., 2008; Meana & Nunnink, 2006). In these situations, low self-esteem about one's body is linked directly to death.

Desirable versus Desiring—Enter Cognitive Distraction

A woman's sexual desire often emanates in large part—or, too often, exclusively—from how desirable she sees herself, instead of what *she* finds desirable.

"I have never stopped to think about what I like in sex. I've come to realize that I have always gauged my sexual response to whether I'm wanted. I get energy and sexy feelings when my partner's turned on by me. I know this leaves me out, but I honestly can't do it differently!"

A woman's view of her body includes not only her feelings about her sexual attractiveness, but her physical condition, her body mass index, or BMI, her facial attractiveness, her weight, her size, and her physical performance in sex. The ability to focus attention on the sexual arousal a woman feels is related not to just one of these factors but to all of them (Seal & Meston, 2007). When a woman likes her body, she can concentrate her self-focus and feel great about herself, her arousal, and her sexual enjoyment. In this situation, if something isn't going quite right in sex, she can use her good body feelings to focus on her sensuality and enhance her sexual response. There is synergy between her sense of her body and her sense of her empowerment in sex. We call this *body esteem*, and it is different from self-consciousness about one's body.

But the reverse is more frequently true—that self-consciousness about one's body creates low body image and leads to "cognitive distraction"—a focus on distracting negative thoughts about the body that can lead to criticalness and objectifying of one's own body. These distracting and negative thoughts cause a woman to feel ashamed of her body—not feeling attractive by cultural standards—and even spectatoring during sex (not being able to get aroused because of sexual self-consciousness and negativity). This ultimately leads to more shame and low or no feelings of sexual arousal, pleasure, or orgasm. Spectatoring has been around for a long time. In men it's focused on performance, but in women it is focused on both performance and attractiveness (Pujols et al., 2010).

Low body esteem leads to avoiding sexual activities (Sanchez & Kiefer, 2007; Dove & Wiederman, 2000) and perhaps eventually opting out of sex and sexual desire (desirability) altogether. And if she is vulnerable to spectatoring, then techniques that encourage a greater self-focus on the body, like sensate focus, may actually make a woman feel more nervous about how she looks, increase her self-consciousness, and interfere with attending to arousal in her own body. Ultimately the goal is to have better body esteem and less distress over one's appearance during sexual activity (Pujols et al., 2010).

There are ways to combat low body esteem, by redirecting attention and practicing mindfulness—techniques we'll address both later in this chapter and in Chapter 13.

Cognitive Distraction, Relationships, and Age

Women have a greater need than men to be found desirable. They are also more influenced by whether they are satisfied with the intimacy in their partnerships. Women's sense of their sexuality is influenced by how they are treated by their partners. When it comes to the day-to-day challenges of life, negative interaction with a partner—called *relationship distress*—concerns a woman more than feelings of personal distress that she may suffer. On the positive side, a woman can have low body-esteem, but if her partner is completely attracted to her and lets her know she's terrific, then her personal distress decreases and she feels better about herself (Pujols et al., 2010). Some sex therapists note that as women age, sexual satisfaction is best predicted not by having a fabulously attractive body but by having quality in relationships and quality of life (Dennerstein et al., 2001; Bancroft et al., 2003). In addition, older women have a smaller gap between their wished-for bodies and their real bodies. They are more accepting of who they really are. In fact, many women feel more positive about their bodies, with less appearance anxiety, as they age.

Feeling good is infectious, and there is a strong association between relationship satisfaction and sexual satisfaction. Those women with satisfaction in these arenas have a better perception of their own sex appeal (Gossmann et al., 2003). Women who feel valued in relationships more often have a positive view of their own sexual attractiveness and pleasure. Quality of life, intimacy, respect, communication, and relationship satisfaction point to sexual satisfaction for women (Koch et al., 2005; Haavio-Mannila & Kontula, 1997).

Keep Away or Come to Me

If an unresolved, unaddressed conflict with a partner exists, the protection of additional weight can express what isn't being acknowledged or explored: *I don't want to make love while there is so much stress between us—so keep away.* Weight becomes a formidable stand-in for the real issues.

At times there are unaddressed psychological reasons that a woman wants to keep her distance from others, at least where physical intimacy is concerned. Weight may be a protection against the perceived dangers such intimacy presents. Weight may give a woman peace of mind—she doesn't have to deal with one more demand or intrusion into her already overburdened life.

If we eroticize women's bodies, it stands to reason that women's partners will have their own responses to bodies that deviate considerably from the standard *du jour*. Both women and men, in straight or same-sex relationships, may respond to their partner's weight or shape by withdrawing their own sexual desire and interest. But sometimes the withdrawal response is a stand-in for other, more complicated relationship problems. A woman's partner may withdraw not because of the weight itself but because of her unresponsiveness. Here's how this looks:

PARTNER A [distraught over poor body esteem]: I'm not desirable anymore because of this weight. If I were, my partner would still show interest in me.

PARTNER B: I can't understand why my partner is avoiding me sexually. I feel shut out. I am very uncomfortable making any sexual overtures at all. All she does is obsess about the way she looks. She isn't into sex with me.

Too Hot to Handle

Being overweight can also neutralize the notion of a woman's sexuality being dangerous. An overweight partner won't stray, won't tempt others. Perhaps both partners are afraid of this possibility, and it gets acted out by maintaining an unhealthy, overweight body. The overweight partner fears her own loss of control should she feel thin and attractive to others. Attractiveness and sexual vitality are intimate internal processes. When this dynamic is present and unrecognized, it can be fatal to any weight management attempts. Neither partner will be able to maintain behaviors supportive of weight loss if the underlying fear is that fat is the only thing that stands in the way of the woman and her rampant sexuality.

CLAIMING OUR BODIES, OUR SEXUALITY

You knew before you opened this book that your perceptions of your body, and the perceptions of women you love of their bodies, have been impacted negatively by all kinds of cultural influences. But have you calculated what this might have cost you in sexual responsiveness and pleasure?

Imagine the sexual energy women could have available to them if they harnessed and directed the resources they expend in useless worry, envy, despair, rumination, negative comparison, and often financial expense to get somewhere that doesn't exist. Women don't just waste the valuable resource of their own energy in this quest. They squander the synergy of the relationship of themselves with others, both women and men.

In this section we outline specific suggestions for exercise, and its imperative role in sexual health, for talking to other women, because a natural outcome of health and self-awareness is outreach and mentoring, and for keeping a perspective about body image and challenging your cognitive distraction and negative thinking when it occurs.

Physicality: We've Come a Long Way

In 1972 Title IX became federal law, mandating that schools provide girls the same opportunities in sports as boys. Title IX was generated for economic reasons. Proponents contended that boys' sports, such as high school and college football, were lavished with money and attention, providing these boys with a later, unfair advantage in the workplace.

Women athletes have strong, lean, taut bodies that come from years of dedicated training. Today's ideal female body is often presented in motion rather than posing prettily. We now have a generation of female athletes who have come on the scene, and many of them have felt the power and freedom that comes from being physically fit. They bring to their adulthood the knowledge of how great it feels to move. In general athleticism is linked to better sexual health. But female athletes can be as self-conscious about body attraction as nonathletes. For instance, many female athletes now wear flawless makeup and designer clothes while dominating their opponents.

Exercise

Not all women are or will be athletes, but exercise is the closest thing we have to a fountain of youth. It is life sustaining. It impacts all areas of health and strength. It keeps us moving and flexible well into our latest years. It helps our bodies maintain nutritional and hormonal balance. It affects mood, and not just because we feel good that we're exercising when we do, but because it regulates important chemicals in the brain.

It is never too late to begin to exercise and reap its benefits. If you are 18 and "too busy to exercise because of school and work," prop your homework on a treadmill and get moving! If you are 80 and your doctor approves, get to the mall and start walking. Exercise should be consistent—three to five times a week for 30 minutes or more. An ideal exercise program includes aerobic exercise, strengthening and balance, and stretching. Your healthcare provider can offer guidelines. Many communities have a recreation center with personnel qualified to offer exercise advice and make recommendations for a balanced routine.

There are sexual benefits to regular exercise:

- Improved pelvic muscle tone enhances orgasm and sexual response. See Chapter 8 for a description of Kegel exercises, which can help maintain muscle control or improve it if the muscles have become lax.
- Physical flexibility contributes to the comfort and pleasure of sex with a partner. The more you can move, the more spontaneous and adventuresome you can be, the less you will concentrate on what you can't do. This can be particularly important to you as you age.
- Exercise is almost an "on" switch for hormones. It reduces fatigue, releases endorphins, and helps your body make the most effective and beneficial use of sex hormones, such as estrogen and androgens.
- Exercise helps your body become fit, toned, and energetic. Seeing the physical benefits of exercise instills pride and confidence that you take into the bedroom. You will also bring the energy that comes from regular exercise and fitness into your love life!

Mentoring Positive Self-Awareness: Talking with Others

No matter the age, women can be their own worst enemies. We have all been with friends, sisters, mothers, and daughters when negative remarks were made about a woman's body or sex life. There is an unfortunate obsession with this trash talk.

"So I told him, 'I have kids hanging on me all day. My body's a wreck. Don't ask
   me to have sex. I couldn't care less.'"
"Other girls might be thinner than me, but the guys know I give great head."
"Look, at my age I'd rather eat than have sex."

We suggest that you not agree with these comments and that you avoid laughing
along with "the girls." Think about standing up to every instance of self-trashing and
sex trashing. This may be easier with older women, who we may see as less vulnerable
than teenage girls. The truth is that teens and young adults are exposed to so much
sexual information that they need very specific messages supportive of their health,
their choices, and their privacy. A girl who feels chronically uncertain about her body,
and hence her appeal, carries this uncertainty into her decisions about sexual behavior. Mixed with this is the dynamic of the young woman being more tuned in to her
desirability than her desire. If we now add to this mix continual overexposure to sex,
from its most banal to bizarre forms featuring truly unbelievable bodies, we have a
recipe for disaster. This is the challenging context in which we want today's woman
to be self-aware, assertive, and discriminating about sexual choices.

What do the youngest of the women among us need? They all need to hear the
stories of women in their lives who have gone through body image crises and physical, emotional, and sexual development and arrived at adulthood feeling positive
about their bodies and sexual health.

If a woman we cared about was going to take a group biking trip far from home
for a number of days, we wouldn't let her launch into the trip with unsafe equipment
or uncertain preparation and plans. So it should stand to reason that she shouldn't
launch into her sexual journey with less preparation and input from the adults who
care about her. A significant aspect of her developing sexuality will be how she feels
about her body. We wouldn't say to her, "Just say no if the road is slippery and your
biking group is going ahead anyhow." Likewise it wouldn't be sufficient to say, "Just
don't pay attention to all of that overinflated perfect-body stuff you see on MTV," or
"Don't waste your money buying all that cosmetic junk."

All teens need exposure to the dilemmas and struggles of women who have
gone before them. They will absorb the ways in which these women solved their own
dilemmas and took their own stands regarding exaggerated focus on appearance and
body "perfection." They will benefit from being exposed to women role models in
their community or the nation or in history whose contributions—not necessarily
their appearances—have been notable and strong.

Challenging Our Thinking: Moving from Punitive to Positive Awareness

Worth a Second Thought

As therapists who do a great deal of couples counseling, we know that if a relationship is even going to approach satisfaction or fulfillment, there is one factor that has

to be present: the ratio of positive to negative statements between the partners must be heavily weighted toward positive comments—probably something like 5 or 6 to 1 (Gottman, 1999). This means for every "I'm really tired of walking over your shoes every time I get near our closet," there need to be five comments that are positive, such as "I love it that you listen to my grandfather's stories of growing up in Iowa" or "Thanks for driving me to this appointment—I'm really nervous about it, and I know it wasn't easy for you to arrange to do this for me." The ratio of more positive to negative comments between partners is more predictive of their happiness and satisfaction with the relationship than their age or how long they have been together.

If this is true for couples, doesn't it make sense that the same applies to us as individuals? Unfortunately, when it comes to self-commentary on body image, the likelihood is high that the ratio is reversed—more negative observations than positive ones. We're talking about the tendency to take notice only of what we consider to be negative about our bodies and emphasizing that to ourselves repeatedly. We install a jury in our heads and appoint ourselves presiding judge, often making harsh pronouncements about our perceived physical shortcomings.

If we applied the five-to-one ratio of positive to negative comments (whether this is statements or thoughts) about ourselves and our bodies, we would be unconsciously training ourselves to notice the positives more readily than we notice the negatives. It takes vigilance to see positives when we're accustomed to seeing negatives. We are not talking about blaming someone for what we don't like about ourselves or not taking responsibility for behaviors that would be healthier if we changed.

Sometimes couples struggle when, as therapists, we ask them to describe the strengths in their relationship. Many times they have come to therapy expecting to focus only on weaknesses. The strengths, whatever they are, are minimized or overlooked completely. As individuals, we too often do this with our physical appearances. We chuckle as a teenager magnifies a zit on her forehead, declaring, "It looks like a beacon!" But we might look in the mirror, take note only of a bulging midriff, and ignore the lovely roundness of breasts or the silkiness of glossy hair. It took conditioning for us to see the negatives first. It will take practice—conscious practice—to change a pattern that is set in place.

Hold That Thought

Alicia, occupying her usual chair in the sexuality class she was attending, listened intently as the instructor talked about "thought stopping." She was emphasizing, at the moment, how it is possible to change one's view of one's body and how often women are prone to negative thinking where their bodies are concerned. Alicia's own thoughts were running rampant—*Now, how am I supposed to feel good about this body? It'll never happen. My stomach is paunchy and has stretch marks, and my thighs are dumpy and dimpled. I feel like two people—one pretty good-looking one from the waist up and one pretty awful from the waist down.*

Gradually, however, through writing in her journal—a class assignment—sharing with the other class members, and listening to the teacher, Alicia's attitudes changed considerably. *I have a right to my feelings about my body, good or bad*, Alicia thought. *Maybe I'm holding on to something that isn't all that good for me.*

Most of us are probably holding on to attitudes that aren't all that good for us. Here are some steps that can help you let go of negative thoughts about your body that you have likely held on to for far too long.

- *Identify* the negative thought when it occurs. Example: Alicia getting dressed in the morning catches a glimpse of herself in the mirror and is swamped by the thought *I hate how my thighs look.*
- *Stop* the negative thought. Do it with words. Example: Alicia can think to herself, *I have a choice about what I think. I will not continue to describe my thighs as awful.*
- *Refocus* your observation. Example: Alicia can think, *I believe I will gain nothing with such self-destructive, negative thoughts. I need to remind myself that I have begun to exercise regularly, and I am proud of this accomplishment.*
- *Substitute* a positive thought for the negative one. Example: Alicia can think, *My legs are growing stronger as I exercise. I can feel the strength increasing every time I work out.*

We don't think of our thoughts as being conditioned into a certain pattern, but they are. Just as our routine of getting up in the morning or retiring in the evening has predictable patterns, so does our thinking. We talked about how negative body imaging might come to be, but why does it continue even when we think we should know better?

Our charge to you is: One more time: *stop that negative thinking.* We know you have heard it before. We take time to reemphasize the point because, ironically, even those who teach positive thinking techniques can tend to hold on stubbornly to their own negative body image, as if this self-destructive thinking were really justified in their personal circumstance.

In Chapter 15 we explain how attitudes and thinking impact our experience of sex. Refer to this chapter for further insight into this issue. Libraries and the self-help shelves at bookstores are loaded with books describing how to modify behavior, beginning with attitudinal changes.

A Perfect Body/Perfect Life?

If we got the "perfect" body, what would happen *then*? Considering the obsession that is often connected with it, here's the way it seems: the traffic lights would forever be green, the bank statements would perpetually show a healthy balance, and love would come with little effort, all because we would be so ornamental. And we could forget about having to work or study hard, or ponder over difficult decisions and life challenges, and of course the medical diagnoses would always be in our favor.

No? Well, what *would* happen?

Consider answering these questions (adapted from Meadow & Weiss, 1992, p. 147):

- "If I had the body I yearn for, men (or women) would . . . "
- "If I weighed what I want, I could . . . "
- "If I had the body I yearn for, my life would . . . "

The answers to these questions can reveal a great deal if you are willing to explore your answers a little more deeply. For example, you might have answered, "If I had the body I yearn for, men would find me sexually attractive and would want to be with me." Now let's explore that further. Do men (or women) find you attractive now? If the honest answer is yes, then what is it they find attractive and what would happen if you felt you were even more attractive? If the honest answer to the question above is no, then ask yourself why. If your answer is "because I'm not thin/tall/pretty enough," then keep going. Ask yourself if you know other women who are as heavy/short/plain as you are and who have still attracted others. If you do know such a woman, what makes her attractive? If you don't, refer back to the discussion on negative thinking to help you see where your thinking has stalled.

The point is that physical appearance may be a factor in attractiveness, but it is not the sum. And physical appearance is not the road to personal fulfillment or lasting relationships. It does not insulate one against pain, disappointment, loss, grief, or illness. There are no shortcuts to intimacy in a relationship, and the work will be just as intense whether you're doing it in your size 6 or 16 jeans.

How Are You Feeling?

Information often tells our head what to think, but emotions often tell our feet what to do. If your car stalls on a railroad track, your brain takes in the information that you have stalled in a dangerous place. It is your emotions, however, mixed with the information, that will most likely get you to take the action and move out of the potentially dangerous situation.

When it comes to feelings, it is important to recognize and interpret the emotions correctly. This may seem obvious, but it often doesn't happen. Emotions are sometimes numbed, disguised, buried, or misinterpreted. This is a bit like having a compass when you need it but not taking the cover off to get your bearings. You can hold the compass at any angle you want to, but with the face of it covered, it can offer you no assistance. You lose the keen advantage of feeling your feelings, understanding them, and using them to help determine behavioral choices.

If our emotions are routinely discounted, ignored, neglected, or subordinated, we lose the ability to trust ourselves. Once that has taken place, we are extremely vulnerable to outside influences. That is, we are more prone to believe or buy into the hype, the seductive promise that is held out to us if only we would believe in the products, the diets, hyperexercise, liposuction, or cosmetics to improve our confidence.

Translating Feelings to Mindfulness

Looking inward at feelings opens another door to the self—the door to mindfulness or meditative practice. The last 10 years have been the decade of the "mindful brain," in which researchers have shown that through a practice of mindfulness, a meditative state of "relaxed wakefulness" (Brotto et al., 2008, p. 1648) and psychoeducation, individuals have been able to tackle many significant psychological concerns, including depression, eating disorders, coping with cancer, and sexual desire problems. In body esteem, mindfulness—based on Zen Buddhism meditation principles (Austin, 1998; Hanh, 1996)—builds on the principles of cognitive-behavioral therapy outlined above. It can be done anywhere at any time but often works best if part of a daily routine. If your level of cognitive distraction is such that you are getting in the way of your sexual pleasure, we suggest you begin with the mindfulness exercises in Chapter 13.

Balance Is Beautiful

Obsession about one's body bleeds away personal power, and anxiety fuels the obsession, which only becomes more disappointing. Obsession is doomed from the beginning: it will fail to deliver. Obsession can be masked as indifference or control. Paralysis—the inability to take important steps for the sake of health and well-being—is one way obsession manifests. If you are in the clutches of an obsession, you are seldom far from thinking about your problem (which could be overeating, overdrinking, or smoking, for example), but your obsession has a short tether. You can't muster feelings beyond powerlessness, so you are left impotent in the face of those problems. You cannot tap into your obsession to find the way to take the action you need to take.

This is not about disregard for healthy standards. Self-pride and self-responsibility are imperative requirements, however, if you want to establish and maintain weight control, a healthy exercise regimen, or some other physical routine. This isn't the stuff of which obsessions are made.

Balance is beautiful. It implies an active, interactive, involved woman—you, absorbed in your life with all of its gifts and pains. It means that you maintain respect for your own boundaries and believe that you, like others who are significant in your life, need time and attention from yourself for yourself. The balance that you strive for encourages moderation and modification where it is needed. Perhaps this is about eating. Perhaps it is about challenging your self-focused negative and disempowering thinking. Perhaps it is about establishing a healthy exercise routine. Perhaps it is about monitoring and managing weight—but on your terms and for your own reasons.

CONTINUING THE JOURNEY IN YOUR BODY

Each woman's sexual journey is personal, though often shared. On this journey no one is immune to feelings of uncertainty and inadequacy. Even having an "ideal" body, however, doesn't provide exemption from these feelings and certainly doesn't assure happiness. We should care for and respect the bodies we have—they are our vehicles in our journeys. Focusing our thoughts toward what we appreciate about our bodies will provide us with the fuel (energy) to keep them in the best condition possible for their journeys.

SEVEN

Illness and Disability

"Even though I was tired, I did pretty well during radiation treatment. I faced some hard days and came through them. When my energy returned, I wanted to make love, but my sexual desire was low and my vagina seemed so dry. I thought my doctor would have some ideas to help with these problems.

"At my next appointment, I asked about increasing my sex drive. My doctor looked uncomfortable and said, 'I saved your life. What more do you want?'

"The 'more' I wanted was to be sexual."

If you are living with illness or disability, your sexuality may be challenged in several ways. For one, your healthcare provider may shut you down when you ask questions about sex, because he or she simply may not know how to answer. Sexual difficulties during illness and disability have multiple causes, and your doctor may not have the knowledge or time or desire to provide you with the customized solution you need. In fact, many women *want* to discuss sexual issues but are afraid their concerns will be dismissed or rejected (Krychman et al., 2006). On top of this obstacle, when you have an illness or disability, you have to cope with changes to your body, self-perception, self-esteem, and identity as well as your social structure and possibly economic status. Then there is the pervasive cultural bias that says if you're sick you are no longer a sexual person; and if you were born with a disability, you're living in a world where sexuality is the domain of the able bodied. In this chapter, we discuss sexual issues in the context of the psychological and pervasive social and interpersonal concerns that you are confronted with in the face of illness and disability.

ILLNESS, DISABILITY, AND SEXUAL VULNERABILITY

When healthcare providers and the public in general consider the impact of illness or disability, they often think in terms of life and death, physical discomfort, disfigurement, and return to work or exclusion from mainstream work entirely. What everyone, except for the person with the illness, often overlooks is the importance of sexuality and how it is affected by the medical condition. Sex is a quality-of-life issue. It gives pleasure to you and can connect you to others even if your body is physically challenged. But how do you make this happen?

First Things First: Using Appropriate Terms

Of course illness and disability often coexist, but just as often they are completely separate entities. Chronic illness is more likely than not to threaten your ability to enjoy sexuality, at least until you adapt to a "new normal." Disability, whether lifelong or later acquired, also presents significant challenges to sexuality. This chapter addresses both the differences and similarities in how your sexuality may be affected, but we urge you to seek out support and information specific to the problems you are experiencing.

Words referencing sexuality and illness and disability deserve careful consideration. The terms *sexual functioning* and *sexual dysfunction* are companions. The first pretty much refers to how well the classic sexual response cycle is working, including sexual interest, lubrication/erection, and orgasm. The focus is primarily on *physical* functioning. Dysfunction, of course, addresses those things that are *not* working, and interventions are designed to fix them (Verschuren et al., 2010). Resources regarding sex, disability, and illness, then, are confined to a definition of what is considered normal, your impairment of function, and what to do. This in fact places everyone with a chronic illness or disability into a *dysfunction* category, because there is some degree of limitation in adapting to and coping with a chronic condition that impacts sexual experience. In contrast, we have chosen to use the term *sexual well-being* in this chapter. *Sexual health* connotes a connection, at least in our dominant culture, with being healthy and able bodied (Browne & Russell, 2005; Verschuren et al., 2010) and therefore is not entirely appropriate to a discussion of illness and disability. Sexual well-being, on the other hand, is just that: how satisfied you are with your sexual experience *now*, in the context you are in, and whether you enjoy the sexual contact you have now, "contact" being defined on your own terms.

Focusing on your sexual well-being rather than dysfunction when you have a chronic illness or disability makes sense in the context of the radical changes that have occurred during your lifetime. Your grandparents or even your parents would have had an entirely different experience and treatment regimen than you. Federal laws have increased accessibility to public places and transportation. Technology has advanced so that specialized surgeons using highly developed instrumentation can perform intricate, delicate surgeries with increasingly effective results. CT and fMRI equipment can provide defined diagnostic information, in many cases almost instantaneously. Rehabilitation medicine and a team approach have changed things so that many conditions in the past that were expected to progress to death fairly rapidly are now controlled. For example, many cancers are currently treated as chronic conditions. These—and so many other advances—have led healthcare practitioners to retool their practices so that the focus is on assisting their patients to improve their abilities and life quality, instead of focusing primarily on their patients' survival (Verschuren et al., 2010). The following are considerations that will help you optimize your sexual well-being whether you have a chronic illness or a disability.

Next: Grieving and Moving Ahead

Maximizing your sexual well-being is difficult if you have not gone through the process of grieving. If you are dealing with a lifelong or later-acquired illness or disability, you and your family are no strangers to grief. Grief becomes a companion to every major life milestone. Adolescence and young adulthood, times that are difficult enough on their own, are deeply affected by chronic illness or disability, particularly around sexuality. Mid-adulthood is a time when most adults pursue careers and life partners. Many envision later life as a time to pursue other interests such as traveling. Sexuality does not disappear because of losses connected to life milestones and compromises due to impaired abilities. In fact, sexuality can become even *more* prominent in these circumstances, with desire for physical intimacy competing with physical challenges.

Hemingway (1929) in *A Farewell to Arms* wrote that the world breaks everyone and that afterward some are stronger in the broken places. This has been our experience of working with women, and those who love them, when illness or disability has disrupted their lives. It's a heartbreaking experience to cope with a disability or to be diagnosed with an illness. But most women don't remain heartbroken; they pick up the pieces of their lives and put them together again. They go on, often stronger in the broken places.

This resiliency is true for your sexuality as well. Your body may have changed, your sexual response may be altered, your energy to make love may be diminished, but you may well choose to find pleasure in your body. You grieve your losses, including sexual losses, and move ahead. You can find ways to become stronger in broken places. Women who've decided to be sexual in their bodies can be very resilient indeed.

In the case of illness, whether you secretly suspected the diagnosis or were caught completely off guard, your first reaction to learning of your illness was probably disbelief and shock. You may have felt betrayed by your body, fearful of how the illness would progress, or pessimistic about your future. People with congenital illnesses and disabilities that create lifelong dependence and limited access to social opportunities are no strangers to loss. One thing is certain: coping with a serious or chronic illness or disability can be an emotional roller coaster that can impact your self-image and sexual identity.

> "I manage my ostomy[1] well, but I still feel funny about it when I'm having sex. I'm not quite ready to have my partner see my stoma."[2]

> "I thought I was doing fine in chemotherapy until the day my hair started coming out in handfuls. I called my husband and sobbed. He came home from work with a buzz cut. I felt like his message was 'We're doing this together.' That night, he initiated lovemaking. It was so reassuring that I cried, this time because I loved him so much."

Even if a life marked by illness eventually turns out to be very good, it will be a different life from before, a *new normal*.

> "Our bodies would twist and bend and become so entwined that it was sometimes hard to figure out which leg or arm belonged to whom. That was before my arthritis. Now just penetration is a major accomplishment. We're doing well; our sex is loving and tender. But I still miss my old body that could connect with such physical intensity."

Sudden-onset disability mirrors the grief of a serious illness. Any compromise to your autonomy such as physical restriction can be beyond shocking at first. If the disability is the result of an accident, there can be a period of time before you and the physicians know how much ability will be retained. The limbo created by this "vigil" is much like awaiting the results of a biopsy or other testing. Recovery or coping with pain alone is daunting. Rehabilitation can last for months or years, and learning your "new body" of necessity becomes your total focus. Everything else may seem like a distraction. If you are partnered, as we've mentioned earlier, your partner is deeply affected as well. The "disbelief" stage precedes or intersects with grief and can last a long time. If, at some time, you were dismayed by the discovery of a gray hair or the presence of laugh lines that don't go away, imagine what it takes to integrate the loss of the use of the hand you write with or the amputation of your right foot due to an accident or diabetes.

Grieving is a necessary part of adjusting to a disability or illness. Grief requires that you admit there have been losses in your life and that you allow yourself to experience all your feelings related to those losses. Grief demands that you get used to things being different in your life and have patience to endure the time it takes for

---

[1] A surgically created opening for discharge of body wastes.

[2] The end of the small or large bowel or ureter protruding through the abdominal wall.

this adaptation. Finally, in grief you must learn to move ahead, despite the aware-ness that your loss and grief will always be a part of you (Worden, 2002).

Changes in physical appearance are one type of loss that can create problems with your sexuality, both because of others' responses and because of your own. If you are born with a congenital illness that will be lifelong, or a physical disabil-ity such as cerebral palsy, sooner or later you and your peers will notice a differ-ence between you and "them." If, for example, you are born with a port-wine skin disorder that covers part of your face, even if you are tall, slender as a model, and gorgeous, that truly insignificant blemish will set you apart, at least initially. Cop-ing with changes in physical appearance far exceeds any issue of a "wounded" self-identity due to illness. Gaining or losing weight, losing your hair, having a body port or shunt, or using prosthetic devices, whether they're wigs or crutches, is an all-out assault on your sense of being sexy. This is even more complicated if you've spent your life in a wheelchair with everyone literally looking "down" at you. Some women refuse to get caught up in social definitions of beauty and sexiness. For other women it's not that clear-cut. It's not just that they think others don't like their bodies. The bigger problem is that *they* don't like their bodies.

It takes grit, confidence, and support to feel and live in your sexy self rather than in the "ill" or "disabled" self you anticipate others will see. You obviously need time to reintegrate your sense of self when there's been an assault to your body. But don't wait too long. Challenge your isolation or negative thinking. Consider joining a support group or getting on the Internet and participating in a chat room for women with your particular concern. If you are partnered, share your concerns and *believe* the feedback you get, which is most likely to be positive when his or her anxiety about *you* has relaxed a bit.

Dealing with Isolation

Professionals who care for you, persons in your support system, family, friends, and neighbors can see you only from their own perspective. The empathy and love from some in your closest circle can transcend that, but most people you interact with are not in that circle. They can and do care about you. They can be and are concerned, but they cannot begin to understand that you are severely nauseated every afternoon or that you have ulcerated sores from poor circulation and a wheelchair that needs replacing. This, in itself, is isolating. Another way you are kept isolated is something we all have done, often involuntarily. To an obvious or subtle degree we keep our emotional and physical distance because you have "it" and we are unconsciously afraid and aware of our own vulnerabilities. We could be *you*. In fact many of us will be faced with challenges at some time of our lives. If you are being avoided, even subtly, you are cut off from normal social interaction and opportunities to develop more than superficial relationships. If your illness/disability occurred later in life, you may see some of the people from your wider social circle "fade out."

Although these responses would invariably be dismaying, there are things within your control that can significantly reduce the negative effects: books, healthcare professionals, support groups, and the Internet are valuable resources for learning ways to improve your quality of life, including your sexual well-being, and reduce your isolation. The process of self-education also tends to push you into meeting other people who are going through the same or similar experiences. Whether it's in face-to-face support groups or chat rooms on the Internet, you'll find connecting with others for information and emotional support invaluable.

Talk to Me

The local news is reporting an earthquake whose epicenter you know is reasonably close to where your son lives in California. The newscaster announces this as an earthquake measuring 4.0 on the Richter scale. Your son answers your cell call immediately and assures you he is fine. The Richter Magnitude Scale actually measures the "shaking" amplitude of an earthquake, but the measurements are usually misperceived by the layperson listening to the news report. What it means is that if the earthquake near your son's home measured 5.0 instead of 4.0, the power, scope, and impact of that quake would have been *10 times* greater than that 1.0-point difference would typically imply.

If you have a serious speech impediment that accompanies your illness or disability, the perception of others who don't know you amplifies the actual level of your disabilities by that 1.0 point, *10 times greater* factor on our metaphoric Richter scale. Avoiders are more avoidant, waitpersons in restaurants likely automatically ask your companion what you want to order, unless they know you, and, inexplicably, people talk louder to you as if that will clear things up. If this applies to you, you have very likely had speech therapy and are very careful about being as clear as possible. Others' insensitivity and impatience are not your fault. If you are in a relationship, before or since your speech problem, you've weathered the particular storms that impact intimacy in these circumstances. Because our culture has created an expectation of such instantaneous response we find ourselves foot tapping if the woman ahead of us in the grocery checkout lane is fishing for change in her purse a bit too long.

Andy has a good friend, Mark, who is severely afflicted with cerebral palsy. Mark is intelligent and independent with assistance. But Andy and Mark have one problem. Mark's speech is significantly impaired. Andy explains that speech *isn't* the problem. "The problem," he explains, "is that I have a 'disability,' and that is that I have trouble understanding you, and I just have to keep working on that." This is a true story but, unfortunately, too rare.

If you are not in a relationship, but hoping to be, pull on every shred of self-confidence you can muster to hold your own, don't be apologetic by posture or gesture. Be as patient as you wish the person you are talking with could be with you. Find ways to practice social confidence—volunteer work, affiliation with religious or community groups, political activism. Many women with speech impairments are in successful intimate relationships.

Facing Fertility Problems

If you are of child-bearing age, the discussion about fertility should definitely be brought up with your partner and your medical practitioner. Some illnesses and treatments may make it impossible or dangerous to get pregnant, or the recommendation may be that you wait for some time posttreatment (as is the case with some cancer treatments). Conversely, your fertility may not be affected, and your attention to contraceptives and safer sex should not inadvertently be overlooked. Some illnesses and treatments will cause infertility. Even if you have had all the children you planned, or never chose to have children at all, the declaration that you no longer have that option can cause real grief. If you were planning to get pregnant, hearing that, in addition to your illness, injury, or disability, you won't be able to carry a child can be devastating. You may not find a support group for this particular route to infertility, but infertility support groups do exist and would easily include you.

Most types of disability do not preclude becoming pregnant, but how to manage getting pregnant may be an issue, and many women with disabilities have difficulty. An added problem is that specialists may not take on a woman with disabilities, paternally or maternally feeling that she may not be ready to add an infant to her burdens. Also, typical infertility evaluations and treatment involve medical procedures that can't be accomplished unless adjustments are made for her (Basson, 1998).

> Haiyan decided to walk the seven blocks to work on that beautiful day: she woke four days later disoriented and in excruciating pain, her husband at her bedside in the ICU. She remained minimally aware for several more weeks but eventually understood that she had been hit by a speeding car, likely a drunk driver, who had run a red light just as she started to cross the street. Her pelvis and femur were crushed. For two years she endured surgery after surgery, physical therapy, depression, and two hospitalizations for infection. Her husband Yang became "disabled" too: not in a physical sense, but because all of his energy and time was spent in the anxious days of Haiyan's surgeries being at the hospital, arranging for transportation when she was at home, filing claims, returning phone calls from concerned others, and attending to numerous other details, not to mention managing to be productive at work and maintaining minimal order at home.

Haiyan and Yang, her husband of 5 years, planned to get pregnant in about a year and a half. The severity and location of her injuries certainly postpone their hoped-for pregnancy indefinitely, and they have been forewarned that she may never be able to become pregnant and carry a fetus to term. Their deep shock and pain over Haiyan's injuries and complications are compounded by the profound disappointment, grief, and loss over their slim hold on hope about conceiving and birthing a healthy baby. This couple joins innumerable couples coping with reproductive fears or losses in the face of their circumstances. For many couples, growing stronger in broken places will include reconstructing their options for becoming parents.

Learning to Manage Pain

Nothing interferes with pleasure faster than pain. In this section, we discuss general pain that results from your illness or disability, how it disrupts intimacy, and ways to reduce its impact on your sexual well-being. In Chapter 8 we focus on genital and pelvic pain, which may be associated with your illness or disability. Many spinal-cord-injured or otherwise wheelchair-bound women have muscle contractures and other problems that make penetrating sexual activity impossible. For women dealing with the side effects of some medical treatments, vaginal drying can cause pain. Your pain might be secondary to your primary condition. There are innumerable things that can cause pain. Whatever your pain source, in addition to reading the material in this book we suggest that you talk to your healthcare provider, check the "Suggested Resources" section at the end of this book, and check websites dealing with your specific illness/disability for other suggestions. Pain is personal and can rob *anyone* of sexual interest.

Being Believed

One of the most isolating parts of being in pain is the feeling that others don't believe you or that they're unable to understand how much pain you're experiencing. If you're in pain, you need support from your healthcare provider, your friends, and your partner. Being believed doesn't necessarily come from putting your suffering on full, open display. Instead, you can take care to educate others about what support or special assistance you'll need to make life easier.

> "Because my pain came and went, I'd forget that my partner couldn't know I was miserable. I'd get irritable about her advances to be sexual when I couldn't even lie down comfortably."

And, believed or not, chronic pain will at times frustrate your partner, no matter how much he or she believes in you. Your partner hopes for a break, just as you do.

Taking Control

The management of your pain requires you to have confidence and believe in your ability to control and cope with it. This may include finding the right healthcare provider, undergoing physical therapy, getting a prosthesis, obtaining educational materials, attending a pain clinic, taking medications, or finding the right chairs, mat-tresses, and pillows to assist you in coping with pain. You may need advocacy if your wheelchair or assistive devices are exacerbating your pain and need to be replaced or recalibrated for your needs. Therapies that can help you cope with pain and/or techniques of self-hypnosis to control pain are very useful. Narcotic medications can dampen interest in sex. You and your physician can discuss current methods of pain control, such as medications that block pain receptors, and ancient remedies such as acupuncture (Basson, 1998). There are other options you can explore as well, more complex than can be explained adequately here. We urge you to remember two things: don't let pain drastically escalate—it becomes harder to control. Also, don't be stoic about enduring sexual pain, sacrificing your own good judgment and best interests for what you presume will be sexual pleasure for your partner.

Experimentation

The management of pain toward the goal of sexual well-being requires experimen-tation. Although there are general rules about what will help with certain kinds of pain, there's no substitute for trying different things and determining what works for you. Too often when sexual activity is discussed or considered, it is implied to be vaginal penetration and genital arousal. An appropriate goal for you may be to work toward having a *positive sexual attitude and feelings* toward yourself and your partner (Verschuren et al., 2010). You may find mornings better than nights for experiment-ing with what feels good. Some women start with a warm bath or shower. Thinking about what soothes and gives pleasure and then incorporating that into intimacy is an important part of managing pain positively. Sex is deeply personal and indi-vidual, as are the ways to connect. It will be important to take responsibility for not becoming overly avoidant about contact with your partner because of the fear of pain. Take control, but don't shut out your loved person.

When It Hurts Too Much to Touch

There'll be times that no matter how positive the attitude, no matter how creative the experimentation, pain still gets the best of you. If that happens, try to keep from making broad generalizations like "It's always going to be like this." Try to stay focused on the present moment. Focus on breathing evenly and try sitting or lying in a way that minimizes the pain. Continue to work with your healthcare provider to find solutions and to learn about new developments in pain management. Reread the section in Chapter 6 called "Hold That Thought." Also see Chapter 13 for sug-gestions for managing your thinking, including a particularly helpful practice called *mindfulness meditation* (and the "Suggested Resources" for information about mind-fulness techniques and practice).

Managing Heavy Menstrual Flow and Incontinence

There are some medical conditions such as von Willebrand's disease or endometriosis where menstrual flow is unpredictable and not easy to manage, not neatly confined to a 5-day period, and/or is copious rather than discreet. This demands lifestyle changes.

A separate situation, but one that impacts sexual intimacy similarly, is that spinal cord injury and neurological disease can result in bowel and bladder incontinence, especially in certain circumstances. The nerves that allow you to control bowel and bladder elimination also are the nerves associated with sexual arousal. If there is nerve damage in the upper region of the spinal cord, genital stimulation can cause incontinence.

If you have heavy or chronic menstrual flow, you can weigh the nuisance versus the anticipated pleasure of engaging in sex during this menstrual time and make your decision knowing what to expect. If your decision is "No way!" it should be discussed in advance and respected.

A decision about engaging in sexually arousing activity when there is concern about bladder or bowel control during the experience requires more discussion, preparation, and, frankly, willingness to approach this with humor and, no pun intended, the ability to go with the flow. It is also unpredictable, raising the anxiety even higher. In these circumstances it would be normal to experience inhibition. We recommend consultation with your practitioners, as well as checking online for others' experiences and recommendations. Discuss with your partner about precisely what you are concerned about happening, how each of you feels about that, and what you need to do to prepare if incontinence occurs. If you are on a controlled schedule for bowel and bladder function, you can certainly plan sexual intimacy around this schedule.

Whether your concern is menstrual flow or elimination control, there are some noninvasive recommendations that can make management easier. Watch the sales and go shopping for deep, dark-colored sheets and large towels that you can spread on your bed. Have smaller towels close at hand. Scented candles, if you wish, can add to your experience. Have a container of baby wipes or larger wet, disposable wipes nearby. Of course what we're describing is not "spontaneous" sex, but you haven't been living a very spontaneous lifestyle recently, and anyway, we believe that in general spontaneous sex is not superior, or even common. Even with the challenges you have, your sexual well-being can flourish in a context of planning, communication, and controlling your environment.

ILLNESS AND SEXUAL WELL-BEING

So far we've been discussing the commonalities of illness and disability—the issues you may have to deal with whether you are living with one or the other. But there are also sexual well-being considerations unique to each. First, let's look at serious illness.

Getting Educated about Your Illness

When a woman is diagnosed with a serious illness, two things are likely when it comes to sexuality: one is that she will be very interested in how illness and treatment are likely to affect her sexually, but she will be reluctant to ask her doctors. Two, education, assessment, and counseling about sexuality are not typically provided, and when they are, they are most often brief and perfunctory (Krychman et al., 2006). Clearly women want and need information about how their illness will affect their sexual well-being. Women want one-on-one, face-to-face discussion with a healthcare provider familiar with their condition. According to one study, women were split between whether they wanted to discuss the information early, before beginning treatment, or after treatment was completed. An opportunity to have one, or ideally more, personal discussions resulted in significantly higher sexual well-being than a control group that had none (Katz, 2005). Lack of information contributes to anxiety and fear. You may have to be your own advocate if an opportunity to discuss what to expect sexually is not offered to you. Recognizing that you, like everyone in a similar situation, will likely be overwhelmed during the early medical appointments, write a list of questions and don't neglect to ask about your body, its functioning, and what sexual response and body changes to expect.

When you are ready to pursue resources on your own, ask for recommendations from the nurse or social worker where you receive your medical care. Some hospitals also have patient libraries with excellent resources. Many illnesses actually have entire support and research networks. For example, the American Cancer Society, American Lung Association, American Heart Association, Arthritis Foundation, Hemophilia Foundation, and American Kidney Foundation all provide information about adjustment to illness, and this network expands continually. Many organizations have excellent booklets about sexual concerns. Internet websites also provide information that relates specifically to your diagnosis or treatment. Women are now "talking" to each other through listservs that have been established for most illnesses and disabilities. If you don't have a computer, you can use one at your local library. They'll explain to you how to obtain a free e-mail address, and you can pick up your e-mail at the library computer.

Reclaiming Your Sexuality: Self-Exploration and Masturbation

As a part of the process of being sexually active during the course of an illness, you need to touch and explore your body, determining what parts feel good when touched and what parts are uncomfortable. Surgical sites, areas around stomas or shunts, and scar tissue often feel uncomfortable, numb, or even painful. It's important to determine in advance what's off limits during sexual activity with your partner.

Self-exploration should include looking as well as touching. If there's been a surgical or other body change, look carefully at the affected area. If it feels too threatening to do this alone the first time, ask your partner or your physician or nurse to be with you. If it's too hard now, go on to some other aspect of self-exploration and come back to this later. The goal is for you to see yourself as a whole person, not as a "stoma" or an "amputee."

Try to be curious about parts of your body that you might not have considered sexy before. Because skin is our largest sensory organ, you can slowly, deliberately touch all of your skin to find areas that feel good. You need to remember that your mind is your most powerful sex organ, rich with sensual memories, images, and fantasies. It may be helpful to review the material on sexual fantasies in Chapter 13.

Masturbation provides a means for you to explore your sexual response and how it may have been altered by your illness. It can also be a valuable source of relaxation and pleasure. Try different positions for masturbating to see which give you the greatest sense of pleasure and comfort. Some women prefer lying on their back; some semirecline with pillows behind them; and some lie on their stomach and increase pelvic pressure by holding a towel or small pillow between their legs. Some women touch just the head of the clitoris; other women like to stroke their inner labia and probe their vagina. Some women rock their whole body back and forth. Some women just move their hands. Some women use vibrators. Some women watch erotic movies. Some read romance novels and masturbate during the "good" parts. Some women heighten their arousal by imagining erotic fantasies. The point is, if masturbation is new to you, feel free to explore, experiment, and enjoy. If it is an "old friend," introduce it to your "new" body.

Overcoming Sexual Response Problems

A woman's sexual response can be affected by the illness itself, by the treatment, by fatigue caused by the illness, and by her self-image. You may find that it's hard to determine exactly what's affecting your sexual response, but you know that *something* is causing things to be different. To determine what to do, begin by checking with your healthcare provider to make sure that sexual activity is not medically risky. If you get the go-ahead, think about what your sexual response was like before the diagnosis. We suggest reading through Part I, "Knowing Your Sexual Story," as a starting point for understanding your sexual response both now and in the past. Next, write down the areas you're concerned about now. Are these changes in desire, arousal, or orgasm? Are you experiencing increased pain? Many women experience diminished self-esteem due to physical changes. Check in with yourself: do you have body-image concerns?

Desire

Illness robs us of sexual desire, either by directly impacting hormonal levels necessary for normal sexual desire or by creating flu-like symptoms and fatigue. Sometimes medications and other treatments have side effects that dampen desire. Some illnesses, like congestive heart failure, compromise breathing and make every movement an effort. If these symptoms are familiar to you, or you simply recognize your loss of desire, the suggestions in Chapter 15 will be useful. In particular, be rested but alert for any sexual experience. If you're sleepy, woozy, or tired, your desire will be affected. Allow yourself the time you need to be ready to experience intimate contact. So many people understandably *want* to rush the process either for themselves or because of concerns for and about their partners. Don't rush, but don't avoid either. When the time is right, look for times of the day when you feel best, perhaps first going for a brief walk or taking a warm shower to enhance your sensory awareness. Make sure your room is comfortably warm. You can purchase small electric heaters to warm a particular space. Dress comfortably and use a semireclining position if lying down places too much stress on your heart or breathing.

Depression is a dampener of desire and is frequently linked with illness. Symptoms of depression can include loss of appetite, changes in sleep patterns (too much or not enough), loss of interest in activities and others, self-isolation, chronic irritability or dissatisfaction, and repetitive thinking of negative thoughts. If you're experiencing depression, counseling may help you overcome not only your depressed mood but also your low sexual desire. In some situations, antidepressant medication may also be helpful. Read Chapter 4 about sexual response, particularly noting that sexual desire and well-being do not spontaneously occur but require you to be intentional; as with recovery, you always have to take that first step.

Arousal and Orgasm

Sexual arousal involves both your sense of excitement and your body's response to sexual stimulation. Normally during sexual arousal, your vagina becomes moist with lubrication, your genital region feels full because of increased blood flow to that area, and you have an all-over aroused feeling in your body. See Chapter 4 for more in-depth discussion of arousal.

Neurological damage, spinal cord injury, vascular damage, chemotherapy, and various medications can interfere with genital blood flow by blocking blood vessels or preventing signals from traveling along the nerves that control vasocongestion (the swelling response in your genital region). Arousal, for purposes of discussing sexual well-being, vasocongestion, and lubrication are significant only in conjunction with your *feeling* sexual excitement. Otherwise it would be like having a beautifully crafted violin but no bow. Anticipating discomfort or coping with fatigue, depression, or worry can affect your arousal. Chapter 15 may help with specific concerns. Some women also report that arousal improved for them once they had completed treatment or finished taking certain medications for their illness. For example, chemotherapy is an anticholinergic (drying) medication that can affect your lubrication and swelling response. You may find that physical aspects of your sexual arousal will improve once you complete your course of chemotherapy. Be sure to read and ask questions about how your illness and treatment can affect sexual arousal. Orgasm may be affected by treatment, medications, neurological or spinal cord damage, depression, distraction due to pain or restricted movement, and other factors. You may find it helpful to reread Part II, "Understanding Your Body," for a better understanding of how orgasm works. The suggestions in Chapter 15 may also be helpful.

DISABILITY AND SEXUAL WELL-BEING

When your parents were kids riding their bikes around the neighborhood, there were no curb cuts. They had to learn to ride so that they could "bump" up the curb when crossing the street. Then, sometime in the early 1990s, curb cuts started appearing, along with ramps to some restaurants and elevators in all newly built buildings. What could this have to do with sex and disability? Good question, with a good answer.

The Americans with Disabilities Act of 1990 quite literally opened doors for persons with disabilities. You can easily locate the original and amended versions of the ADA on the Internet for a fuller understanding of the scope of this act as an agent to prevent discrimination against people with disabilities, increase accessibility and transportation opportunities, remove barriers, and require reasonable renovations in businesses to accommodate special needs.

The relatively new accessibility mandated by the 1990 law has eased social and sexual barriers for many. Young women (and men) with disabilities don't even remember a time when accessibility was so poor that persons with disabilities were basically housebound. Today it is hardly a novelty to see a handicapped person on the same bus you're on or at the same party you are attending.

Exclusion and Inclusion

People with disabilities have more social and workplace access than ever before. Able-bodied people in long-term relationships or marriages with men or women with disabilities are not uncommon. We aren't referring here to couples where one person incurs a disability in the course of their relationship, but where the relationship flourishes when "abled" and "differently abled" have eyes only for each other (sighted or not) and not for the handicap. Their parents and friends are clapping at their weddings or commitment ceremonies.

There is definitely variability in that acceptance. If you have a disability, you've reckoned with the prejudices of others who may dismiss you without knowing you. You may have had unnecessary social limitations imposed on you by well-intended parents who didn't want you to be hurt, physically or emotionally. You may have been overprotected or ignored, assumed to be asexual.

Invalid can have two meanings, one of them being *not* valid. For a lesbian woman with a disability, both meanings, unfortunately, tend to apply.

> As a queer activist, I've always thought that I've been very aware of injustice and oppression in the world. . . . I try to always keep in mind how necessary it is to be visible as a lesbian. A little over a year ago when my partner became disabled, I began to learn that I didn't really know anything about invisibility. I learned about an entire population of people that are ignored, left out of most discussions regarding their own lives. I learned that disabled lesbians are not only invalidated and marginalized by the larger society, but are ignored and avoided by able-bodied members of the queer community as well. (Taylor, 2001)

If you can advocate for yourself, maintain some independence even if you need daily care-provider assistance, and are active some way in your community, you are less likely to be marginalized. The dividing line is very thin and not static nor definable, but somewhere on this continuum persons with severe enough disabilities or people in institutional or controlled settings are "meant" to stay in an asexual niche. Their expression of any sexual needs are distorted by others, viewed as deviant, and responded to with disdain or worse (Browne & Russell, 2005).

Your disability could be congenital, a disability you were born with, or acquired at any time in your life. *When* is important. Your problem can be expected to stay at about the same level it is currently, or to progress, such as with multiple sclerosis, where loss of function is anticipated, but not in any way that you can predict and prepare for. You may live 4 miles from an amazing rehabilitation facility and be surrounded by family and peer support, or you may live in an isolated environment where rehabilitative medicine is difficult to access and "support" comes primarily through the Internet. You may have a partner who loves you, or who leaves you, or you may have no partner at all. But, living with disability, you have had to continually adapt, drawing from your inner resources in ways that might be unimaginable for those who haven't faced such challenges. And you've done it, even though you've had to manage the negative stereotypes that too frequently leave little room for the "world" to embrace your sexuality.

Developmental Issues and Sexuality Information

One of the complications of sex education in any form, except for discussions of hygiene, pubertal development, and the basics of reproduction, is that for sex education to have any real meaning, you must have attained autonomy and discriminating decision-making skills. Women with congenital disabilities are vulnerable to abuse and exploitation (for that matter, *all* persons with disabilities have a higher incidence of exploitation). Compliance has been rewarded over independent decision making, and social segregation is not unusual. The result can be a lack of good information about sexual health and protecting oneself from sexual exploitation as well as insecurity about making informed sexual decisions.

If your disability had a late onset and you achieved some of the mastery skills of adulthood, your situation presents one set of problems but sidesteps others. You have had little or no preparation for a new level of dependency. This can result in rage and depression. Sexually you don't "know" this new body and likely are repeatedly frustrated and surprised by the physical limitations and changed sensations. You will be helped by reading this book as well as locating additional information in the "Suggested Resources" section.

Helping an Adolescent Girl Negotiate Disability and Sexuality

Adolescence is a devastating time to suffer a disability through injury, accident, or illness. The typical portrayal of a "normal" teenage girl is that she is examining every centimeter of her body, exaggerating "flaws," and trying on every outfit of clothes she owns, discarding them in tears before she settles on something to wear in order to leave the house. This is a stereotypic, inflated portrayal of reality, but there is some truth to it. She is peer oriented, and this is developmentally appropriate. This insecurity brings with it a sense of dread as well as a sense of belonging, or hoping to belong. Adolescence is not a time when a secure, grounded sense of self exists, even if you're the prom queen type. Where sex is concerned, girls are being cautioned by their parents or guardians at every step, negotiating that unsettled place of becoming desirable, and *wanting* to be, and potentially being in the confusing place of being the one setting limits in a "romantic" encounter. Girls experiencing a disability at this portal to adulthood are just, at this moment in time, *constructing* their sexual self-esteem; they certainly can't *draw* from previous life experience to make adaptations.

Girls at this stage are a work in progress in the best of circumstances, and now they must form their self-image in the foreign country of disability. Peer support is essential, and face-to-face, preferably in a group. If this is physically impossible, Skype or some form of video cam can facilitate direct contact. Timing will be important: too soon, and a sense of isolation may be reinforced. The teen herself should not be the only person determining when outside help and peer support is needed. As we've stressed throughout this book, seek help and check it out. The assistance should be competent, experienced, and compassionate. The blow of a teen disability affects everyone in the environment. You can't tap one metal tube on a wind chime without creating a "concert." Everyone may need help with this: the young woman deserves respect for her sexuality, and sexual well-being is as every bit as important to address as any other feature of her disabling condition. Ignoring it even while other major adaptations are being made can have lifelong ramifications.

Adults who become disabled after having been sexually active and able bodied have challenges that go far beyond coping with lost sensation or mobility. It takes a long time for someone to integrate the reality of having sustained irreversible damage and never being "herself" in the same way again. This is not "denial" or "not facing reality." You've heard that men and women who've had a limb amputated have "phantom" pain in that limb. This isn't psychosomatic: the central nervous system is actually trying to reconfigure to the new situation. Sudden-onset disability is like that. People will describe having dreams of themselves as able bodied months to years after the initial event. Women who've experienced a sudden disability—even if their appearance remains almost unchanged—will most often admit, when questioned, that their sense of attractiveness has plummeted from their pre-injury perception.

Congenital Illness or Disability

Lifelong disability severe enough to require ongoing assistance with toileting, bathing, dressing, and other daily activities presents specific challenges. You've had to struggle for your own definition of independence within a life framework of physical dependency and frequent resistance to your independence from others. In your day-to-day social life, you were likely "protected" from the forays into horsing around with other kids while growing up, learning from mistakes. You weren't protected from peer exclusion, though. The result of these types of social separateness is isolation. Isolation can lead to (and very often does) an overidealized and unrealistic fantasy life about relationships. Unfortunately, these fantasies aren't of much use in the real world of complicated real relationships. With no or little real time, no developmental experience with opposite-sex interactions with their thrills and disappointments, new relationships years and years later may be like suddenly being exposed to a North Dakota winter storm without adequate outerwear: no protection.

Facilitated Sex

The term *facilitated sex* refers to assistance that may be required for people with disabilities to enjoy masturbation or partnered sex. Physically disabled individuals often employ personal care assistants (PCAs) to do everything from helping them manage a cup of coffee to assisting them with menstrual hygiene. Protocols and boundaries for personal care services have been established for some time, but assisting with sexual activity is a "new frontier" (Tepper, 2009). A PCA's duties may include facilitated sex—assisting a couple, both with severe disabilities, to position for sexual intimacy, giving them privacy, and returning when summoned—and/or *facilitated masturbation*, in which the PCA positions the employer with a vibrator, perhaps setting up some erotic material on a video device, and giving her privacy.

Questions that have yet to be answered include how far the facilitation can go and who makes the decisions.

At this point in time facilitated sex *does not*, in our dominant culture, include hand-over-hand masturbation, where the caregiver's hand is over the hand of the other person, providing the movement and friction for orgasm. Facilitated sex also does not currently include PCAs staying in the room, or entering the room, when sexual privacy is requested. A PCA is likely to balk at assisting an individual, especially a woman, to hire a person for sexual activity. The question of consent is hotly contested in the disability community: for instance, what happens with a long-term couple where one has lost mental function, say, to Alzheimer's disease, and cannot consent or refuse to have sex with the partner?

The fact that the person with the disability employs the PCA, rather than the PCA having the person with a disability as a "client," is significant in that it implies that the disabled person has control over the details of the job description. This definition of their relationship is technically true even if the person with a disability is profoundly handicapped. The idea that control resides with the employer was borne out in a study interviewing persons employing PCAs. The interviewees revealed that they considered *themselves* rather than the PCAs the ones to manage the boundaries (Browne & Russell, 2005), despite the fact that in reality the PCA has the most "control" in such a situation. The PCA can refuse by ignoring a request, or by considering the request deviant, because of his or her own moral values, or out of embarrassment. Also, the PCA's employing *agency* may have some rules about such facilitation, superseding the individual's desires.

Madison is a woman with severe cerebral palsy, and Shirley is her longtime PCA. Perhaps Madison would like to ask Shirley to assist her with masturbation. But would doing so raise boundary issues, and if so, how? Who establishes the boundaries, Madison or Shirley? The most likely scenario is that Madison will be too embarrassed to ask in the first place—and so might a couple wanting to request facilitated sex, or one partner of the couple. Some may ask leading questions to get a sense of where their PCA would stand on such an issue. But if disabled individuals do ask, and fail to get a positive response, they are likely to abandon the request, even if they appropriately feel that sexual well-being is a part of personal care.

All of these issues, taken one by one, are managed differently in different cultures and countries. Disabled women (along with their partners) will need to break new ground on many of these issues, depending on societal attitudes and their own.

Sexual Response

The effects of congenital illness or disability, or neurological or spinal cord injury, on sexual response are so varied that your rehabilitation and medical teams will be the best initial sources for information. The section on illness in this chapter offers some general information and suggestions that may apply to you.

One interesting fact about spinal cord injury that may escape your information sources regards orgasm. Depending on the extent of the injury, a woman may retain the ability to lubricate if she becomes sexually excited. Even more interesting, about 50% in their sample of women continue to be orgasmic even with complete injury, as reported by Beverly Whipple, Carolyn Gerdez, and Barry Komisaruk (Whipple et al., 1996).

PSYCHIATRIC CONDITIONS

If you have a psychiatric condition, you may also feel that people treat your sexuality as if it were nonexistent, or a symptom to treat. In fact, your sexuality is important and deserves your attention. Some psychiatric problems don't impair thinking and judgment, others impair thinking intermittently, and for some, judgment is impaired all the time. During times of impaired thinking you may make poor decisions regarding taking care of your sexual self or avoiding sexually dangerous people and situations. If you know there are intermittent periods when your judgment is impaired (for instance, with major depression, bipolar disorder, schizophrenia, or active psychosis), then these are times you will need others to help keep you safe.

Whether or not you are in a relapse, avoid isolating yourself from others who can be a positive part of your life. This may include family, friends, coworkers, and neighbors. Many communities have local chapters of the National Alliance for the Mentally Ill (NAMI), a remarkable self-help group. NAMI also has an excellent website (*www.nami.org*) for education, support, and advocacy.

You may find that your medications have sexual side effects. Antipsychotic and antidepressant drugs can negatively impact all phases of a woman's sexual response. We want to stress, however, that even though sex is an important quality-of-life issue, mental stability has to take precedence. Little can be gained by alleviating the negative sexual side effects of medication if your well-being is placed in jeopardy due to unchecked psychiatric symptoms. Psychiatrists have respect for, and awareness of, the negative side effects of medication and will work with you to manage symptoms and minimize these side effects.

Developmental Disability: A New View for the Families

A developmental disability is a disorder that occurs during childhood or adolescent development and is expected to impair a person's ability to function independently in adulthood. Sometimes a developmental disorder is due to one condition, as in a child with Down syndrome. Sometimes it is a cluster of disorders. An example would be Debby, a woman born with cerebral palsy linked to brain damage at birth. Debby has a seizure disorder, can't walk, and is moderately cognitively impaired. Debby's cluster of problems would be categorized as a developmental disability. Debby will need to have supportive care all her life. Her education, mobility, cognitive ability, self-care ability, and potential to earn a living are permanently affected by her cerebral palsy and intellectual disability. Her ability to make discriminating choices about sexual activity will also be affected, although Debby, like all women, will be a sexual person throughout her life. Debby will need the support and guidance of the people who love her throughout her life. She'll also need their respect for her sexuality as a woman and her need to be educated about sexual functioning and sexual choices that her disability will permit her to make.

Cognitive Impairment

Throughout this book we say that sexuality is a process of growth, development, and experience and that the way a woman experiences her sexuality depends on biological and social factors as well. Cognitive impairment, one of the most common developmental disabilities, places an adult woman in double jeopardy: she has cognitive impairments that make her dependent in ways other women aren't, and others view her sexuality primarily from the perspective of her perceived vulnerability. Her emerging sexuality, usually first apparent at puberty, is often met with vigilance and rigid control. Debby's parents' greatest fear is that she could become pregnant if someone takes advantage of the fact that she is easily influenced or manipulated.

There are two responses often seen when others equate a woman's sexuality with vulnerability. One is overprotectiveness, which actually has the effect of creating more vulnerability. The other is a denial that allows parents, family members, friends, teachers, and neighbors to see women with mental retardation as living in adult bodies but with a child's mind. Because it can be so disturbing and confusing to deal with the sexuality of an adult with a cognitive disability, it becomes easier for families to support the *perpetual child* than to deal with the *developing adult*. Society—collective social attitudes—follows suit.

Debby might be cognitively impaired, but she isn't stupid. She knows that adults in her domain are uncomfortable with her curiosity about sex. Her interests and exploration of this fascinating subject become covert.

In Chapter 1 we talked about the fairy tale of Sleeping Beauty. This fair and vulnerable young girl is doomed from the beginning of the story. Her parents want to protect her from pricking her finger on a spindle and falling into a 100-year sleep. They make every possible effort to keep her from even knowing what a spindle is. Still, the parents fail in their total protection of Sleeping Beauty, even though they go to great lengths to ensure her safety. We wouldn't have much of a fairy tale if Sleeping Beauty's parents had given her a safe-spindle education from the time she was small, so that when she finally did encounter a spindle, she would have some way of making a discriminating decision about touching it or, better yet, how to use it appropriately.

As sex therapists and educators we support more, not less, sex education and counseling for adults with developmental disabilities and cognitive impairment. Parents of adolescents and young adults with mental retardation have to face their fears and resist the urge to be overly protective. Because so much of childhood and youth is a rehearsal for adulthood, it is imperative that persons with developmental disabilities learn to make as many choices as possible as early as possible. This will help them make more discriminating decisions throughout their lives. We also encourage those who have a relationship with a child with cognitive impairment to envision that person's adulthood. Sometimes it takes courage to think beyond childhood and imagine an adult. There is no better way to begin those steps toward supporting adult life than by seeing a woman as a sexual human being throughout her life.

An adult woman with a developmental disability should have a complete physical, including a pelvic exam, to assure that she is in good health and to address any medical problems, including problems with menstruation. Never, under any circumstances, mislead a young woman to think she is "going to the mall," or "out for ice cream" if the real destination is an office for a pelvic exam. The opposite approach is best—preparing the woman for everything she can expect, to the best of her ability to comprehend. Misleading her will inevitably lead to mistrust, fear, and anxiety over every future medical appointment, and maybe even about that *real* excursion for ice cream. If the woman cannot understand the purpose of a pelvic exam and expresses distress, ultrasound may be substituted. If a woman is not sexually active, her risk of cervical cancer is greatly reduced and she may not need annual pap and pelvic exams. Check with your healthcare provider about a gynecologist or "specialty" clinic that offers individualized health care for persons with developmental disabilities.

Sexuality education should be provided. Self-care in personal menstrual hygiene, a discussion of conception and contraceptives, and an understanding of sexual function (including desire, arousal, and orgasm) are important components of sex education for any woman with a developmental disability who is capable of directed self-care. A discussion of masturbation and the meaning of self-pleasure is a further example of teaching a woman with developmental disability how to care for herself. This discussion can include an explanation of "public" and "private" with regard to sexual self-expression and should be combined with an assessment of her living space to make sure she has privacy in which to masturbate. Women who are living independently or in group settings should also be taught about types of sexual interaction, from brief to committed partnerships. These conversations should be ongoing dialogues rather than one-time events. Many websites and books discuss sexuality concerns for the developmentally disabled. A good place to start is The Arc of the United States (formerly the Association for Retarded Citizens) at *www.thearc. org*; The Arc and other helpful organizations are listed in the "Suggested Resources." Sex education and training will also be important for group-home staff to ensure that they can respectfully handle sexual concerns as they arise.

THE LAST WORD: ADAPTING AND YOUR RELATIONSHIP

The Best Predictor of Your Recovery of Sexual Well-Being

If you are in a committed relationship, recuperating from a serious illness or mastering a disabling condition, nothing—*nothing*—will be more important to your sexual well-being than the strength of your relationship and how things were sexually before your physical world changed. This claim is well documented and supported. Couples transcend catastrophic losses, as we said at the beginning of this chapter, and they often grow stronger in broken places. We haven't minimized what you may experience and what you have experienced, and we are not inclined toward inflated positive reassurance. Some of the "broken" may never be repaired. One person writes: "When I first learned of my partner's disability, I wept for days. She is an amputee, right arm and right leg. I couldn't believe that there wasn't some way to undo it. I grieved for the loss . . . constantly waking up at night with the shocking realization that nothing would change her loss" (Taylor, 2001). Your kidney cancer may mean long-term dialysis; the wheelchair for your MS may not see the day when it is folded up into the corner of the garage. But if your relationship is strong and your earlier sexual experiences together were positive, you have a foundation that won't be demolished, as well as tools to rebuild sexual and sensual pleasure.

A Word, but Not the "Last Word," If You Are Single

We know your relationship might not have survived, leaving you with not only a health crisis but a broken heart. We can't know why this happened. We do know that it means more than recovering, recuperating, rehabilitating, and adapting to the "new normal" of you. This is a time to rely on your inner circle of close people to manage the myriad challenges you face. If you have been single throughout the most acute challenges of your illness or disability, you know how to manage life independently. Of course you may need tailored professional support for environmental, self-care, transportation, and other changes. If disability is a new companion to your identity, as life stabilizes you are facing new social challenges. The Internet is a source for dating advice and dating sites. Surfing the Internet and joining your local support systems will reinforce that your social opportunities are not confined to people with disabilities. How do you meet potential future partners? For the most part, like everyone else.

Wise Advice

Women who have experienced the trauma we've described throughout this chapter are frequently prepared and willing to share their experiences and advice about sexuality and body-image reconciliation. Sex therapists, medical researchers, physicians, and a wide range of specialists contribute to the growing body of knowledge about sexual well-being and recovery. Reliable Internet resources can be accessed instantaneously. But any resource you use must be evaluated and "filtered" according to your own circumstances, your values, and your needs.

What Is Sexual Well-Being?

Sexual well-being is reconnecting to your sexuality, feeling positive and comfortable in your sexual self. Note: This definition does *not* refer to specific sexual activities, but rather to your attitude and openness (Verschuren et al., 2010). If you find yourself avoiding your partner's touch or permitting touch when your anxiety is high and muscles are tense and you don't want to be doing what you're doing, it is time to back up. Talk to your partner. See Chapter 12 for advice about discussing a sexual issue. The two of you may need outside assistance—medical advice, support, sex therapy—through this difficult period. It may take time for you to identify sexuality as a positive part of you and to achieve sexual well-being.

Your Partner's Sexual Well-Being

It is not uncommon, nor surprising, that your partner's sexual well-being could have been affected in conjunction with your illness or disability. This is not your fault, and nothing that you could have done would have changed your partner's concern and worry about you. Your partner may have developed a sexual dysfunction such as sexual avoidance or erectile problems. Initiate discussions acknowledging the stress of caregiving and how worry about hurting you influenced these problems. Set a "recovery timeline," and if problems persist, seek professional help, preferably with a sex therapist, at the same time ruling out medical problems your partner may be experiencing.

A Good Marriage Improves Everything

First, know that research on couple relationships in illness/disability circumstances is done on married couples, infrequently at that, and rarely on live-together partners or gay couples. But the evidence is that women in strong relationships live longer and experience more life satisfaction. Of course there are stormy seas, but when the storms subside, those relationships help. It may not be the predominant outcome, but some couples even report their relationships strengthen when they navigate a serious health issue. They've made it through the eye of the hurricane, recognized that survival is not assured, and reprioritized what is most valuable. Access media and you are continually reminded to take care of your physical health. Your relationship health is a significant factor in your longevity and well-being, too. This is cautionary: don't take your relationship for granted, and even if no illness or disability is on your horizon, at some time and in some way your relationship will be challenged by a crisis. The state of your relationship will be one of the most powerful factors in how effectively that crisis, chronic or acute, is mastered.

Sex Is Not a Performance

What is the first thing you think of when you hear the word *sex*? The automatic response for most is sexual intercourse. Throughout this book we strive for a much broader definition, and you likely would have answered the "What is sex?" question differently than most. However, almost all of us have to push the words *sexual intercourse*, the default response, aside to access our more expansive definition. When it comes to illness and disability, an altered concept of sex is imperative. That does not mean inferior! As sex therapists we've seen women who have been grateful that their illness has meant being more reflective, more open, more humorous, more intentional, and more experimental about sex. The following are some tips. They won't all work for you, of course, but you may gather some ideas.

• *If your body changed, how about your sexual environment?* There's a chance that during the journey you've been through your bedroom has been "assaulted" too. Closets neglected, detritus from who-knows-what ignored. How about a new beginning? You can unapologetically call upon those women who have been saying "If there is anything I can do . . . " and create a new environment, with them doing the work. You don't even have to do the organizing or all of the decision making. This is not a frivolous suggestion: organizing your personal space, changing things a bit or a lot, can help with your adjustment and your attitude.

• *Too self-conscious right now?* Throughout the book we discuss negative body image. However, if you are adapting to any of a myriad of body changes from dark circles under your eyes to disfigurement from burns, you can take things slowly. Being naked with your partner is a wonderful feeling, but that might take time, too. Having intimacy with clothing on or being partially nude is fine. Silky material can feel wonderful for both of you. Very soft, warm, low lighting adds ambiance and reduces self-consciousness.

• *Sensual is sex, too.* Sight, sound, taste, smell, and touch connect us to ourselves, to others, and to our world. A loss of one or more of our senses is a body crisis, and yet our amazing selves find ways to compensate to some degree, sometimes a remarkable degree, by the increase of acuity of other senses. Touch we'll discuss separately. If you can hold your partner and look into his or her eyes for a few minutes rather than seconds, your experience of intimacy can deepen by the moment. You can be imaginative with sound and taste; subtle is best. Smell is one of the most powerful and connecting senses we have. Hold each other if possible, avoid using perfumed products, and snuggle so that you can take in the wonderful and unique scents of your partner. Talk softly and gently about what this brings up for you.

• *Touch.* Your skin is your largest sex organ, replete with innumerable nerve endings. Planned and pleasing massage is a sexual activity. It stimulates oxytocin, one of the hormones of sexual arousal. It results in internal as well as external feelings of sexual well-being (Castleman, 2004). Whole body massage is the most desirable—slow, warm, and sensual. Advance discussion with your partner should make clear that massage isn't "foreplay" (there isn't such a thing in sex), but is sexual within itself. Because of physical limitations, whole body massage may not be possible, but rubbing bodies together and nuzzling can have similar results.

• *Flirt: You can do it!* You don't have to be like a supermodel, slinking down a runway, to flirt. You don't have to be coy or bat your eyelashes if this feels absolutely absurd to you. Make an unexpected phone call or send a message to your partner, expressing something romantic, but within your comfort zone. When you are together, say at dinner, lean forward and be attentive, telegraphing your love and openness. Maintain eye contact and quiet the background noise as much as possible. What you are communicating to yourself and to your partner by flirting is "I'm here, and I'm still me!"

• *Erogenous zones.* If you've gotten good sexuality information, rather than just symptom-based information, you have likely been introduced to the fact that many parts of the body are nerve rich and can be extraordinarily erotic with stimulation. We usually think of erogenous zones as being from the neck down, but actually the face, ears, and neck are highly sensitive. See Chapter 12 for information about the special, intimate, sexual advantages of kissing.

• *Ready to heat it up?* Time for new batteries for your vibrator, or giving thought to which one to buy (see Chapter 13 and the "Suggested Resources" for further vibrator information). Pleasure and fun are the goal here. Experiment where on your body and your partner's body vibration and pressure feel just right—not too much. Remember, even with spinal cord injury you may be able to achieve an orgasm. Try stimulating the G spot if it is physically possible. Overstimulation, however, leads to numbness or discomfort rather than deep pleasure. Stay very present when you are experiencing arousal. During your illness, accident, or medical treatment, you may have learned the very effective coping mechanism of dissociating from the pain or procedure you were going through. With sexual arousal, your nervous system is "excited," too. Of course it is a different excitation, but it can be disturbing when you have worked so hard so often to remain calm.

Nonintercourse can be great fun. Naked or wearing whatever feels right, your male partner with an erect or partially erect penis, or your female partner using a dildo or not, you mimic the movement of intercourse (Castleman, 2004). Use lots of lubrication and, with your legs closed and your partner's penis between your legs, the movements of your bodies together replicate intercourse. There can be variations, including your legs open and your partner's penis rubbing against your vulva but with no penetration. If mobility is significantly impaired, the two of you can move together with the abilities you retain, loving each other with adaptability, but mostly with love.

EIGHT

When Sex Causes Pain

There are few circumstances more daunting to a woman's sexuality than to have her experience of sex repeatedly associated with pain. If you are coping with such pain, you know what we mean when we say that this invisible condition affects your everyday life and many decisions you make. For example, if you have chronic burning pain in your vulva, something as simple as being invited to a concert becomes a challenge. Because of the pain, you have to factor in how long you can sit and what you can wear to make the discomfort manageable. If you are in a relationship, it is likely that you and your partner have found yourselves avoiding sex or even situations that could lead to sex. If you are not in a relationship, you may avoid the possibility of entering one—it becomes too painful to contemplate.

The bad news—as if you needed any more bad news—is that diagnosing the cause of chronic sexual pain is often difficult. If sometime in the past you sought medical treatment for sexual pain, chances are you were told that no physical abnormalities could be identified and that the problem may be psychological. And, unfortunately, without proper diagnosis and treatment, your chronic sexual pain probably didn't resolve itself.

The good news is that this trend is changing. Your healthcare provider is more likely today than in years past to take your experience seriously. We are now learning a great deal more about what causes sexual pain and how to treat it effectively. If you question whether you're getting appropriate care for your sexual pain, get a second opinion. You as a patient are in a better position than ever before to advocate for yourself. There is a wealth of information available on the Internet that can help you educate yourself about sexual pain, available treatments, and centers that specialize in this problem.

The majority of sexual pain for women falls into one of three categories. When pain during sexual activity occurs in the visible portion of the genitals, we refer to it as vulvar pain. Internal or vaginal pain occurs inside the body during vaginal penetration or thrusting. Pelvic floor muscle pain occurs in the muscles that wrap around the opening of the vagina and is triggered by vaginal penetration.

Many factors can cause or aggravate pain, so a thorough medical work-up is important. Sometimes the pelvic muscles become lax and internal organs begin to prolapse (slip down) into the vagina or even up against the vulva. General bacterial infections, STIs, masses on the uterine ligaments, tubes, or ovaries, and endometriosis can all be sources of pain. Sometimes medical conditions such as interstitial cystitis or irritable bowel syndrome cause pain during sexual intercourse or even attempts at penetration. Gynecologic cancer can be a cause of sexual pain, but usually only during the later stages of the disease. Sometimes pain can be associated with sensitivity to certain soaps, shampoos, fabrics, medications, douches, or topical ointments. Regardless of the cause, the first line of defense against painful sex is a thorough medical evaluation.

VULVAR PAIN

Chronic pain, burning, rawness, stinging, or itching in the vulva is called *vulvodynia*. If you have this condition, you might feel discomfort only when you attempt sexual activity, or the pain might be constant (or intermittent) and not restricted to sexual activity. For some women sexual arousal by itself, without penetration or even physical contact, can cause pain because of the vasocongestion that occurs in the genital region.

If you have experienced vulvar pain, you may be familiar with the term *vulvar vestibulitis*—a subset of vulvodynia that happens in a very specific part of the vulva. The vulvar vestibule starts at the hymenal ring and blends with the labia minora. There is a line of keratinized skin where the vulvar vestibule meets the labia minora called the *Hart's line* (Haefner, 2000). Within this area, some women have distinct points of tenderness. The cause of vulvar vestibulitis is not known. It is not a STI, so it's not something you can pass on to your partner.

Because vulvodynia has many possible causes, it is important to have a gynecology specialist evaluate the problem. Seek medical help as soon as you can. Pain is a neurological process that follows neuronal pathways. It is a bit like a path in the woods: at first the path may be hardly noticeable, but if it is traveled enough, it becomes clearly worn. Pain is like that. The longer it is present, the more entrenched it becomes.

Pain amplification occurs because the nerve endings in the vulva become hypersensitive and the central nervous system (think "brain") becomes sensitized to pain (Webbe et al., 2010; Meana & Lykins, 2009). This amplified pain is distressing, and the distress actually increases the experience of pain (Ehrström et al., 2009). Over time, some women develop increased fearfulness or phobia about vulvar touching or engaging in any kind of penetration (Binik, 2010). That is when pain turns to suffering. Suffering is the experience of pain with the addition of emotional anguish. Suffering is often heightened by the fear that nothing more can be done—suffering leads to helplessness and can even be traumatizing.

Your situation does not need to be viewed as hopeless. If you have had long-standing pain, check the "Suggested Resources" list for books and websites that provide a wealth of information on treatment options and symptomatic relief for vulvar and pelvic pain, including information about mind–body syndrome and mindfulness techniques.

In addition to getting appropriate medical care, a cornerstone of recovery from chronic vulvar, internal, or pelvic pain is education and support. Join a chat room on the web and share ideas and concerns with other women. If you don't have a computer, go to the library and use one there. It will help you feel less isolated even as you find ways to advocate for quality care. Your partner also needs support and education, as described later in this chapter.

If you have vulvodynia, you may fear that sex will never again be pleasurable. Not so. Even in cases where pain is acute, a number of medical treatments are proving to be helpful. For example, vulvar pain can often be relieved by tricyclic anti-depressant medication. The treatment seems to work by interfering with the nerve transmission of pain in the part of the brain where pain is perceived and processed. It is outside the scope of this chapter to offer prescriptive recommendations about medication and other medical treatments, but specialists who treat the problem will have many ideas. Instead, we will offer some self-help ideas for decreasing the discomfort of vulvodynia and minimizing sexual difficulties.

Relief for Pain and Itching

Measures that effectively relieve pain and itching differ from person to person, but some common recommendations include:

- *Clothing:* Use only white, 100% cotton underwear, not synthetic underwear with a cotton crotch. Avoid close-fitting clothing. Wash underwear in mild soap and put it through an extra rinse cycle.
- *Chemicals:* Be alert to chemical irritants that may be present in soaps, shampoos, panty liners, and so on. Use a gentle soap on the rest of your body, but avoid using soap on the vulva.
- *Hygiene:* Keep the vulva dry, but rinse often. Warm water cleanses the vulva adequately after urination. Cornstarch can also be used to absorb moisture.
- *Diet:* Watch your diet. There may be a correlation between oxalates in the diet and vulvar pain. Oxalates are a by-product of oxalic acids, which are present in some plant foods (nonanimal products) such as coffee. Many women find that cutting back on foods containing oxalates and taking calcium citrate

(which decreases calcium oxalate formation in the urine) decreases vulvar pain and itching. You can learn about the low-oxalate diet on the Internet or from your healthcare provider. We recommend that you follow this diet under medical supervision. Over time you will be able to determine which foods, in particular, aggravate your vulvar condition and should be avoided.

Vulvar Pain and Sex

Couples coping with chronic sexual pain are naturally at a loss for what to do. The frustrating and intrusive association of pain with sex often means that nongenital sensual pleasure is lost as well. The default mode for many couples dealing with vulvar pain is to avoid all physical contact because of the fear that sexually stimulating activity is expected to follow.

If you have become touch avoidant because you have been coping with vulvar pain, openly discuss this with your partner. This is not an easy conversation, but it is one of the most important you will have. Explain to your partner that vulvar pain is preventing your enjoyment of sexual activity. The pain is idiosyncratic from woman to woman. Some women can tolerate penetration but not vulvar touching; other women have difficulty with intercourse, any kind of vaginal penetration, and touching on the vulva (Binik et al., 2002). Incidentally, you can reassure your partner that there's no research that shows that a couple's interactions cause this problem (Davis & Reissing, 2007). Couples with vulvar pain are as psychologically healthy as couples without vulvar pain, but they have more difficulties with sex.

It will not work for your partner to take an avoidant "hands-off" approach or be overly solicitous—"Oh, don't think about my needs." In either instance, a partner can end up being hostile because needs of her or his own are not being addressed and eventually the denied feelings come out. It is better for couples to learn a facilitative approach—problem solving and talking honestly about the challenges and possible paths through this problem together. This kind of conversation can feel awkward in the moment but leads to better long-term adjustment than denial of the problem and avoidance of feelings (Desrosiers et al., 2008). Consider inviting your partner to come to a medical appointment with you so that both of you can talk with your healthcare provider (Connor et al., 2008).

Accept together that sexual interaction is important to you as a couple. Brainstorm about other types of sexual activities that could be substituted for those that cause pain. If speaking openly is awkward, consider using sex therapist Aline Zoldbrod's excellent book *Sex Talk* (Zoldbrod & Dockett, 2002) to jump-start the conversation. There are lots of ways to be sexual; try to think of what "script" will work for the two of you. This will involve grieving for you both. Don't be surprised by a sudden upsurge of sadness from either of you regarding this challenge. You can work toward better solutions only if you honestly face your loss.

Reintroduce holding, hugging, kissing, and massage, making clear that these pleasurable activities are not to be associated with any additional expectations and are complete unto themselves. Touching and caressing should be valued for their own merits and not seen as an inevitable prelude to genital sex.

If you decide to have sexual activity with your partner while you have vulvar pain, there are a number of things you can try to decrease the discomfort. It's essential to realize, however, that you should never feel forced or pressured into having sex. A grit-my-teeth-and-get-through-it approach will almost always backfire in the long run; it can cause you to be fearful and avoidant of sex, and your partner, in turn, will feel confused, unfulfilled, and perhaps even guilty. If you decide to try the following suggestions, make sure it's because you *want to*, not because you feel you have to.

- Educate your partner about your condition.
- Learn about your own pain responses. Are there times of day when you have less pain? What parts of your vulva produce pain upon touch? Are there sexual positions that cause less pain?
- Figure out what still feels pleasurable. For example, do you enjoy having your breasts and upper thighs stroked as long as the vulva is off limits? If your clitoris is a sore spot, is it pleasurable when you avoid the clitoris and stimulate inside the vagina?
- Check with your gynecologist about occasionally using a topical anesthetic (e.g., lidocaine) to temporarily numb the skin.
- If you have pain with sexual arousal, try using an ice pack on your crotch (for no more than 20 minutes). You can also use the ice pack during or after sex.
- Urinate before and after having sex, rinsing yourself with warm water after urination.
- Make certain that you decide in advance which activities will and will not be included during sex and remain in control of those activities.
- Use added water-based lubrication such as Slippery Stuff. Information about ordering lubricants online can be found in the "Lubricants" section of Chapter 15. Avoid lubrication that has additives, including fragrances.
- Use vitamin E oil or olive oil. Some women find that the oils contain fewer irritants.
- If you decide to have intercourse, have your partner first put one finger into your vagina, then two fingers. Massage the pelvic muscle by gently rubbing the area at the vaginal opening. When it's time for penetration, guide the penis in and control the amount and intensity of movement. Your partner should never push. Have penetration for just a minute. You don't have to thrust. Then have your partner withdraw his penis and go on to other sexual play. Slowly build up the intercourse time over many sessions of lovemaking.
- Never override your experience of pain. If you are in pain, *stop.*

After sexual contact with your partner, cuddle and communicate. Talk about at least one thing that went well, but avoid talking about disappointments or frustrations. You are trying to build a repertoire of success. Later, when you're dressed and in a neutral setting, you can analyze what went right and wrong and what to do next time.

Think about developing a plan to cope with vulvar pain that will include increasing your knowledge, finding a good healthcare practitioner, and finding pain relief that works for you. Respect yourself for all that you are doing to stay sane and cope. Consider journaling about how this affects your life and how you will cope creatively (Connor et al., 2008). Include in your plan how you and your partner will manage vulvar pain and will establish your own shared intimacy, including physical pleasure that works for the two of you. At first you may feel alone and isolated, but hopefully over time you will consider turning outward and connecting with others who also have vulvar vestibulitis syndrome (VVS).

INTERNAL PAIN

Whereas vulvar pain is experienced in an area of the body (vulva) that we can see and touch, with internal or vaginal pain the sexual pain is experienced inside the body, in places we can't see but can certainly feel. It's pain that does not necessarily occur in the vagina but is triggered by a penis, finger, or sex toy inside the vagina. Sometimes this type of pain is called *pelvic pain* or *deep thrusting pain*.

Causes of and Treatments for Internal Pain

Lack of Arousal

A common cause of sexual pain is vaginal dryness. The excitement phase of the sexual response prepares the vagina for penetration by providing lubrication for the genitals (see Chapter 4 for more about sexual arousal). You can tell if you are aroused and lubricated by the vaginal opening, which becomes somewhat swollen and slippery. Lack of adequate lubrication can cause friction, leading to pain, irritation, and rawness at the opening of the vagina. The walls of your vagina can also be irritated by penetration if lubrication is insufficient.

If you try to have vaginal penetration without enough stimulating activity to produce lubrication, penetration can be uncomfortable or painful. It's important that you gauge the timing of penetration not simply by your partner's desire but by your own readiness for penetration. You might want to try deep breathing and other mind–body techniques described in Chapter 13.

Lubrication can be compromised by several physical factors, such as medication side effects, low estrogen due to aging, or hormonal changes during nursing. If this is the case in your situation, you can compensate by using a supplemental water-based lubricant such as Slippery Stuff. Different types and brands of lubrication last varying lengths of time and have different viscosities or textures. Stay away from anything with additives. You want this lubricant to be mild. You can order lubrications from several of the websites (like *www.goodvibes.com*, *www.drugstore.com*, or *babeland.com*, or *pureromance.com*) listed in "Suggested Resources."

If you are having problems with sexual arousal, see Chapter 15 for additional ideas.

Pelvic Inflammatory Disease

PID is an infection in the uterus, fallopian tubes, or ovaries. As with any infection, PID can range from a very mild condition to a severe medical crisis requiring emergency treatment and hospitalization. Because STIs can cause PID, you are at greater risk of developing this condition if you have been sexually active with several partners. Douching also can increase your risk of developing PID, because some of the douche fluid may enter the uterus and because douching temporarily removes the important mucous lining of the vagina, creating more chance for irritation or infection.

Because there are many possible causes of PID, including STIs, and because PID can lead to infertility, it is important to get medical treatment as soon as you suspect that you might have this condition. If you experience pain inside your lower abdomen when your cervix or uterus is jarred by sexual intercourse, and this happens over a period of time and not just as an isolated incident or two, get a medical evaluation. Other symptoms of PID include persistent abdominal pain, backache, fever, and a vaginal discharge that differs from your normal discharge.

Your medical care provider will order lab work such as blood tests and mucus smears. Sometimes a diagnostic laparoscopy is indicated (a common surgical procedure in which a tiny camera is inserted into the abdominal wall to see and treat what is going on inside the body). PID is often treated with a carefully monitored antibiotic regimen.

A Tough Hymen

A hymen that doesn't give way easily to finger or penis penetration can cause pain during penetrative sex. It isn't common, but sometimes the hymenal tissue is rigid and tough, and a simple surgical procedure may be necessary to correct the problem. The medical term is *imperforate hymen*. If you suspect the opening to your vagina isn't as elastic as it should be, a pelvic exam will reveal whether there is an imperforate hymen. For more information about the hymen, see Chapter 3.

Uterus in the Wrong Position

Sometimes the internal organs or genital tract isn't in the correct position. A tipped uterus is an example of such a condition. If you consistently have a feeling of pressure or pain in your lower back and tenderness in the abdomen during intercourse, you may have a tipped uterus. You can experiment with sexual positions to see if a different one leads to more comfort during intercourse. Chapter 14 describes four common positions for intercourse.

We spoke earlier in this chapter about a prolapse, where the pelvic muscles become lax and internal organs can slip out of place; the cervix and uterus may even protrude into the vagina. If you have a prolapse, it will be very easy for your healthcare provider to make this diagnosis. There are both surgical and nonsurgical measures that can relieve this problem. If you continue to have pain after medical treatment for a prolapse, and experimenting with sexual positions does not help, consider seeing a sex therapist.

Muscle and Skeletal Problems

Muscle or skeletal problems can be a source of pain with sex. (Here we're talking about muscles other than the pelvic floor muscles, which we discuss in the next section.) Scoliosis (curvature of the spine) is an example of a musculoskeletal problem that can cause discomfort during penetration. The discomfort may be due to spasms in the lower back muscles that have been working to compensate for the scoliosis. Another example would be a muscle strain in the abdominal wall that is aggravated during intercourse. The oversensitive muscles may go into painful spasms when there is vaginal penetration and thrusting.

Musculoskeletal problems can be difficult to diagnose. If you have chronic pain with sex and have had extensive diagnostic tests that fail to turn up any explanations for your pain, an evaluation by a physical therapist may be in order. In many cases physical therapy can help relieve symptoms arising from musculoskeletal problems. You may also benefit from biofeedback procedures discussed in the next section. Also review the material on illness and disability in Chapter 7.

PELVIC FLOOR MUSCLE PAIN

Pelvic floor muscle pain (PMP) is also known as *vaginismus*. Pelvic floor muscle pain is a more accurate term than vaginismus, however, because the pain involves the musculature in the pelvic floor, not in the vagina. (See Chapter 3 for more information about the pelvic floor muscles.) These muscles can tighten near the vaginal opening and make penetration by a penis, finger, tampon, or any outside object painful or impossible. If these muscles contract involuntarily, there can be a painful spasm. In other cases, the pain does not come from muscular spasm but from the tightness around the vaginal opening caused by the muscular contraction. The penis or any other object trying to penetrate the constricted opening to the vagina can cause bruising of surrounding tissue, making it very tender or painful to touch.

Pelvic muscle pain can be primary, meaning a woman has always experienced muscle spasm when penetration has been attempted; or secondary, meaning the onset of PMP followed some event like an infection or trauma.

"I had yeast infections one after another for a while. It made intercourse uncomfortable at first, and then downright painful. The thing is, even after the infections cleared up completely, I still had the pain. I had no idea what was wrong, and my doctor wasn't much help. She said I was clear of infection and to just relax."

It is very common for pelvic muscles to tighten or spasm involuntarily following some form of vulvar or internal pain. It's the body and mind's way of protecting you—trying to avoid further pain by avoiding further penetration. Unfortunately, though well intentioned, this attempt at self-protection inadvertently becomes the cause of further pain.

Pelvic muscle pain can *really* hurt. Women who chronically experience PMP report that the pain is excruciating. It is often described as a burning sensation. Anyone who has had a severe and sudden cramp in a leg muscle knows how painful a muscle spasm can be. PMP sets up a cycle of pain and dread so that any attempts at penetration, or even circumstances in which penetration might be expected, create anticipatory anxiety. This anxiety can make it difficult or impossible for you to relax in sexual situations. The anxiety may also trigger, or contribute to, further muscular contractions—which lead to further pain—which leads to further anxiety. And so the cycle continues.

Most women with PMP experience muscular pain as soon as penetration is attempted, though some don't feel pain until penetration has been achieved. A rare few experience the spasm not at penetration but at withdrawal. Some women experience extreme muscle tightening without an accompanying painful spasm. Regardless of the pattern, PMP is tenacious. It doesn't usually go away spontaneously, but it *is* treatable.

What causes PMP? This is a little like trying to say what causes a fever. PMP is a symptom, not a disease. When pelvic muscle pain develops in response to another painful condition, such as after a vaginal infection, we can easily understand the connection. Pelvic muscle pain can also develop (though rarely) after a sexual assault or sexual abuse. We have seen pelvic muscle tightness develop after injury—even minor injury—to the pelvic area. An example would be a girl falling on the crossbar of a bicycle and perforating her hymen so that she bleeds. The injury is more fright-ening than serious, but because PMP is a protective reaction, it becomes a reflexive response when the vaginal area is "threatened" again at a later time, even if the "threat" is consensual intercourse.

When pelvic muscle pain is present but not easily explained, healthcare profes-sionals can assume that there must be a psychological cause. It is certain that pain with sex will always have psychological components. Feelings of alienation, isola-tion, and loss are common and normal psychological responses to chronic pain. The challenge in many cases is to determine whether the psychological distress develops because of the pain or whether the pain develops because of underlying psychologi-cal issues.

Treatment of PMP

Physical Therapy and Biofeedback

Physical therapy (in combination with medical care and sex therapy) is the most effective way to treat PMP and is almost always helpful as an adjunctive therapy for vulvar and internal pain as well. The best person to provide this treatment is a physi-cal therapist who has been trained specifically in the rehabilitation of the pelvic floor muscles. A physician referral is often required for this specialized treatment.

Why is this treatment so effective? If you have chronic pelvic pain, you may have learned to shut off the conscious sensations from these muscles, so you have difficulty identifying the muscles and exercising any voluntary control over them. In addition, the muscles may be chronically tense, chronically weak, or in a chronic state of spasm. The physical therapist can help you identify these muscles and gain better control over them. As you learn how to tense and relax these muscles, you can gradually relieve the chronic muscular tension and allow penetration without undue tightness or discomfort.

Physical therapy for PMP often includes biofeedback. Biofeedback is a treatment using a monitoring device that gives you feedback on how your actions are affecting a biological process like heart rate, blood pressure, or muscle tone. As you try dif-ferent strategies to influence or control a body response, the biofeedback equipment provides information about your success. With this feedback, you can fine-tune your thoughts and actions until you develop good control.

For PMP, the biofeedback component of treatment uses a stimulation sensor that measures the degree of tension in the pelvic floor muscles. After you have been completely prepared and are comfortable, a tampon-like device called a *periometer* is inserted into your vagina. If you are uneasy about any penetration, the therapist works at your pace, never overriding your reluctance. The sensor stimulates the pelvic muscles to contract, and you and the therapist get immediate feedback on a computer screen about how the muscles are working. The therapist trains you to gain voluntary control over the pelvic muscles, then prescribes a home program for you to follow. This method works very well not only for patients who have overly tense pelvic floor muscles but also for patients with interstitial cystitis, vulvar pain, urinary incontinence, and some forms of vaginal or pelvic pain.

If you don't have medical insurance that would cover such treatment, don't give up. A consultation/evaluation session with a physical therapist can be invaluable and is worth saving up for a visit or two. The physical therapist can recommend inexpensive periometers that you can purchase and use at home. In one or two sessions, the therapist can teach you how to insert the periometer and how to program this biofeedback device to improve your muscular control. Additional information is located in the "Suggested Resources" section on pain.

Physical Therapy and Ultrasound

In some cases a physical therapist may use ultrasound treatment to help with chronic PMP and tension. This treatment may precede biofeedback. Ultrasound is a painless, nonintrusive treatment that has been used extensively by physical therapists for patients with injuries, muscular pain, and muscular spasm. More recently, therapists have discovered that this treatment can rehabilitate pelvic floor muscles. Ultrasound introduces sound waves deep into tissues. It is sometimes referred to as "deep heat." It increases blood flow, promotes healing if there is trauma to the tissues, and helps to relax tightened muscles.

Kegel Exercises and Dilator Therapy

One of the problems women have with PMP is that they become unaware of how to exercise voluntary muscle control. Kegel exercises involve consciously squeezing and relaxing the pelvic floor muscles so that you gain voluntary control over these muscles. One way to identify how to control and relax these muscles is to experiment when you urinate. When you start to urinate, try to stop the stream of urine. When you can do this, you are contracting your pelvic floor muscles. When you stop trying and the urine stream resumes, you have relaxed the pelvic muscles. Once you've identified the muscles, practice contracting and relaxing them (Kegel exercises) when you're not urinating.

The goal of Kegel exercises is not to tense the muscles but to learn to relax them and exert voluntary control over them. When you contract the pelvic muscles, you are tensing them. To release the tension, stop contracting and push slightly, as if you were attempting to expel urine or a tampon. This is, in part, how you relax the pelvic muscles. Pay particular attention to what it feels like when you relax the muscles. These exercises should be practiced several times a day. Kegel exercises are best learned under the guidance of a physical therapist or healthcare practitioner during a pelvic examination so that you can be certain you are properly contracting and relaxing the correct muscles. Kegels can also be used to help strengthen muscles that have become too "relaxed," as with urinary incontinence.

Using your improved muscular control from the Kegel exercises, you can use vaginal dilators to train or retrain your body to allow penetration without involuntary muscular contractions. Vaginal dilators were originally designed for patients who had undergone surgery or radiation treatment for the vagina. They are cylinders with rounded tips that come in sets ranging in size from very small, about the size of a tampon, to large, approximating the size of an erect penis. Depending on the manufacturer, the dilators can be made of a plastic material that is rigid or flexible and rubbery. Dilators can be ordered through your healthcare provider. They are also available at *www.vaginismus.com*.

Dilator therapy is usually done alone in the privacy of your home. You begin by inserting the smallest dilator and keeping it in place for several minutes, commonly 10 to 20 minutes. This is repeated 3 to 5 times a week. Once you have comfortably mastered the smallest dilator, you move up one size and repeat the process until you can accommodate the largest dilator without difficulty or discomfort. You should clean the dilators with soap and water after each use.

Two important points: First, if you have pain when inserting a dilator, stop. Dilator therapy won't be effective if you are in pain, so proceed slowly and at your own pace. Second, the use of dilators can be a highly effective treatment for PMP, but we emphatically state that dilator therapy should be directed by a sex therapist, physical therapist, or healthcare practitioner. The practitioner or therapist can explain how to use the dilators, indicate when to graduate to the next size of dilator, and monitor your overall progress. Too many women have been given dilators and marginal instruction. Without ongoing guidance, the dilators often end up discarded in a dresser drawer, and the woman remains frustrated and confounded.

Mind–Body Syndrome and Mindfulness Techniques

In the last 2 decades there has been an explosion of research about the interaction of the mind, the body, and interpersonal experiences. This research has focused on greater understanding of neural circuitry and changes that can be brought about by practicing focused attention on a regular basis. Psychotherapists now think about psychotherapy and healing in larger frameworks than "talk therapy" alone. One of the important findings is that real pain is exacerbated by the mind's interaction with the pain and that the mind can assist the body in coping with pain. There are thoughtful discussions of this in several helpful books that are listed in the "Suggested Resources." They directly address pain and its interaction with mind–body systems (Kabat-Zinn, 2005, 2006; Sarno, 1999; Schubiner & Betzold, 2010; Siegel, 2008, 2010). Mindfulness exercises are described in Chapter 13.

Botox and Electric Stimulation

Healthcare providers are adapting treatments used with other chronic pain diagnoses to help women with vulvar pain. The first is Botox. Given while a woman is sedated, botulinum toxin (Botox A [BTX/A]) injected at the site of pain has proven effective as both an analgesic and a muscle relaxant. Botox blocks neural pathways that signal pain, an effect that significantly decreases pain and allows women to proceed with physical therapy, dilator or insertion therapies, or gentle vaginal penetration during sexual activity (Butrick, 2009). However, Botox can be drying, and additional lubricant will be necessary with any penetration (Pacik, 2009).

There is increased interest in noninvasive electrical stimulation (called *e-stim* or *ES*). E-stim is now integrated into treatment for urinary incontinence and other physical therapy conditions. It works by using a surface probe to apply a small amount of electrical stimulation to the muscles to "reeducate and reactivate" the muscles. The affected muscles respond with more muscle tone, less muscle irritability, and better muscle reflex accuracy to the stimulation. When the surface probe was applied to pelvic floor muscles for women with vulvar pain, it improved muscle responding and seemed to provide progressive desensitization to pain (Nappi et al., 2003).

SEX THERAPY

Even when there are physical reasons for pain, psychological and relationship issues should not be overlooked. Research has continually demonstrated that pain management is best accomplished when there is a multidisciplinary treatment approach that addresses not only the physical cause of the pain but also the impact of the pain on the individual and the couple. In many cases of sexual pain, treatment with a sex therapist can be very helpful. See Chapter 16 for suggestions for how to find a qualified sex therapist. Just as physicians specialize in one aspect of medicine or another, sex therapists tend to specialize. Make sure your potential sex therapist has had experience working with chronic sexual pain.

A sex therapist can help you and your partner understand the symptom you are experiencing, where it is located in your body, the common relationship strains that may occur, and treatment strategies for overcoming the symptoms. Your sex therapist will be alert to whether the symptom of pain keeps some balance or serves some purpose in your relationship. For example, one couple coping with PMP disclosed that they were at odds with each other about when to try to get pregnant. The husband urgently wanted to begin a family, but the wife was not ready to take this major life step. In this case the symptom—chronic PMP—served a purpose; it kept the couple from dealing with their underlying conflict about pregnancy. Although the conflict didn't cause the symptom in the first place, there certainly was a covert reason the wife might not have been completely eager to resolve the problem.

Combined Therapies for Vulvar Vestibulitis Syndrome

Most healthcare providers, including sex therapists, think that the wisest path is a combined approach that integrates medications like tricyclic antidepressants, pelvic floor physical therapy, and psychological counseling (Reed et al., 2008; Weijmar-Schultz et al., 2005). Cognitive-behavioral therapy (CBT), individually or in a group, has been found effective (ter Kuile & Weijenborg, 2006) but must be integrated with a patient, empathic approach since this is a very challenging diagnosis. The bottom line is that nothing will be gained by "prescribing and minimizing"—rather, respectful, thoughtful, and consistent treatment should be the gold standard of care.

FINAL THOUGHTS ON PAIN MANAGEMENT

One of our patients said that having chronic sexual pain made her want to divorce her genitals. Compensating for pain can certainly make you want to live anyplace but in your body, and for this reason you may find yourself becoming further and further disconnected from the pleasures and benefits of movement and touch. We want to encourage you to live and move and relax in your body again. Massage therapy is a good place to start. It reminds you of sensations of connection, pleasure, and relaxation. Then select a form of exercise that you enjoy: biking, walking, swimming, dancing, yoga, martial arts, aerobics at your gym. Experiment with ways to relax and enjoy pleasure in your body, even if it doesn't come directly from your genitals. Sexual pain can be a challenge, but it doesn't have to prevent you from taking care of your sexual self.

NINE

Sexually Transmitted Infections

Sexually transmitted infections (STIs; also referred to as *sexually transmitted diseases—STDs*) are germs that can be viral, bacterial, or parasitic. They are transmitted during sexual contact, entering through a mucous membrane (mouth, vagina, inner labia, anus) or small tears in the skin. STIs are perpetuated by denial and stigma, and the only way to stop them is with the naked truth.

STIs are quite common, and some do not actively cause disease in the person carrying the infection but can still unwittingly be passed on to someone else. Most can be either cured or managed with a "get on it" approach and smart health care. STIs are diagnosed in 19 million Americans every year, with young people aged 15–24 representing almost half of that number (Centers for Disease Control and Prevention [CDC], n.d.). The worldwide numbers are even more mindboggling. The World Health Organization (WHO, 2007) estimates that in the age group of 15–49 there are more than 340 million new cases of curable STIs each year. These are the bacterial and protozoal STIs and do not include the incurable viruses HIV/AIDS, herpes, and genital warts.

In many countries public health initiatives including active education, prevention, and treatment are having a significant impact on the incidence of some STIs. In the United States, however, STIs are not addressed adequately in the classroom, in the media, or in the legislatures. Everyone groans when the PowerPoints with the magnified slides of pubic lice or chlamydia flash on the screen, but no one discusses how to have a *conversation* with a new partner about STIs. On TV, unprotected, casual sex may occasionally result in an unwanted pregnancy, but rarely an STI and never a dialogue. Teaching how to talk about STIs remains oddly sidelined in the United States while other countries—just visit YouTube and type in "condom ads" and the country of your choice—are openly promoting safer sex.

STIs exact a particularly harsh toll on women. And because women are more susceptible biologically—the inner labia and the vagina contain mucous membranes that are more permeable than skin—globally they are five times more likely than men to get an STI from unprotected genital-to-genital contact (United Nations Population Fund, n.d.). Women also experience a wider range of physical complications, including infertility, pelvic pain, ectopic pregnancies, and cervical cancer. Worldwide, 40% of women with untreated but curable chlamydia or gonorrhea will develop PID, a condition that will lead to one in four of those women becoming infertile (WHO, 2007, p. 1).

Sadly, it is quite typical for a woman to experience shame or a loss of self-esteem if infected. Anyone can get an STI, the same way anyone can get strep throat. Nonetheless too often the reaction to STIs is a moralistic judgment that someone who had unprotected sex just got what he or she deserved. Let us be clear as we begin this chapter: a woman with an STI is a woman with a medical problem who needs medical care, education, and support to care for herself. Spare her the moralizing; she doesn't need or deserve it.

STIs: FROM THE INCONVENIENT TO THE LETHAL

STIs refer to the more than 30 organisms (WHO, 2007) that can be sexually transmitted between partners, with results ranging from mild embarrassment and inconvenience to severe disability and death. Some STIs are bacterial and are curable when detected early and treated with appropriate antibiotics. Other STIs are caused by a virus, like HIV/AIDS, genital warts, and herpes. With the exception of the viruses HPV and hepatitis B, we have yet to come up with a vaccine that can protect people from viral STIs. Researchers hope one day to have vaccines to prevent the transmission of herpes and HIV. A third type of STI is caused by neither bacteria nor a virus but by fungus, protozoa, lice, or mites. These STIs can be cured or at least have the severity of the symptoms controlled.

Some STIs, like syphilis and gonorrhea, are almost always transmitted by sexual contact. Other STIs, like HIV or hepatitis B, can be transmitted in nonsexual ways such as sharing an infected hypodermic needle or receiving a tainted blood transfusion. And some STIs can result without any transmission whatsoever. For example, many women have yeast cells lying dormant in their genital area that can become active in response to pregnancy, birth control pills, antibiotics, diabetes, or spermicides containing nonoxynol-9. Their resulting yeast infection is not caused by sexual behavior, but it can indeed be transmitted sexually to a partner. Many STIs can be transmitted from a pregnant mother to her unborn child.

Table 9.1 summarizes 11 of the most common STIs, listing symptoms, means of transmission, possible complications, and available treatments. For more detailed information about each STI, consult the "Suggested Resources" at the end of this book.

TABLE 9.1. Sexually Transmitted Infections (STIs)

STI	Symptoms	Transmission	Complications	Treatment
		Bacterial STIs		
Gonorrhea	• Vaginal discharge, painful urination, or unusual vaginal bleeding • Often symptomless • Can be confused with yeast infections	• Genital sexual contact • Mother to newborn during vaginal delivery	• Can affect urethra, anus, vagina, cervix, and uterus • Spontaneous abortion or premature delivery • Untreated, can develop into pelvic inflammatory disease and broad systemic reactions like arthritis, skin disease, and heart damage	• Antibiotics
Chlamydia trachomatis	• Vaginal discharge, painful urination, or unusual vaginal bleeding • Often symptomless, up to 75% of infected women are unaware they have this STI	• Genital sexual contact • Mother to newborn during vaginal delivery	• Chronic inflammation of the cervix, rectal inflammation, pelvic inflammatory disease • Infertility • Ectopic pregnancy • Premature delivery	• Antibiotics
Syphilis	• Primary phase—ulcer at point of infection • Secondary phase—rash, low fever, aches and pains, sore throat, swollen glands • Following the above phases, the person can be symptomless for years, yet internal damage continues	• Genital sexual contact • Mother to fetus • Skin contact	• Paralysis • Blindness • Mental deterioration • Death	• Antibiotics

Viral STIs

Hepatitis B	• Jaundice (yellowing of skin and whites of the eyes) • Fever, headache, joint pain, skin rash, and dark urine	• Infected semen, vaginal secretions, blood, or saliva coming in contact with mucous membrane or breaks in skin • Mother to fetus • Breast-feeding	• Cirrhosis • Liver failure • Liver cancer • Death	• In some cases, an acute infection resolves and the virus clears • For a chronic infection, no cure; supportive measures include antiviral medication and abstinence from alcohol • Inoculate partner with hepatitis B vaccine
Herpes simplex virus type 2 (HSV-2)	• First outbreak (primary) is usually the most painful, often with flu-like symptoms—fever, swollen glands, general stiffness, aches and pains; local symptoms include itching and burning, herpes sores (roundish, watery bumps) on genitals, cervix, buttocks, anus, or inner thighs • Recurrent episodes, symptoms usually milder and more local, marked by herpes sores	• Occurs when body is shedding the virus, which comes in contact with mucous membrane or breaks in the skin • Shedding can occur even when sores are not visible ("silent shedding") • Contact with towels, bedding, or clothing • Mother to fetus	• During primary outbreak, spontaneous abortion, premature birth, and low birth weight	• Zovirax for symptom relief, not cure

(cont.)

205

TABLE 9.1. *(cont.)*

STI	Symptoms	Transmission	Complications	Treatment
Human papilloma virus (HPV; genital warts)	• Warts may be visible on genitals or anus, or microscopic and unseen inside the vagina or on the cervix	• Genital sexual contact • Contact with towels, bedding, or clothing (possible) • Mother to child during vaginal delivery	• Cervical cancer	• Many HPV infections are cured by body's own immune system • Removal by freezing, cauterizing, laser treatment, or surgery • Topical treatments with caustic chemicals • Alpha-interferon injections
Human immuno-deficiency virus (HIV)	• Initially symptomless or mild flu-like symptoms • After initial symptoms, often symptomless for a long period of time, yet still highly contagious • In later stages, weight loss, fever, diarrhea, and opportunistic infections	• Infected semen, vaginal secretions, blood, or saliva coming in contact with mucous membrane or breaks in skin • Mother to fetus • Breast-feeding	• Breakdown of body's immune system, allowing opportunistic infections • Tumors • Mental deterioration • Death	• Maximizing healthy lifestyle • Antiviral medications, such as AZT, that slow replication of HIV cells
		Other STIs		
Candida albicans (yeast infection)	• Genital itching • Inflammation of the vulva • Genital soreness, burning, swelling, pain during intercourse, painful urination • Vaginal discharge	• Genital sexual contact • Can occur without transmission from someone else	• Usually none, other than disruption caused by symptoms	• Monistat, Mycelex, Femstat, Nystatin, Nizoral • Wearing loose-fitting clothing, cotton-lined underwear

	Symptoms	How Transmitted	Possible Health Effects	Treatment/Prevention
Trichomoniasis (protozoan; a parasitic infection)	• Often symptomless • Itching, painful intercourse, burning or painful urination, frothy gray or yellow-green vaginal discharge • Fever • Symptoms may only occur during, or immediately following, menstruation	• Genital sexual contact • Damp towels or clothing recently used by an infected person • Mother to fetus	• Usually none, other than disruption caused by symptoms	• Metronidazole (Flagyl) or tinidazole
Pubic lice (crabs; different from head and body lice)	• Genital itching • Inflammation of the vulva • Small blue spots from louse bites • Pubic lice may also be found in armpits or eyelashes	• Genital sexual contact • Contact with objects (clothing, towels, and bed linen) infested with pubic lice or their eggs	• Usually none, other than disruption caused by symptoms or secondary skin infection due to scratching	• Over-the-counter preparations that kill lice and their eggs • Permethrin cream • Lindane shampoo (not recommended for small children or pregnant women) • Thorough cleaning of clothing, towels, and bed linens • Use of disinfectants for nonwashable items
Scabies (mites that burrow under the surface of the skin)	• Intense itching, red rash, welts, pustules • Most often infest the hands or wrists, but also genitals and other parts of the body below the neck	• Genital sexual contact • Any close body contact • Contact with objects (clothing, towels, and bed linen) infested with mites	• Usually none, other than disruption caused by symptoms or secondary skin infection due to scratching	• Lindane lotion or cream • For infants, young children, and pregnant women: sulfur ointment • Thorough laundering of clothing, towels, and bed linen

Human Papilloma Virus and the New Vaccines

The most common STI virus is human papilloma virus (HPV). Worldwide there are about 300 million new carriers of HPV every year (WHO, 2007), and it is estimated that half of all sexually active men and women will contract HPV during some point in their lives. HPV is easily transmitted and is often "silent"—because many people will have no obvious symptoms, a person may never know she or he has HPV. There are 40 genital strains of HPV, and the immune system clears most spontaneously from the body. About 15 strains of HPV, however, cause genital cancers; the most prevalent is cervical cancer, the second most common cancer for women in the world (Kawana et al., 2009).

The good news on HPV is that the development of HPV vaccines (like Gardasil and Cervarix) is projected to eventually reduce the number of new cases of cervical cancer. Gardasil is given in a series of three injections for vaccination and is best given before a girl or young woman becomes sexually active and is exposed to HPV. It protects against HPV strains 6, 11, 16, and 18. If a young woman is sexually active but has not been exposed to HPV, she can still be vaccinated with Gardasil. Cervarix, a one-shot vaccination, is effective as long as a girl or woman has not been exposed to the most common cancer-causing strains—HPV 16 and 18.

Although these vaccinations don't protect against all strains, they are estimated to provide 60–75% increased protection against HPV (Kawana et al., 2009) and represent a significant step forward toward the day when we have a vaccination for all strains of genital HPV (Madrid-Marina et al., 2009). The additional challenge will be making current and future vaccinations accessible for all women. In some countries like the United States, the vaccinations and cervical pap tests are paid for by insurance or and available through public health departments. Vaccinations and pap test screenings are expensive, however, making it difficult for resource-limited countries to provide them to all women.

ONE MORE TIME: SAFER SEX

STIs are spread by physical contact. Bacterial and viral organisms enter the body through a mucous membrane. The mucous membranes are warm, moist, and more permeable than other areas of skin. Mucous membranes include the mouth and parts of the vulva, urethra, vagina, and anus. Most sex education programs now stress using a barrier, such as a latex condom—either the male or female version—for sexual activity involving genitals.

STIs are transferred from person to person. Animals don't give humans STIs, and doorknobs, toilet seats, or other objects are rarely transmitters because bacteria and viruses are fragile and require fresh, warm fluid to survive. They die quickly when they remain outside the human body. Exceptions do exist, however, as noted in Table 9.1.

STIs affect people of any age. The greatest risk factor is feeling "It can't happen to me." Younger people can mistakenly think that oral sex isn't risky and, because they're not having intercourse, "What's the big deal?" Older people forgo condoms because they foolishly think they're too old to worry about pregnancy and that STIs happen only to younger people. This proves once again that magical thinking and the myth of invulnerability know no age.

There are other myths that cut across all age groups. The myths about romance, spontaneity, and nice partners not having "dirty diseases" are some of the biggest problems. Some women refuse to be realistic about safer-sex practices, often not insisting on STI testing and latex barriers because they're afraid of being judged. It's a double bind—a woman who is assertive about safer sex is often perceived as either too uptight or way too loose.

No matter what age, each woman must empower herself to speak to her partner about safer sex. It's about care and health and, ultimately, self-love. If a woman cannot find the words, her greatest problem may be that her self-esteem is so low it can literally kill her.

There are a number of strategies to help women become more comfortable with taking precautions. For example, learn from the experiences of other women you know. Women have a long history of confiding in each other, so ask family and trusted friends what they say when insisting on safer sex. Discover your "voice"— your ability and right to speak up without embarrassment or shame regarding safer sex. For practice, try making the following statements out loud, over and over again, until the words come out with confidence:

> "I have an STI. It's not the end of the world, but we have to be careful when we have sex."

> "I want to be sexual and safe: I always use condoms and latex barriers."

> "I had an STI and want to avoid being part of that 'food chain' again. Let's use condoms."

You can also read everything you can find on the subject and become informed not only about HIV/AIDS but about other STIs as well and where to get condoms and testing. Check out medical clinics, family practice physicians, family planning clinics, and public health clinics.

Finally, don't throw out the passion and fun. Getting turned on and getting it on should include sex and latex.

Latex and Nonlatex Barriers: Condoms, Oral Sex Dams, and Gloves

The goal of safer sex is to minimize direct contact of the woman's genitals, anus, or mouth with the partner's body fluids and genitals. Barriers that prevent or reduce the exchange of body fluids are the most common means of protection. Of these barrier methods, condoms are an excellent source of protection during vaginal or anal penetration. For vaginal penetration, remember the female condom too. The newer female condoms are easier to handle and protect the inner labia as well as the vagina. Gloves are another type of barrier that can be used for penetration of the vagina or anus. For latex-allergic individuals, seek out the nonlatex versions of condoms and gloves sold at pharmacies or online.

We don't recommend dental dams because they are too small and it's easy for them to slip out of place. For oral sex, either mouth-to-vulva (called *cunnilingus*) or mouth-to-anus (called *anilingus* or *rimming*), use oral sex dams—they are made for sex and are larger (usually 6 × 8 or 6 × 10 inches) and come in colors and flavors. Unless you are lucky enough to live near a safe-sex store, you'll probably have to go online to purchase these items (see our web resource recommendations at the end of the book).

Nonmicrowavable plastic food wrap has also been suggested as a more economical and easier-to-use barrier. Although its effectiveness has not been proven conclusively in controlled scientific studies, it is a frequent choice because of availability. Become comfortable handling barriers before you need them. Practice sliding male condoms onto bananas or putting on a female condom. Lay a piece of latex flat across your palm and see how creative you can be with your tongue and lips. If you feel silly practicing, remind yourself how practice makes perfect. Why not bring better sex technique to your sex life while taking care of your body?

Women Having Sex with Women: Be Smart about Safer Sex

Whether lesbian, bisexual, or trans, having sex with a woman also carries risk for transmission of STIs. It is a myth that women with female sexual partners don't need to practice safer sex. Lesbian, bisexual, and trans women have had a much harder time getting accurate information from healthcare providers about their sexual health and safer-sex techniques. This has led many women to downplay or ignore the need for protection (Marrazzo et al., 2005). The fact is that STIs don't discriminate on the basis of where the body fluids come from. Mucous membranes or tiny cuts or tears in the skin are equally permeable to semen, saliva, or vaginal mucus. The sharing of vaginal mucus from person to person is also the sharing of bacteria and may cause an increased incidence of this STI for same-sex partners (Marrazzo et al., 2010).

Safety and Empowerment

A word of warning for all women: seriously consider the relationship of drugs and alcohol to sex. A woman "under the influence" doesn't do her best thinking, and neither will her partner. "Getting high and getting off" can lead to disaster. In the United States, studies show that college-age women who binge drink are at the highest risk for getting STIs (Lindley et al., 2008). You can help yourself by getting educated about drinking and sex, planning for sex, and staying sober. Survivors of trauma may use drugs or alcohol to dissociate from their bodies. If you find yourself in the triangle of drinking, drugging, and dissociating, go to a clinic and tell a healthcare provider you need help. Your life is worth it.

We wish we could say that all women can be empowered to negotiate safer sex with a partner, but it is not true. Many women coping with economic, social, and cultural injustices have unprotected sex and hope for the best. We wish that every woman could be treated with respect and would have sufficient power to have control over condom use (Crepaz et al., 2009). If you have a partner who refuses to wear a condom, suggest less risky behaviors as alternatives, like oral sex (you'll still be at risk for gonorrhea, herpes, and HPV, but you have a much lower risk for HIV/AIDS) and manual stimulation. Rubbing skin against skin can be very sexy and creative. Of all the sexual activities possible with a partner, mutual masturbation offers the least risk. Vaginal condoms are another option if cost is not a concern.

In the future, we hope there will be more options, both socially and medically, for women protecting themselves from STIs. Sex educators know that we need gender-specific education in teaching women how to negotiate condom use with partners. Research on vaccines continue. Scientists are also working on microbicides—substances applied topically that would boost the skin and mucous membrane's ability to fight off STIs (McGowan, 2008).

Being thoughtful about precautions doesn't have to diminish sex in life. Like buckling up when driving your car or wearing a life vest while boating, the pleasure you take in something you enjoy is hardly affected by being safe—taking precautions can actually lead to more enjoyment over time by preventing mishaps or tragedies.

The "Doesn't Work" List

Not so long ago, spermicidal gels with nonoxynol-9 or octoxynol-9 were recommended. Data now show that they don't protect you from STIs, so take them off the list.

Vaginal and anal douching are still practiced by many women before sexual activity. But what you don't know can hurt you. Douching, even with water, removes the all-important mucus that lines the walls of the vagina and anus. Once the mucus is "washed off," the walls are even more permeable and susceptible to STIs as well as small cuts or abrasions (Carballo-Diéguez et al., 2008).

In some cultures, women insert herb or plant material that is known to dry out the vagina, thereby increasing friction during "dry" sex. A mucus-dry vagina is a vagina that is more susceptible to both STIs and small cuts and tears.

IF YOU GET AN STI, IT'S NO TIME TO DENY

Typically the first reactions to learning you have an STI will be depression, fears of rejection, and concern about your health (Vozina & Steben, 2001). You may even just try to ignore the whole thing. Denial is not a luxury you can afford when it comes to STIs, however, because when you have one, you need treatment. If you don't currently have a physician or nurse practitioner, call your local hospital, public health department, or community mental health agency and ask for a list of local healthcare practitioners. If keeping costs down is important, ask if there are local agencies that care for women's medical needs at low or no cost, such as a women's resource center, a public health clinic, or a family planning agency. You can also ask the healthcare providers to whom you are referred about the possibility of a sliding fee scale. If you feel yourself going into "hiding mode," ask your partner or a close friend to help you make the calls or go with you.

Remember that early and consistent health care, including taking all medications prescribed and returning for follow-up appointments, is important for effective treatment. You will feel more inclined to pursue the treatment you need if you are confident that the healthcare provider will treat you with the respect you deserve. Simply put, don't consult any practitioner who treats you as if you're the problem. You should be treated with sensitivity and respect. Your examination and treatment for an STI should maintain your privacy; so call ahead and ask about confidentiality. For some STIs, like HIV or syphilis, the law requires healthcare providers to get a more thorough medical history, including the names of your sexual partners so that they can be notified of possible exposure. In some situations, you won't be required to give the names of sexual partners if you agree to contact them yourself. If you decide to handle it yourself, be sure to follow through. Others' health, fertility, and well-being are at stake, and you're only doing what you would want to have done for you.

When you go to your appointment, consider taking someone with you for support (to reduce any feelings of loneliness or shame) and as a second set of ears to listen to medical recommendations. The laws in all states provide that minors can receive testing and treatment for STIs without their parents' permission, though in some states physicians aren't prevented from telling a young woman's parents that she was treated after the fact. So if you are underage, ask the clinic ahead of time about its policy regarding confidentiality and how billing or any follow-up occurs.

Questions and concerns about STIs aren't easy to bring up with a partner, but remember the old sex education caveat: when you go to bed with someone, you're going to bed with every partner with whom that person has had sex. Women who won't sit down on a public toilet seat for fear of "getting something" are often willing to have sex with a new partner without first talking about STIs, simply because they're too embarrassed to raise the issue. What's wrong with this picture? We believe that if a woman feels she can be naked with someone, she should be prepared to ask some pretty bold questions beforehand.

COMMON SEXUAL CONCERNS

Let's say you discover you have an STI. What happens next? After education and early treatment comes a period of adjustment in your sense of self. At first you may feel that you will never ever have sex again. Some women find they become more inhibited and less spontaneous about sex. You may feel ashamed or disgusted with your body and yourself. Women can isolate themselves, worry about rejection, and further isolate—a cycle that leads to depression for many (Goggin et al., 1998; Goldmeier, 2001) as well as a decrease in their own desire and arousal. Some women report that because of their experiences they no longer find sex as pleasurable or even stop having sex (Vozina & Steben, 2001). You may feel angry with the sexual partner who knowingly or unknowingly transmitted the STI.

Acknowledging this diagnosis as a loss and allowing yourself to feel anger and grief are a very real part of adjustment. Then comes the process of fitting this new reality into the rest of your life.

Whom to Tell and When

> Heidi was falling in love with Jenna. They had a great time together, sharing countless hours talking, laughing, and cuddling. Jenna made it clear she wanted to move forward in the relationship, and Heidi did too, but how to tell Jenna about the genital warts? She'd have to tell her soon, but she didn't know what to say. She was really scared Jenna would dump her.

> Deanna was stunned when she had a herpes outbreak after becoming sexually active with Carlos. Her first outbreak, and she didn't know where she'd gotten it. She wondered if Carlos had been a "silent carrier" and didn't know it. Now she had to tell him, not only about her herpes but that he needed testing too. Their relationship was so new, she wondered if they'd stay together.

Sorting out whom to tell about your STI and when is like those Russian nesting dolls—there are issues within the issue of getting the STI. If you are involved with only one person and got the STI from that person, immediately tell him or her. In some situations, the STI might have become symptomatic during the current relationship, but may actually have been acquired earlier. A healthcare practitioner will need to see your partner to determine whether he or she is carrying an undiagnosed or untreated STI.

We'd like to say that all partners will respond with kindness, but that's not the case. Sometimes partners get frightened and angry. At that point you are dealing with not only your own diagnosis but also the strain in your relationship. None of this is easy to get through, and you will need support and education as well as treatment. If support from a partner or friend isn't sufficient, seek out a support group meeting, an Internet support group, or professional counseling. Ask your healthcare provider for referrals. In some cases, couples do break up because of the STI. Many couples hang in there; they keep talking and eventually sort out that the STI is not the end of the world.

If you are single, you'll be faced with issues related to timing and honesty: thinking about what to say and when to say it to a new partner. It's dishonest not to tell a sexual partner about an STI. Moreover, in the case of HIV or AIDS, not telling the partner is a felony in many states. But do you tell your entire STI story to every person you date? It's such a dilemma that some women just retreat from any relationship involvement at all.

Here's what we suggest. First, think about what you'd like to get out of this relationship. Is this just for fun and friendship, with no anticipation of sexual involvement? In this case you don't need to tell your partner anything about yourself sexually, including whether or not you have an STI. But what if you're not sure where the relationship might go? If you're not looking for sex but not opposed to it either, tell your partner about your STI once you know the relationship is getting physically intimate. When the relationship moves to intimate touching and kissing, when you or your partner says, "I don't want to rush this, but . . . " or "Why don't you stay?," it's time to be straightforward about the STI. The cues that a relationship is heating up might be different, but they're usually pretty unmistakable. The cue says "I want to get physical with you." That's when you need to tell your partner, "Look, I think this is terrific, but we need to talk about me physically. I've had genital warts [or whatever the STI is], and we need to make sure that we're careful so that you don't get it. I can tell you how we can best manage it. Let's talk."

Will this be easy? No, because nothing about STIs is easy. Will this cool some hot romances? You bet. Will this discussion look like an Oscar-winning scene on the silver screen? Probably not. People tend to stumble around when they're explaining things. They backtrack and repeat questions they've already asked. It's part of getting accustomed to the new reality. All we can say is, if it chills the relationship permanently, then the relationship wasn't meant to be. As in the rest of this book, we're promoting honesty as the best route to meaningful relationships, whether they're brief or long lasting. The relationship you have with yourself is the most important one you'll ever have.

Rejecting Your Body

If you get an STI, you may very well withdraw from any sense of connection to your body. You may describe it as divorcing yourself from your genitals, being mad at your body for betraying you, or denying the importance of your natural sexual responses. When a person is frightened, it's normal to take a fight–flight stance, being either angry or withdrawing. But because you have only one body and need to live in it for a lifetime, it makes more sense to address the hurt, bewilderment, and grief through education, counseling, and support. Then you can figure out how to move on and feel whole again.

Guilt and Shame

If you were exposed to hepatitis at your workplace or to malaria on a vacation, no one worth loving would say to you, "You should be ashamed that you got hepatitis [or malaria]." Instead, others would feel bad for you and express their concern. It's one of the meaner aspects of human nature that we tend to blame people for anything that goes wrong for them sexually, whether it's an accidental pregnancy or an STI. Although the Salem witch trials were conducted over 300 years ago, when it comes to sexual behavior, people are likely to put women on trial for their troubles, saying "She should have known better" or "It serves her right for doing what she did." To make matters worse, remember that because her genitals contain more mucous membranes and can retain body fluids from another person for a longer time, a woman is more at risk than a man for contracting an STI.

Someone once said that "guilt is the gift that keeps on giving," and shame seems even more generous. Even if others don't taunt us or shake their heads behind our backs, we chastise ourselves: "I should have known better." If you are diagnosed with any STI, talk to a healthcare provider, counselor, or other supportive person about the diagnosis. You can be sorry that it happened. You can be sad that it will cause adjustments in your sexual relationship with another person. You can be angry that life is not always fair. But remember that you're not a bad person because you have an STI.

Continuing to Be Sexual

People often associate safer-sex techniques with casual sexual relationships, not long-term monogamous relationships. Many couples, however, face the prospect of having to use safer-sex techniques for the rest of their lives.

> "I used to love having a lover go down on me—but that was before I found out I was HIV positive. Oral sex dams are better than nothing, but there are times when I really feel cheated."

> "I'm finally in a relationship that works, but it feels like a condom will always come between us."

If you are in a committed relationship and have an incurable STI, you and your partner have an important decision to make. Do you nurse your bitterness, feel sorry for yourselves, and remain focused on what you can't do? Or do you decide to continue being sexual, focusing on what you can do and looking for creative ways to heighten eroticism in your relationship?

With an estimated 65 million Americans with incurable viral STIs, you and your partner are certainly not alone in facing this dilemma. Like countless other couples in the same situation, it will be important for you to put your challenges in perspective. Sex is wonderful, but no smart person ever said it was simple. Keep talking to each other about your sexual interests, your desire for physical closeness. Allow yourself to grieve that sex will not be as it was before and that a sad experience has happened in your life. Grieving allows you to fully acknowledge what you have come through and where you are in your life now. Stay educated by reading about how other couples enrich their sex lives. Remember that the Basson model of sexual responsivity begins with a willingness and motivation to be sexually active (see Chapter 4). Make informed decisions, be creative, and keep sex a vibrant part of your relationship.

> "Latex barriers and hygiene—a small price to pay for the hot sex we're having. The precautions have become automatic, and we stay focused on the passion."

> "When I met my partner, I was up front about my herpes. We used condoms religiously, and the sex was great. When we made our relationship permanent, we discussed whether we wanted to keep using a condom if I was asymptomatic. At first, I felt really awkward—I'd feel horrible if I passed herpes on. But my partner said it wouldn't be the end of the world if it happened and was willing to take the chance. Since then, we've been careful whenever I have a flare-up, but otherwise, we just don't worry."

LIFE AFTER LOSS: THE STI ISN'T THE END OF THE WORLD

With loss comes grieving, and being diagnosed with an STI usually triggers grief—a normal reaction. Adjustments to the infection come with time, education, and support. Reading widely, asking questions of healthcare providers, and seeking out others who've lived with a similar STI can help you make the adjustment from fear to empowerment. Resources to assist you in this adjustment are listed at the end of the book.

One final note about your health care: it matters. If you don't have adequate medical coverage, then call the public health department or family planning agency in your community for referrals to low-cost or free services. STIs may change your life, but they don't have to rule your life.

TEN

Trauma

Trauma leaves a scar that can disrupt every aspect of life, including sexuality, whether it comes in the form of being robbed, witnessing a murder, being the victim of sexual abuse, or becoming disfigured as a result of an illness, accident, or surgery. Although people vary widely in the severity of their response to trauma, it's not uncommon for women to feel alienated from their bodies following a traumatic experience. In this and other ways, trauma can most certainly affect a woman's sex life.

In this chapter we discuss how trauma can impact your sexuality and your sexual relatedness to your partner and describe ways to overcome posttraumatic responses. Chapters 13, 14, and 15 provide additional suggestions for sexual resilience and overcoming sexual difficulties. You, perhaps with guidance, will determine when you are ready for these suggestions and exercises. Your first step is to take charge of your body—becoming aware of your body's sensations and feeling control over yourself and your circumstances. If these suggestions make you feel pressured, tell yourself to focus first on reducing anxiety and panic. Remember that you are building a sense of your sexuality from the inside out. Go gently and at the pace that is right for you. If you find any of the suggestions in this chapter too difficult or if you need additional help, consider seeing a sex therapist. Chapter 16 provides useful information about sex therapy and finding a qualified therapist.

The suggestions we offer in this chapter should not be viewed as a substitute for obtaining professional help in the aftermath of a traumatic experience. Counseling can give you insight into why you continue to feel upset, numb, or anxious following a traumatic event. It can provide you with emotional support and psychological understanding that can help you feel better about your life.

In addition to counseling, you may find it valuable to read more about trauma. The websites *www.trauma-pages.com* and *www.traumacenter.org* provide excellent information and refer you to other informative websites, books, and articles. In addition, we list several books about trauma and sex in our "Suggested Resources" section at the end of the book. All of this material can help you better understand what happened to you and provide ways to reclaim your life.

THE IMPACT OF TRAUMA ON YOUR SEXUALITY

Trauma and the Treatment of Posttraumatic Stress Disorder

By definition, trauma is a shock that follows a disastrous or terrifying experience. Your brain and nervous system interpret the traumatic event as a life-or-death crisis. Whether the trauma is physical or psychological, something that happens directly to you or something you witness, one event or a series of events, sexual abuse or something else entirely, your body immediately goes into a self-protective mode, preparing you to defend yourself, flee from the danger, or stop feeling. Unfortunately, even after the real danger has passed, the traumatized mind and nervous system continue to respond, sometimes for years, as if the threat still exists. Designed to protect you from feeling overwhelmed, this self-protective mode often interferes with your experiencing the fullness of your life.

The aftermath of trauma is often referred to as *posttraumatic stress disorder*, or *PTSD*. PTSD creates adjustment challenges for individuals who have suffered personally devastating experiences ranging from war to domestic violence. Clinicians and researchers alike are engaged in concerted efforts to better understand what happens to the brain and body after trauma and design better methods of treatment. We know the brain is susceptible to being both hurt and ultimately healed interpersonally (Siegel, 2010). Brain scanning shows that the neural wiring related to both hypervigilance and dissociation can be helped by mindfulness techniques (psychological strategies described below), psychotherapy, and healthy self-regulation and self-soothing.

PTSD often leads to sexual difficulties. Women have lower rates of sexual interaction (Anticević & Britvić, 2008) and higher rates of sexual problems of all types after PTSD (Schnurr et al., 2009). In addition, research now points to the ways in which maltreatment and neglect in children from birth to age 5 lead to dissociation, anxiety, and depression in adulthood (Kaplow & Widom, 2007; Brown et al., 2009). Unfortunately, many of the medications for PTSD-related depression, anxiety, and dysregulation can also contribute to sexual problems (Schnurr et al., 2009).

Research about treatment for PTSD shows that it is important to address sexual problems and concerns separately but concurrently with treatment for trauma (Chudakov et al., 2008).

Impact on Your Sexual Behavior

If you have experienced a traumatic event, you may have noticed that one of your self-protective mechanisms is to continually reorder the priorities in your life in an ongoing effort to put things "right." In the face of terror, normal interests and pursuits lose importance. Sex and pleasure may fall by the wayside. In this state of preparedness and protection, your brain may be continually vigilant and assessing for any further threat. This vigilance makes relaxation or an erotic focus during lovemaking very difficult. It can also make you overly reactive and irritated with certain sounds, noises, or touch—like the slurpy sound of kissing, the slippery feel of vaginal lubrication or semen, or anything rubbing against your skin. Any unexpected sound or shift in your partner's movements or emotions is monitored for signs of possible danger.

> "We lived with my grandparents, and my grandfather would have explosive rages when he was drinking. You didn't know when it would happen. Now I don't like things to ever get out of control. Whenever emotions run high, or even when my partner gets sexually excited, I withdraw because I can't tell what could happen next. Am I a freak? I hate unpredictability."

Being constantly on guard means that your body is often in a state of hyperarousal: a racing heart, lack of regular sleep, anxiety, nervousness, tension, panic, and a strong startle response. Your body is responding as if it is about to encounter a lethal threat at any moment. Not surprisingly, this constant state of internal agitation can drown out any erotic stirring.

> "I can't tolerate being touched on my shoulders or back. That's where the mugger grabbed me. If my partner accidentally reaches for me from behind, I have a panic attack—my heart races, my knees buckle, and I can't breathe. I am constantly on guard when having sex. I have to orchestrate every touch and movement in order to have sex. Should I give up on trying to be sexual?"

A traumatic experience not only affects how you think about safety and predictability in the world but also can deprive you of self-confidence. You may no longer trust your emotions, and you may try to suppress any intense feeling, including passion and sexual arousal.

Women can also "check out" during sex (or other perceived "dangerous" situations), going numb and not feeling in their bodies. This is the opposite of hypervigilance but has the same sexual result—sex is not easy, and it's not pleasurable.

Sexual Trauma, Triggers, and Self-Esteem

When a traumatic event involves sexual abuse, factors related directly to the sexual abuse may interfere with normal sexual response. If the sexual abuse was mixed with love and special attention, you could feel confused and have difficulty accepting the possibility that you may have "allowed" the abuse to occur because it brought you the attention that you craved. In addition, if you were abused as a child, it is confusing to feel both love and rage toward a person whose position in your life may have been so important—be it a grandparent, sibling, mother, father, or stepparent—yet who had wreaked so much havoc. If you experienced arousal and even orgasmed during the abuse, you may feel ashamed that your body responded sexually. It's not surprising that such confusion and shame often spill over into future sexual situations.

Following a traumatic experience, certain cues or reminders often remain in the memory and trigger unwanted flashbacks, emotional numbness, or panic. In the case of sexual trauma, a trigger could be a person who reminds you of the abuser, a place similar to where the trauma occurred, or any smell, touch, taste, sight, or sound that your memory associates with the trauma. The trigger may be quite specific, like having a certain part of your body touched, or general, like anything that has a sexual connotation. You usually know your triggers, but occasionally new triggers can catch you off guard. Your response to triggers will usually be worse when you are fatigued or upset. Research suggests that over time the brain becomes more reactive to ever lower levels of anything that resembles the original trigger. This process, called *kindling*, means that you can become panicked at increasingly lower reminders of the original stimulus.

> "While we were having sex, my hair got caught under my partner's elbow. The sensation of having my hair pulled triggered a flashback to being raped. I was terrified. The rapist had yanked me by my hair to keep me from moving."

To complicate a painful situation even further, women who are having sexual difficulties following a sexual or nonsexual trauma often condemn themselves for being numb or overreacting. Researchers are not entirely sure why the range of possible responses to a traumatic experience is so broad, but if you are having a troublesome response to a trauma, keep in mind that everyone has different amounts of fear and horror that are tolerable before the body and mind begin to take desperate measures for self-protection. Suffering trauma does not make you weak or inadequate. And you can make efforts to reclaim your sexuality after a traumatic experience. We believe it is important that you do so, because it's a step toward reclaiming predictability and pleasure in all areas of your life.

Confusing and Distorted Responses to Sexual Trauma

In dangerous situations human beings have an innate tendency to fight, flee, or freeze. In many cases of sexual trauma, a woman may "flee" through sexual avoidance or emotional disconnection or may suddenly find herself in attack mode, especially if startled or pressured. Another aspect of trauma is the "freeze" response, in which panic leads to the inability to move at all.

If you have suffered sexual trauma but are not sure of its effects on your behavior, attitudes, or sexual response, the following descriptions may lead to a better self-understanding.

Genital Swelling

In laboratory research, scientists have studied the sexual response of volunteers who were shown different images on a screen. While viewing the pictures, the research subjects were connected to sensitive monitors that measure blood flow and swelling response in the genitals. Although the male volunteers became aroused only to the specific sexual acts they reported as arousing, women tended to get physically aroused even when not subjectively or sexually interested in a particular theme, for instance, a rape scene. When the women were asked if they experienced arousal when viewing the pictures, they reported arousal only to those sexual activities that were sexually interesting to them. They were unaware that their genitals responded to pictures they did not find attractive at all (Suschinsky et al., 2009). What is happening here?

Researchers hypothesize that there may be many reasons that a woman doesn't experience subjective arousal even though her genitals register arousal. She may be tired, momentarily distracted and not focused on arousal, or not aware of her genital sensations. Another possible reason that women don't report arousal when viewing slides that are not experienced as subjectively arousing is that women's genital swelling and lubrication serve as a protective response. Women's genitals, especially the vagina, are vulnerable to tearing and other injuries if attacked. If assaulted, it is beneficial for a woman to lubricate and have genital fullness, because genitals that are engorged with blood are less likely to be torn or damaged. So viewing a rape or assault scene may be the height of "turn-off," but the genital arousal "turns on" as an instinctual protective mechanism.

Women who have been beaten or raped may feel confused or even guilty if they lubricated, felt arousal, or even had an orgasm when assaulted. It's important for women to know that this response is based on instinctual genital swelling, which causes sexual pleasure and satisfaction but also is designed to protect their genitals from perceived danger (Suschinsky et al., 2009).

> "I could never understand why I had orgasmed when raped, when I can't reach orgasm with my partner during lovemaking. It was helpful to learn from my therapist that this was a body protection mechanism. I stopped feeling humiliated about the orgasm."

Increased Vulnerability and Impulsive Risk Taking

Women who have been victims of sexual abuse, as either children or adults, may later engage in behaviors that are impulsive and can be sexually risky. Let us be very clear: this is not about a woman "wanting" or "inviting" abuse or trauma. Rather the impulsivity is a very common human attempt to overcome painful memories by "facing down the fear," and in more dangerous situations, to literally be numb—dissociated—when terrified. Sadly, this response can lead to nights of excessive drinking and "hooking up," which can expose women to STIs or even further sexual abuse. In fact, because the brain starts to unconsciously "tune out" when a person is terrified and vulnerable, each time a sexual trauma occurs, the likelihood of later being exposed to further unwanted, unprotected, and risky sexual behavior increases, as does the likelihood of further incidents of sexual abuse.

You may ask, "What is going on here? How can lightning strike twice in the same place?" Women who have been sexually traumatized more than once ask the same questions and tragically and mistakenly conclude they are somehow responsible for their abuse. Contrary to their unwarranted sense of shame, however, this impulsive pattern of risk taking is not a reflection of a character flaw, but the result of unconscious mechanisms that strive to protect a person from anxiety or fear.

When a person is sexually abused, the brain reacts in ways not entirely understood, ways meant to protect a person from being helpless, but as you will read in the following sections, ways that ultimately can be self-defeating. In some cases, the impulsivity is an attempt to prove something, like "I can handle sexual situations." In other cases, the impulsive risk taking may be due to an "I don't care" attitude, resulting from depression, despair, or self-loathing: "I am sexual only to be an object for someone else's use." Regardless of the cause, all too often adult women who have been sexually abused have additional tragedy unjustly heaped on their initial trauma. Sometimes what results is not abuse per se but a "bad experience," like unprotected sex that fortunately does not lead to STIs or pregnancy.

If you have had additional traumatic experiences after an initial abuse, this is definitely a time to get into therapy. We know this will not be easy, but with help you can tackle this pattern.

Lack of Sexual Desire

Many women who have been sexually abused find that they have little or no interest in sex. Their lack of sexual desire may be an attempt to flee from or avoid something that was frightening and dangerous. Sometimes this lack of interest starts immediately following the sexual abuse, and sometimes it appears years later, after a long period of normal sexual activity. In Chapter 4 we discussed the hormonal influence of new relationships and how our hormones emerge in special ways to enhance our attraction and *reduce our fear levels*. But this hormonal enhancement has an early expiration: after a year or two it abates.

The delayed emergence of this defense mechanism (fleeing danger by avoiding sex) can be perplexing. It usually happens in cases where other defenses were first used to minimize the horror of the sexual abuse, only to eventually become ineffective. In some cases, the delayed emergence of low sexual desire can be due to the psyche's defensive response to what it mistakenly interprets as a repeat of an earlier trauma. For example, conflict in a relationship, in the unconscious mind, could seem uncomfortably similar to an earlier sexual assault. The current conflict could differ night and day from the past trauma, but the mind might pick up on some common denominator like betrayal, anger, or fear and sound the alarm to protect against a repeat of past harm. Chapter 15 provides a detailed discussion of low sexual desire, its causes, and ways to overcome it.

Sexual Aversion

Following sexual trauma, some women do not simply lose their interest in sex; they become disgusted and frightened by anything sexual. Sexual aversion is often a phobic reaction that can be traced back to earlier trauma. Because of the trauma, sexual cues trigger a strong emotional reaction. The aversion to sex serves as a way of avoiding or fleeing from sex. If you have a sexual aversion, you may react negatively to specific sexual cues like the sight of an erect penis, or you may find all aspects of sex, including nudity, hugging, and kissing, distasteful. An aversion can vary from a moderate dislike and anxiety about sex to the extremes of panic, disgust, and revulsion. Even the thought of these sexual behaviors may trigger a negative emotional reaction.

> "At first I thought I could cope with my disgust by avoiding certain sexual activities. As long as I didn't do the things that were done to me as a child, I felt I'd be okay. Unfortunately, my aversion got worse and I found myself wanting to hit and kick my partner anytime I was touched, as if I was being assaulted."

Although both low sexual desire and sexual aversion serve as a means of avoiding or fleeing sex, they are different forms of self-protection. When a woman has low sexual desire due to past trauma, sexual cues produce no response. She unconsciously seeks protection by not responding to anything that could reactivate the buried pain. In cases of sexual aversion, the pain is often closer to the surface. Rather than experiencing no response to sexual cues, a woman with a sexual aversion experiences strong negative emotions. Feelings of disgust prompt the woman to avoid sex, which is a way to avoid a recurrence of the earlier trauma.

Similar to low sexual desire, sexual aversion may first occur right after the trauma or may appear later in your life, even after a period of safe, pleasant sexual experiences. Relationship problems, a life crisis, or even hormonal changes due to various causes can trigger sexual aversion in some women as a delayed reaction to an earlier trauma. Something as mundane as disappointment in your partner for being nonresponsive to your needs can become unconsciously associated with earlier trauma or neglect, resulting in a late onset of sexual aversion.

Sexual aversion has elements of anxiety and panic, which may respond well to medication. If you are in therapy, discuss with your therapist how medication might help you.

Dissociative Sex

Dissociative sex represents a third type of protection against sexual conflict or the impact of earlier trauma. Rather than losing sexual desire or pulling away from sex out of disgust, you may mentally distance yourself from your body during sexual activity. Sometimes this distancing, or dissociating, is achieved by using alcohol or drugs. Maybe you experience yourself going off into a trance-like state during sex. Or perhaps you feel disconnected from your body during sex, as if your partner is making love to someone else's body. In all these instances, mentally removing yourself from a sexual situation represents a desperate attempt to avoid reexperiencing the trauma of the past.

> "I go through the motions of having sex, but I'm not really present in my body. I know I'm touching and being touched, but I'm not into it."

Dissociation can range from having mild nonsexual daydreams during sex to totally blanking out so that you have no recall of what happened during sex. The latter response is rare, quite dangerous, and falls beyond the scope of this book. If your dissociation is so severe that you lose all recall, contact a therapist. If you don't blank out but do become emotionally distant or numb during sex, you may find the suggestions later in this chapter useful. You may also find it helpful to read Part II, "Understanding Your Body," if you have not already read it, and Part V, "Developing Sexual Comfort, Confidence, and Satisfaction," for additional exercises that will teach you how to stay present in your body.

Sexual Compulsion

Some women who have been sexually traumatized will take or make any sexual opportunity they can. Their vigilance isn't in place for self-protection, but for the next sexual hit. Sex becomes a compulsion over which they have little control.

> "I had sex with any guy anywhere. I was known as the campus slut, and I didn't care. As long as I was having sex, I felt powerful and desired. Afterward, I would get scared I wasn't loved and go looking for sex again."

If you have a sexual compulsion, sometimes called a *sexual addiction*, you probably find yourself in an endless cycle of seeking sex to numb or overcome painful emotions, only to feel more miserable after each sexual encounter. It may be that you masturbate 10 or 12 times a day but feel only exhaustion or temporary pleasure if you attain orgasm. Perhaps you pick up multiple partners at bars, but the sex is disconnected and you feel lousy afterward. Maybe you go to chat rooms and engage in online sexual activity, feeling only emptiness in the aftermath. Your attempt to gain control over sex ends up leaving you out of control. You may also be more susceptible to chronically drinking or getting high before having sex. You may expose yourself to countless dangers, including relationship conflicts and the risk of physical harm.

The possible motivations for sexual compulsion are countless. It may be a way of reenacting the trauma—creating it over and over—in a futile attempt to master it. The compulsivity may be an attempt to prove that you are no longer afraid of getting hurt by anyone, that you're on top of the sex game. Perhaps by making sex so meaningless you might be trying to prove that what happened years ago was no big deal. Sex may temporarily make you feel wanted or powerful. After seducing others and making them desire you, however, you feel powerless and bad about yourself until you repeat the pattern. Compulsive sex can also be a way of devaluing yourself. Because others abused you in the past, you may feel that you don't deserve to be treated well. Regardless of the reason, compulsive behavior takes over your life.

Sexual compulsion is a complicated and dangerous reaction to trauma. It is frequently impulsive. If you suspect that you have a compulsive sexual disorder, we recommend that you seek out an individual therapist or a professionally led group for women with sexual compulsion to help you disengage from this pattern. This can get better.

Trophy Sex

Usually when we hear references to sex and trophies, we think of men in pursuit of sexual conquests. Trophy sex can also apply to women, however. It may be a response to sexual trauma, although just as commonly it is driven by different psychological needs. If you find that you get a rush from the hunt and capture of another person, you may be engaging in trophy sex.

Consider the following scenario. Your search for a sexual conquest begins with an awareness—however vague—that you are dissatisfied and perhaps depressed. You set out to make something happen and feel your first rush of excitement when you identify your prey. Then you begin the game of teasing seduction to capture his or her attention. In the end, much to your delight, you have the person eating out of your hand. You've won—you have another trophy for your mantel. The only problem is, once you've won, you're no longer interested. You may even feel burdened if the conquest shows up again.

> "Men can be real bastards, but when you know how to handle them, they're harmless. I've had professional athletes, famous lawyers, an obscenely rich CEO, even an actor from one of the daytime soaps lusting after me. They were like putty in my hands—I can seduce anybody."

If this scenario is familiar or makes you laugh uncomfortably, you may be engaging in trophy sex. The sexual hunt may be an attempt to overcome feelings of powerlessness and exploitation you've had in earlier life experiences, often with men. Ultimately, trophy sex is without satisfaction; you're enjoying not the sex but the conquest. As in the case of compulsive sexual behavior, trophy sex may be an attempt to fight back in response to earlier experiences of abuse. By sexually conquering others, you may feel that you are conquering your perpetrators, past and future. Although in extreme cases trophy sex can be compulsive, where your sexual behavior is driven and largely out of your control, more often trophy sex is under your control but driven by a self-defeating motivation—conquest rather than pleasure or intimacy.

If you're aware of this pattern in your sexual activity, try using the suggestions later in this chapter to stay present in your sexuality. If you continue to find yourself drawn toward trophy seeking, we recommend that you get counseling to help you gain greater insight into factors prompting this behavior and ways to engage in healthier sexual interaction.

Nonsexual Complications

Although not all women who have experienced trauma will react in the ways described above, the impact of trauma can be quite profound in other ways. Women who experienced sexual abuse may have more challenges with relationships in general and more sexual dissatisfaction as adults—whether or not they experience a specific sexual problem. Women who have been sexually abused are more likely to describe themselves in negative terms, view their bodies in a poor light, and think of their partners as uncaring and overcontrolling. Even in consensual sexual interaction, they can often have negative feelings of shame, disgust, fear, and anger when sexually aroused.

A Cautionary Note

Although low sexual desire, sexual aversion, dissociative sex, sexual compulsion, and trophy sex may be the by-products of sexual trauma, these problems can also have many other underlying causes. If you engage in any of these behaviors but have no recollection of previous sexual abuse, don't assume that you must have been abused. Work with a therapist to explore why you are resorting to self-defeating sexual behavior.

Helpful Therapies

There are a number of therapy modalities that are particularly effective with the challenges we've outlined here. First and foremost, if you decide to engage in one of these therapies (or in any therapy), make certain that the person is accredited, experienced in that modality, and licensed to provide the treatment. The American Psychological Association endorses eye movement desensitization and reprocessing (EMDR) for people in acute distress. A structured, safe, specific treatment is implemented and is highly effective in reducing autonomic responses to triggers. Biofeedback can help with one of the primary problems of trauma: overarousal of the central nervous system. Biofeedback at times uses measurements, such as measuring heart rate or skin temperature, to demonstrate to the client and therapist that hyperarousal is occurring. Techniques for relaxing these responses is guided, but controlled by the patient, who can actually *see* the results. CBT (cognitive-behavioral therapy) is designed specifically for the client's needs and for self-help. There are even computerized CBT sessions. Prolonged exposure therapy begins with psychoeducation, followed by breathing exercises to reduce anxiety. "Real-world" experience is incorporated in guided, gradual, safe exposure to places, people, or things that you may have avoided because of their association with trauma. For example, for someone who was assaulted in a grove of pine trees, the first step might be, in a safe environment, to hold, touch, and smell a small pine branch. You can see where this could go from there.

CREATING SEXUAL SATISFACTION

Overcoming trauma involves learning how to feel safe again and becoming empowered with sexual knowledge, self-assurance, and the skills needed to keep unwanted emotions in check. This is how you open yourself to experiencing sexual pleasure unencumbered by posttraumatic symptoms.

Be Present in Your Body: Awareness and Mindfulness

Sexual activity requires you to be fully present in your body, aware of your body's responses, so that you can enjoy the pleasure your body can produce. Dissociating, being distracted by intrusive thoughts, or experiencing agitation during sex prevents you from being present in your body. You can learn to be present in your body by *taking control* of your body, learning to *soothe yourself*, and *defusing triggers*.

Take Control

Taking control means making sure you feel safe and your partner is supportive and respectful of your goals. Start by checking your environment to make sure it is safe, comfortable, and pleasing to your senses. Purchase items for your bedroom that create a safe, comforting, and pleasing ambience. Do this yourself—relying on your partner perpetuates the pattern of not being in control.

Make an honest assessment of your current sex life. Are you engaging in sexual behavior that puts you at risk or makes you feel uncomfortable (e.g., having sex with strangers or performing oral sex reluctantly)? If so, tell yourself that you're taking a break from that behavior. If the activity involves a partner, tell your partner no and explain that you don't like what you've been doing and that you're taking steps to feel more comfortable with sex. If you feel awkward talking to your partner about sex, take a look at Chapter 14 for suggestions.

Soothe Yourself

In your attempt to create a better sex life, you may experience emotional numbing or hyperarousal, especially anxiety. There are excellent books on understanding anxiety and learning soothing responses to counteract anxiety and panic (see "Anxiety" in "Suggested Resources"). Soothing responses such as deep breathing, positive self-talk, calming imagery, muscle relaxation, and body movement can help you stay present in your body, decrease anxiety, clear your mind, and take control. The term *mindfulness* is a reference to these healthy ways of noticing the movement of your body and your breathing and of staying aware from moment to moment without rushing or disconnecting from the present.

To learn how to soothe yourself, try the following four steps. First, start by practicing a breathing technique that you can use when you experience anxiety, panic, or numbing. Focus on your breathing. Take slow deep breaths from your diaphragm (some women think of this breathing as coming from their belly) while counting backward from 100. Another way to focus on breathing is to breathe in, hold for three counts, breathe out, and hold for three more counts. Repeat this sequence 10 times. If you experience breathlessness, try harder to exhale all the air in your lungs before breathing in. Not exhaling deeply enough can lead to shortness of breath.

Second, once you've brought your breathing under control, you are ready to talk to yourself with a clear mind. Tell yourself that numbing and hyperarousal are normal responses to trauma triggers and that you can tolerate them and remain aware of your body. We call this *positive self-talk*, a useful technique for soothing. If you need suggestions for how to talk to yourself positively, see Chapter 15 for ways to challenge negative thoughts with positive ones. This step will take time to perfect.

Third, practice picturing soothing images in your mind. Examples of mental images that many women find soothing include a sun-swept seashore, billowy clouds, mountains, birds in flight, or a field of wildflowers. Some women use prayer, meditation, or a positive statement like "I am a loving and good person" as their soothing mental activity.

Fourth, as you picture your soothing image, notice where you feel muscle tension. Reduce the tension by first tensing the muscles further and then relaxing them.

Practice these four techniques for 10 to 20 minutes a day, until you feel you can do all four with some confidence. Pay particular attention to your breathing. Don't hold your breath—keep breathing and accept that it takes time to learn to do this.

Once your initial soothing responses are working, try additional soothing techniques involving movement and sensory awareness. Because trauma may have caused you to feel frozen with terror, it's important to learn to move your body and respond to sensory cues. In the presence of numbing or hyperarousal, you can find relief from these uncomfortable sensations by focusing on body movement and sensory experiences—things that keep you grounded in the here and now rather than snapping back to the terrifying past. Start by moving your body in ways that feel good to you. This may be standing, walking meditatively—or raucously—around the room, stretching your arms above your head, swaying, stomping, stooping, or moving from side to side. You can rock your body as if you're in a rocking chair, tilt your pelvis back and forth, or practice Kegels (see Chapter 8). *Any* form of movement that is comfortable and natural for you can be helpful. Becoming absorbed in how the joints in your little finger allow you to bend it can bring you back into your body.

Next, pay close attention to your sensory experience. Touch, taste, or smell something that pleases you; listen to music or the sounds of nature (if any) around you; gaze at the trees outside your window.

> "There are times when I'm suddenly overwhelmed by fear and dread. It feels like I'm suffocating. I've learned to calm myself by breathing slowly, reassuring myself, and moving around. When I can get a clear image in my mind or focus on something concrete around me, I feel grounded. It's like I get a grip on things, and the scary feelings seem to drift away. I have a fish tank in my apartment. Watching the fish always calms me down."

Self-soothing requires practice, but it is worth it: self-soothing becomes the cornerstone for creating positive sexuality. It also serves as an effective tool to combat posttraumatic symptoms by freeing you to stay present in your body and to focus on pleasurable sensations of any kind.

Defuse Triggers: Taking Charge

Triggers run the show unless you take charge of your sexual life. As you move through these exercises, remember: anything involving changing brain and body response takes time. If you tend to be impatient, go easy on yourself.

It's important to know your triggers if you want to overcome them. Make a list of the different experiences that trigger dissociation, numbing, aversion, or hyperarousal during sex. Consider people, places, things, forms of sensory stimulation, fantasies, and types of touch or physical activity in compiling your list. Write your list of triggers as negative statements, such as "I don't like to be touched" or "I don't like kissing." Now write how each trigger makes you feel. For example, if being touched makes you feel anxious or angry, write those words next to your trigger statement.

I don't like to be touched.   *Being touched makes me angry.*

As you do this, you may find that just thinking about the triggers can lead to a trauma response like dissociation or hyperarousal. If this happens, *use your soothing techniques as you write.*

Next, read aloud your list of triggers and feelings. Now write a take-charge statement next to every trigger. "I don't like to be touched" can be paired with "I will decide who touches me and when." "I don't like kissing" can be paired with "There are a lot of activities I like that don't involve my lips!"

Developing this list of positive statements helps you lessen the power of triggers to elicit posttraumatic reactions by giving triggers more links, more possible responses, than just reexperiencing the trauma. The positive statements can actually compete with traumatic recall when triggers are encountered.

Another way some women face triggers and minimize them is by using their imagination. They will write the negative trigger statement several times, each time making their handwriting smaller. They imagine shrinking the writing into a tiny pinpoint and sending it away from them. Or if they view themselves as scared and helpless, they conjure up another image of themselves as a stronger, more powerful person coming to the aid of the frightened self. They see this stronger person helping the scared person. They repeat to themselves, "I'm safer now; I'm stronger now; I'm in charge now."

As you continue using these strategies to defuse your triggers, you will become more adept at staying present in your body. Using these exercises may help you think of other ways to use imagery and mindfulness to take charge of your body.

Predict and Modify Your Reactions to Sex

Once you've established how to remain present in your body, you're ready to predict your reactions to sex and plan strategies for change.

To begin, make a list of sensual or sexual activities you'd be interested in trying. Your list might look like this:

Alone: *Rub my hand gently over my other hand and arm.*

Alone: *Masturbate for five minutes.*

With my partner: *Try French kissing.*

With my partner: *Try massaging each other's butt.*

Next, think about possible negative reactions that could occur with these activities. Be as honest as you can and write the possible reactions next to each sexual activity. For instance:

Gently rub my arm.	Negative reaction: I don't like how my skin feels.
Masturbate for 5 minutes.	Negative reaction: I start to dissociate.
Try French kissing.	Negative reaction: I jerk my head away and feel nervous.
Try massaging each other's butts.	Negative reaction: I hold my breath.

Think about how you could counter each negative reaction by using the soothing techniques you've learned. Write down the technique next to the reaction. If at any time while you're writing you experience a negative reaction, practice the techniques you've learned. For example:

Negative reaction:	I feel sick to my stomach.
Soothing:	I breathe evenly and deeply. I begin self-talk. I tell myself that I can concentrate on how smooth and soft my skin feels. My stomach settles down, and I stay focused on the pleasant tickling sensation.
Negative reaction:	I start to dissociate.
Soothing:	I breathe evenly. I begin self-talking, telling myself to stay present, and I concentrate on my fingers touching my skin. If necessary, I get up and walk around the room and then come back and try again.
Negative reaction:	I jerk my head away and feel nervous.
Soothing:	I breathe evenly. I look at my partner and tell [him or her] that I feel nervous but that I want to continue by first kissing [his or her] cheeks and closed lips. I stay in control of the movements.
Negative reaction:	I hold my breath.
Soothing:	I practice breathing evenly. I take my partner's hand and guide it across my butt. I continue my self-talk, telling myself this is something I want to do for me.

Predicting and modifying your responses will take time and planning. Reread the discussion about triggers and try to think about how each type of trigger might apply to your sexual activity. Think of soothing responses that include breathing, positive self-talk, soothing images, muscle relaxation, and movement.

Setting positive goals for sexual activity is another way of modifying negative reactions. If all you expect from sex are negative reactions, chances are that's exactly what you'll get. But if you set goals like pleasure, satisfaction, calmness, or closeness to your partner, you can counteract possible negative reactions by putting positive expectations in their place. Remember you are in the driver's seat and that makes these new experiences profoundly different from the trauma or neglect in the past.

Revisit your list of three sexual activities that you are interested in trying. Next to each activity, write a positive goal. Try to be realistic when setting these goals. For example, an intense orgasm might be great at some point in the future, but for starters, perhaps feeling calm during lovemaking can be a positive improvement.

Activity	Positive goal
Alone: Rub my arm gently.	I can touch myself and experience a pleasant sensation.
Alone: Masturbate for 5 minutes.	I can touch my body sexually and stay calm.
With my partner: Try French kissing.	I can initiate intimate contact face-to-face and stay present in my body using my soothing techniques.
With my partner: Try massaging each other's butt	I can touch and be touched while breathing evenly and being aware of my ability to enjoy some physical contact.

Negative reactions to sex may never disappear entirely, but their impact will be minimized by your prediction and active control of them.

Practice, Practice, Practice

Being present and predicting/modifying reactions build islands of safety in your sex life, which gives you more control. Now it's time to build an island of pleasure also. Over time, practicing new goals for sexual activity and controlling your response to triggers will bring you both pleasure and a sense of empowerment.

To begin, test out your predictions and remedies by experimenting with various types of sexual activity, perhaps starting with the activities you listed in the previous section. Later you can expand your list of the sexual activities you'd like to enjoy, arranging them from the easiest to the most difficult. Remember to tell your partner about the changes you're seeking.

We suggest you find a way to practice the first sexual activity on your list at least several times a week. You may find it helpful to start your practice with sensory touch, getting comfortable first with your sensory response by yourself and then moving on to masturbation and partner touch. If you feel unsure about masturbating, read more about it in Chapter 13. If you don't have a partner but would like to be in a relationship, then perhaps you'll want to start by making a list of ways to begin to meet people and gain confidence in forming relationships.

As you gain confidence through practice with masturbation, try increasing the intensity of what you're doing. Intentionally try to lose control: go faster, be noisier, let the intensity of the vibrator get stronger, and let your fantasies get a little wilder. Remember to keep remaining in the present. If you start to feel anxious, remember to soothe yourself. If necessary, return to the previous level of activity that was comfortable and continue practicing that until you're ready to move to something more challenging.

After you gain confidence by yourself, you can add sex with your partner. Decide what sexual activities you want to try and tell them in advance to your partner. It helps if your partner is also learning about his or her own sexuality while you're working on your own. Encourage your partner to masturbate and to be positive about sexuality as well.

The two greatest barriers to successful practice are negative self-talk and setting goals that are too ambitious. In Chapter 15 we describe ways to challenge negative thoughts. Reread your list of desired sexual behaviors and break down your goals into smaller, more manageable ones. For instance, if learning to kiss your partner on the mouth is a goal, but it proves to be too overwhelming right now, start with kissing the back of your hand or your forearm. Notice your response to moving your lips moistly over your own skin. When that's comfortable, explain to your partner that you'll begin cheek to cheek, by rubbing skin and enjoying the sensation. Build up slowly to kissing on the mouth. *The Sexual Healing Journey* (Maltz, 2001) and *The Survivor's Guide to Sex* (Haines, 1999) give effective step-by-step suggestions for how to introduce new sexual activities at a slow and comfortable pace.

Practice takes commitment. You may find it helpful to ask a good friend to serve as your check-in to keep you practicing; decide on a way to report to your friend on a regular basis. Or, if you prefer privacy, keep a journal in which you note your progress toward your goals. If practicing is too difficult to do on your own, consider counseling to help you reach your goals.

Take a Break

What about taking a break from practicing if you feel too overwhelmed? Although time away from practice might be all right for a brief period, be careful that it doesn't become avoidance. Avoidance is usually driven by fear of experiencing negative reactions or shame over not being able to overcome them. Throughout this book, we've encouraged you to take responsibility for your sexuality, including your healing. If you find that you are taking a break not because you're turning your attention to other areas of growth but because you're avoiding your sexual discomfort, we encourage you to take responsibility by seeking counseling. Because fear and shame are both profoundly isolating and disconnecting, the sense of restored connection you'll feel through counseling will help you overcome your avoidance and feel more empowered about your sexuality.

What about Pressure from My Partner?

As you work on healing and creating sexual satisfaction, your partner will not always be on the same page. Sometimes you'll both be able to recognize a current stressor that keeps the two of you from finding your balance. And remember, just as you've had challenges in your life, so has your partner. Even if his or her family and past history look perfect compared to the difficulties you've survived, it simply isn't so. Everyone has baggage, and no one is perfect. As your self-awareness grows, one pitfall is that you could perceive your partner's desire and need to be close to you as undermining your growth process. There is much responsibility inherent in personal growth; evaluate your responsibilities carefully so that you don't use your reactions as another form of avoidance. Be ready for those moments when you feel you've mastered an incredibly difficult trigger and shared this with your partner and then he or she does something you feel is insensitive, like touch you in just the way that sets your teeth on edge. This does not mean your partner is Cruella de Vil or the star of *Animal House*, but it does mean you'll both have to own up to working on the bumpy parts. If you want a deeper look at couples communication, dynamics, and even neurobiology, we recommend books, CDs, and websites for couples to improve communication. You'll find them in the "Suggested Resources" at the back of the book. Chances are your partner has an equal amount of work to do. And if you feel you cannot navigate this alone, we encourage you to seek a couples therapist with expertise in this area.

Empower Yourself

Your sexuality can make you feel powerful or powerless. The goal of your work in creating a sexual life is to feel your own empowerment. Sexual activity should always be consensual, meaning that you agree to, and accept, the activity. If you're having sex with a partner, make sure you know exactly what kind of sexual activity you want with this person. Make clear what you want and set limits for what you don't want sexually. Have sex only with partners who practice safer sex.

If you find you can't ask for what you want or can't set limits, you probably aren't ready for partnered sex. Continue the earlier exercises designed to help you be more present in your body and predict/modify your negative reactions. Practice out loud in front of a mirror or with a friend what you want to say to your partner when you feel ready for partnered sex. If your sex life doesn't seem consensual and under your control, we recommend that you see a therapist to help you regain control.

This chapter can be the beginning of change for you. Keep reading other books on sexuality and overcoming trauma. Continue to work on creating your sexual life. Many women also find it helpful to exercise regularly, practice yoga, dance, do body work, or martial arts. Other women find sensory experiences healing, like massage, gardening, painting, or working with clay. These experiences support your efforts to take care of yourself and, because they are body experiences, contribute to a more positive sexuality. You may find individual therapy extremely helpful.

Restoring safety, pleasure, and empowerment to your sexuality takes time. You may want to start a sexual acceptance journal in which you record your experiences as "being present," "predicting," and "practicing." Give yourself permission to celebrate your successes by using "I" statements when you write your accomplishments. For example, your successes might read like this: "I like my sexual fantasies," "I like to masturbate," and "I like oral sex with my partner." Review your journal frequently.

Creating a sexual life after trauma takes courage, patience, and self-love. The more positive sexual experiences you have, in which you are in control and grounded in your body, the better you will feel.

PART IV

Creating a Better Sexual Relationship

Many women enter sexual relationships with the expectation that sex, the most natural thing in the world, will come naturally to two people who love and desire each other. As one woman said, "I figured that my responsibility for good sex with my partner was to show up and not have a headache." Another put it this way: "I was naïve enough to think that just because I wanted to have a good sex life, it would fall out of the sky and into my bed." Unfortunately, sexual relationships don't work like that. Sustaining a satisfying sexual relationship, especially one that fosters mutual growth, requires honest communication, knowledge and exploration, experimentation and practice, generosity, understanding, and even a healthy sense of humor. When you have stars in your eyes, it's not easy to see the rigid gender scripts, cultural myths, sexual ignorance, and stigma that can stand in the way of your having the best possible sexual relationship with your partner. And when you've been together "forever," habit and entrenched expectations (or disappointments) can blind you to the possibilities for a fulfilling sexual future.

Part IV begins with a discussion of men and their sexuality. We certainly realize that not all sexual relationships are heterosexual, but the majority of our readers have been, are, or will be in a relationship with a man. They can benefit from understanding how their male partners function sexually. We then move on to explore the sexual challenges facing all couples—lesbian and straight—and ways to enhance a sexual relationship. Exercises to help couples improve their sexual communication and to open up new, exciting dimensions in their lovemaking can be found in Chapter 14.

Chapters 11 and 12 are dedicated to helping you create a better sexual relationship, no matter what your ages or how long you've been together. By understanding your partner better, having accurate information about sexual behavior, developing effective communication skills, and avoiding the pitfalls that all too often challenge a sexual relationship, you will be able to experience more fully the pleasure that comes from making love. The first step toward achieving these goals is to uncloak the myths and misconceptions that blindside so many sexual relationships. Chapters 11 and 12 address some of the most common ones our clients bring to us, often in the form of questions such as:

- "Is a man supposed to come that quickly?"
- "If men really do have a stronger sex drive than women, why do I want to make love so much more often than my husband?"
- "What's a normal size for a penis?"
- "Does a man who's circumcised feel more pleasure?"
- "If my partner is having trouble getting turned on, does that mean I'm not sexy?"
- "Why don't we feel in love like we used to?"
- "Why does my partner get so defensive when I offer helpful feedback?"
- "If I think my partner is involved in cybersex, what should I do?"
- "As a lesbian, won't my partner and I have an easier time communicating since we're both women?"
- "Straight or gay, what are some strategies to improve a relationship?"
- "I get too reactive when we argue—how can I calm myself down?"
- "How do we start talking about sex with each other?"

ELEVEN

Male Sexuality

Understanding your partner and his or her sexuality is an essential ingredient for achieving sexual satisfaction in a relationship. Whereas lesbian women are usually only as mystified by their partner's sexuality as they are by their own experience of sex, heterosexual women are often somewhat clueless about what makes their partner tick, especially in the bedroom. Sometimes their knowledge of male sexuality is limited to the popular myths floating around, or to biased, and often distorted, explanations provided by their partners. Misinformation is anathema to leading a healthy sexual life and enjoying a happy sexual relationship.

NEWS FLASH: MEN AND WOMEN ARE DIFFERENT

Although men and women have identical anatomical structures for the first 6 weeks after conception and are born, raised, and educated in the same environments, their experiences differ dramatically. When women are frustrated, for example, they may find relief in tears; men may erupt into anger. When a little boy is hit by a pitched ball, the mother wants to nurture and console; the father insists that it will toughen him up. When women encounter conflict, they want to "talk it out"; men may swagger, posture, and bump bellies. Women can embrace; men settle for a handshake. When a special moment occurs between two lovers, women might say, "I love you"; men might think, or even say, "Let's screw." When lost, women will ask for directions. There are men, on the other hand, whose pictures appear on milk cartons because after 10 years they're still driving around searching for their destination.

Obviously these examples are stereotypical and admittedly unfair, but there's enough truth here to highlight something we all know: men truly are different, not superior or inferior, but different from women. Yet as different and mysterious as men might be, it is usually a man who becomes a woman's life-mate. It's often with a man that a woman faces the joys and challenges of life—leaving home, pursuing a career, raising a family, grieving losses, and growing old. Understanding men and their sexuality is therefore important, because it can help women to better love them, live with them, and be sexual with them.

Throughout the remainder of this chapter we will attempt to remove some of the mystery about men and their sexuality. Because this is a book about sex, we're going to restrict our focus to men's sexual behavior. We'll look at how their bodies respond to sexual excitement and how their sexual ability is affected by worry, illness, and age. We encourage you to check the resource list at the end of the book for suggested reading on personality and behavioral differences between men and women and ways that men and women can relate to each other in more effective, respectful, and loving ways.

MALE SEXUAL ANATOMY

An understanding of male sexual anatomy is a prerequisite to understanding male sexuality. Once we understand the parts, we can make better sense of how they respond and work together in sexual situations.

Penis

The penis is often the epicenter of a man's sense of manhood, potency, and sexuality. It's made up of muscular and spongy tissue wrapped by an elastic sheathing. This organ performs two very basic and important functions. By means of the urethra, a tube that runs from the bladder to the tip of the penis, the penis allows the man both to void his bladder and to deliver semen to a woman's womb. Because of this latter function, for thousands of years the penis has had a mythical significance in many cultures around the world. Phallic symbols have often served as sacred icons in early religions that revered fertility, that mysterious process that participates in the power of creation.

The shaft of the penis consists of three tubes, or cylinders, two of them resting on top of the third (see Figure 11.1). The top two cigar-shaped tubes are called the *corpora cavernosa*, and the bottom tube the *corpus spongiosum*. The urethra runs through the bottom tube, from end to end. These tubes consist of spongy tissue, small smooth muscles, nerve fibers, and blood vessels. They're wrapped in a tough, elastic sheathing called the *tunica albuginea*. When the penis is aroused, the corporal bodies become engorged with blood, which expands the tunica the way air inflates a rubber tire. Just as the rubber stretches to its natural limit and the tire becomes solid, the tunica stretches until the shaft of the penis becomes rigid.

The *tunica albuginea* surrounding the bottom tube is thinner than the sheathing surrounding the upper corporal bodies. When erect, the bottom tube is not as rigid

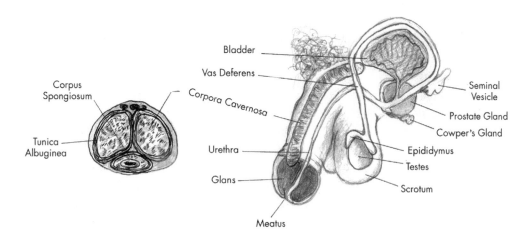

FIGURE 11.1. Male sexual organs.

as the upper tubes, which is why it's called the corpus spongiosum, or the spongy body. During an erection, the corpus spongiosum looks like a ridge protruding along the underside of the penile shaft.

The end of the corpus spongiosum extends past the two upper tubes and forms the head of the penis, called the *glans*. During an erection, the glans becomes engorged with blood and grows larger in size, but unlike the rest of the penile shaft, it has no sheathing and will remain soft and spongy. This quality makes the glans a natural cushion for when the penis thrusts back and forth inside the vagina during intercourse. At the tip of the glans is the urinary opening of the urethra, called the *meatus*.

The place where penile skin meets the glans is called the *coronal ridge*. In newborn and uncircumcised males, skin extends from the coronal ridge forward to cover the glans (inner foreskin), folds over and doubles back over the glans (outer foreskin), and continues back along the penile shaft to the abdomen. The foreskin is connected to the underside of the penis, just behind the glans, by a ridge of skin called the *frenulum*. This ridge or fold of skin is similar to the ridge of skin stretching between the underside of your tongue and the floor of your mouth. The frenulum pulls the foreskin over the glans when the penis is flaccid. The glans, coronal ridge, and frenulum have many more nerve endings than the shaft of the penis and are very sensitive to stimulation. During an erection the foreskin tends to retract, especially during intercourse, making these sensitive areas (glans, frenulum, and coronal ridge) more accessible to direct stimulation.

In a circumcision, the folded-over foreskin is cut away just beyond the coronal ridge, leaving the glans of the penis permanently exposed. Circumcisions are performed for cultural, religious, cosmetic, and health reasons. Today in the United States, there is a robust debate about the advantages and disadvantages of circumcision. Proponents argue that circumcision decreases the risk of developing infections and contracting STIs. Opponents object to infants being subjected to the traumatic pain of a surgical procedure without the benefit of anesthesia. They point out that good hygiene and safer-sex practices reduce the reported risks of infection, some of which appear to be based on questionable scientific data.

Men have also wondered whether there are sexual advantages or disadvantages to being circumcised. It's a classic case of "The grass is always greener on the other side of the fence." Uncircumcised men have wondered whether absence of the foreskin makes intercourse more pleasurable for men who are circumcised. Circumcised men have wondered whether the foreskin makes it easier for uncircumcised men to maintain ejaculatory control. In truth, no evidence supports differences in the sexual experience of circumcised and uncircumcised men. Actually, when an uncircumcised penis is erect and inserted in the vagina, the foreskin is pulled back so that the glans is stimulated in the same way as the glans of a circumcised penis.

What about Size?

While discussing the penis, we may as well address the age-old question about size. Rarely will you meet a man who, in his heart of hearts, does not wish that his penis were a little, or in some cases a lot, bigger. Men are hounded by the belief that to measure their manhood, you must measure their penis. They worry that anything less than a gargantuan appendage will disappoint and fail to satisfy their partner.

The average length of a flaccid penis is between 3.5 and 4 inches. The average length of an erect penis is between 5 and 7 inches. Size of a flaccid penis can vary depending on external temperature, mood, and even body weight. The penile shaft does not stop where it connects with the torso but actually continues internally and anchors to the pubic bone. When a man gains weight, more of his penis ends up inside of his body. Also, a shorter flaccid penis will expand proportionately much more dramatically when erect than a longer penis does.

Does Size Make a Difference?

Yes and no. These days the politically correct answer is: size makes no difference. But this is not totally accurate. Even though men often wish they had a larger penis, an extremely large penis can be problematic. On occasion we see couples who are distressed over not being able to have pain-free intercourse because of the excessive girth of the man's penis. For them, size definitely *does* make a difference, but unfortunately a negative one.

Size also makes a positive difference for some women. They enjoy the feeling of surrounding and containing a penis that stretches the vaginal opening. They report that it's pleasurable when they feel like the penis "fills them up." Although this pleasurable feeling depends partially on adequate muscle tone around the opening of the vagina, the girth of the penis will also contribute to the "filled-up" sensation. In addition to girth, the length of the penis makes a difference for some women, who enjoy the sensation during intercourse that occurs when a penis is long enough to stimulate the cervix directly.

In a survey of 25,000 women taken by MSNBC and *Elle* magazine, 84% of the women were totally satisfied with the size of their partner's penis, and 2% wished their partner were smaller. The remainder expressed the wish that their partner was larger. Interestingly, more than 25,000 men participated in the same survey, and almost half expressed the wish that they had larger penises, even if they perceived themselves to be average sized or better (Lever et al., 2006).

So if size can make a difference, does this mean that a woman has been short-changed if her partner is not well endowed? Or that a man with a small or average-sized penis cannot be a good lover? Absolutely not. Sexual pleasure is the result of multiple factors. The presence or absence of any one particular sensation will not make or break the sexual experience. Although direct stimulation of the cervix or feeling stretched by penile girth can be pleasurable for some women, the major source of genital response is stimulation of the clitoris and nerve endings within the first 2 to 3 inches of the vagina. These highly erogenous areas, including the G spot, are well within the reach of even an unusually small penis. This is why it's not surprising that national surveys show that the majority of women downplay the significance of size. Research also shows that sexual arousal and satisfaction for women are dependent on much more than direct stimulation of the genitals. Affection, emotional intimacy, and communication are equally critical ingredients for a woman's sexual pleasure.

The Scrotum: What's in the Sac?

The scrotum is a pouch of loose, wrinkled skin that is lined by a thin layer of muscle called the *tunica dartos*. Hanging below the penis, the scrotum has two compartments, one for each of the testicles. The testicles are oval glands measuring about an inch wide and an inch and a half long. The testicles produce testosterone and sperm. Testosterone is an important hormone for sexual desire, sperm production, and the development of secondary male characteristics. If a man loses his testicles before puberty, he will be sterile as an adult; he will likely have little interest in sex; his voice will not deepen; and he will not develop the pattern of body and facial hair characteristic of adult men. Damage to the testicles after puberty can lead to sexual and reproductive problems. Fortunately, most men need only one functioning testicle for normal development, sexual response, and reproductive capability.

Starting with puberty, sperm production is continuous throughout the remainder of a man's life. Fifty-thousand sperm are produced every minute in the testicles, but it takes more than 70 days for the sperm to mature fully. On the back, upper surface of each testicle, 5 to 7 yards of tiny tubing are tightly coiled back and forth into an oval structure called the *epididymis*. After sperm are manufactured in the testicles, they move to the epididymis for storage and maturation. When a man becomes sexually aroused, as many as 500 million mature sperm are moved through the *vas deferens*, a tube connecting each testicle to the urethra. When a man has a vasectomy, the vas deferens from each testicle is severed, which prevents sperm from passing from the testicles to the penis.

Sperm need to be manufactured and stored at about 2 degrees lower than normal body temperature. This is why the testicles, unlike ovaries, are positioned away from the torso. It's probably advantageous that sperm can't survive very long at normal body temperature. Otherwise, once they are deposited in the vagina, they would be free to set up housekeeping and wander around until they could impregnate an ovum. Pregnancy rates would be incredibly high, arguably at a rate that would be maladaptive for the species.

As the thin muscle lining of the scrotum expands and contracts, the testicles are positioned farther away from, or closer to, the torso, thereby regulating temperature. When a man comes out of the shower or a hot tub, his scrotal sac looks distended—the body is trying to cool the testes by removing them from heat generated by the torso. On the other hand, during exercise, sexual arousal, or when a man feels anxious or threatened, the testicles are drawn up closer to the torso, protecting them from being fully exposed to possible harm.

It's normal for one testicle to hang lower than the other. This uneven positioning provides protection for both testicles by preventing them from being squeezed together between a man's legs.

Seminal Vesicles

Males have two *seminal vesicles*, which are small glands located behind the bladder. The opening of these glands joins with the vasa deferentia (plural for vas deferens) and connects to the urethra in the prostate. When a man orgasms, the seminal vesicles contract, secreting a fluid rich with fructose that helps nourish the sperm. Fluid from the seminal vesicles makes up about two-thirds of the *ejaculate*, which is another name for semen emitted, or about to be emitted, during ejaculation.

Prostate

The prostate is a muscular gland that surrounds a man's urethra at the base of the bladder. The portion of the urethra running through the prostate is called the *prostatic urethra* and is where semen collects for ejaculation. At the top of the prostate, where it joins to the opening of the bladder, a circular band of muscle, called the *internal urethral sphincter*, squeezes shut during orgasm to prevent ejaculate from going up into the bladder. At the other end of the prostate, another circular band of muscle, the *external urethral sphincter*, tightens as the prostatic urethra fills with ejaculate. This action allows semen to collect in the prostate just prior to ejaculation.

Secretions from the prostate gland combine with sperm from the vasa deferentia and fluid from the seminal vesicles and make up about a third of the ejaculate. Even though there may be as many as 500 million sperm in an average ejaculation, sperm make up only a minuscule part of the ejaculate. For that reason, men do not experience any noticeable change in their ejaculation after a vasectomy.

When a man ejaculates, the internal urethral sphincter squeezes shut the opening of the bladder, and the urethra and pelvic musculature go through a series of contractions to expel the semen from the prostatic urethra. Because the bladder is shut off and the external urethral sphincter is relaxed, the semen can go in only one direction—down the length of the shaft and out through the tip of the penis.

Some men develop ejaculation problems when the prostate is damaged. A common treatment for an enlarged prostate that is blocking the free flow of urine through the prostatic urethra is called a *transurethral resection of the prostate* (TURP). During this procedure, an instrument is threaded through the urethra, and excess tissue inside the prostate is clipped. If, in the process, damage is done to the opening of the bladder, it may not close properly during orgasm. If this happens, during ejaculation semen will seek the path of least resistance. Rather than going down the length of the penis, the semen will go into the bladder. The man will experience the pleasurable sensations of orgasm, but he will have a dry ejaculation, called *retrograde ejaculation*. With this condition, he may notice white fluid in his urine when he voids after sexual activity. This is perfectly normal; the retrograde ejaculate is voided from the bladder during urination. Diabetes can cause similar problems by interfering with the nerve fibers that control the opening and closing of the bladder during sexual excitement.

If the prostate is surgically removed, a man will still be capable of experiencing an orgasm, but he will not ejaculate. With the removal of the prostate gland, the vasa deferentia and seminal vesicles no longer connect to the urethra. Prostatic fluid, seminal fluid, and sperm are no longer available to create ejaculate.

Cowper's Glands

The Cowper's glands are two small glands that connect to the urethra below the prostate. During sexual arousal, these glands secrete a mucous substance into the urethra that protects the sperm cells by neutralizing any acidity that may remain in the urethra from earlier urination. The discharge from the Cowper's glands also serves as a lubricant for the glans of the penis.

SEXUAL RESPONSE

It's easiest to understand the male sexual response if we divide it into the same categories of desire, arousal, and orgasm that we used for women.

Desire

Sexual desire, or the slang equivalent—"being horny"—is a *receptivity* to sexual activity and a *responsiveness* to sexual stimulation. Signs of sexual desire can include sexual thoughts, sexual fantasies, seeking out opportunities for sexual activity, or enjoying sexual interaction. For men it often but not always precedes an erection and ejaculation. Just as is the case for some women, on occasion a man may not experience sexual desire (interest) until he first becomes sexually aroused. Men, like women, can become aroused and orgasm without sexual desire, but the presence or absence of desire will greatly influence sexual frequency and satisfaction.

Hormones and neurotransmitters play an important role for men in generating sexual appetite. Research has shown that the frequency of sexual thoughts and fantasies increases and decreases in tandem with rises and drops in *testosterone* levels. Testosterone is one of a number of steroid hormones that can alter a "sensory threshold," which refers to the lowest level at which a stimulus can trigger a response. If a woman's flirtatious smile is normally a sexual cue for a man, he will be more likely to pick up on it and respond to it if his testosterone level is in the normal range. If his hormone level is below normal, he may miss or ignore the cue. Research also suggests that testosterone levels increase genital sensitivity to stimulation. Testosterone therefore affects sexual desire not only by increasing the chances of a man picking up on a sexual cue but also by increasing the probability that he will respond physically.

As for neurotransmitters, the brain requires a balance of sexual excitation and sexual inhibition. Without this balance, a person could be either sexually out of control or sexually inert. Prolactin and serotonin tend to inhibit sexual drive, whereas dopamine and norepinephrine tend to stimulate sexual interest. Dopamine in particular appears to play an important role in exciting sexual desire. While testosterone appears to drive lust in general, dopamine appears to play a role in finding the object of desire attractive, if ever so briefly, and prompting the pursuit of sexual pleasure.

Is there a gender difference in sexual desire? Are men biologically driven by a stronger sex drive than women? If you give any credence to all the corny jokes about men who think with their penises and women who have perpetual headaches, you might believe that men are innately more highly sexed than women are. It's not true. Both women and men are capable of having strong sex drives. If there is a gender difference when it comes to sexual interest, it's not that biology makes men want sex more than women do but rather how our culture conditions women and men differently.

Throughout this book we have touched on how culture can inhibit the development of a woman's comfort with her sexuality. Our dominant culture tends to evaluate the significance of sexual behavior differently for women and men. Most men, for example, have been programmed to interpret having sex as the ultimate evidence of their desirability and masculinity. Early in life, having sex is equated with conquest; only losers can't "get any." Men learn that having sex increases not only their prestige but also the worth or value of any occasion during which it occurs. A date, a special evening, or a vacation is always best if there's sex; without sex, the event is less than perfect.

That's not necessarily the case for women—at least, not as often. Sex can be great, but for many women it's not as critical an ingredient for making an event or occasion special as it is for most men. Being sexually desired by a man can be nice, but it isn't necessarily a compliment. Women are well aware that men have been conditioned to seek sex for sex's sake, and they certainly know that sexual attention may not always be a sign of affection. For many women, being held, respected, and listened to—not sex—signal that they're special, cherished, and desired. None of this is intended to imply that men enjoy sex more than women or that men have an innately stronger sex drive than women. But men and women tend to assign different roles to sex, and that difference can give the impression of a general difference in desire. Even though social stereotypes suggest that men are always ready for sex, in truth, men, just like women, have sexual appetites that fluctuate according to not only hormonal levels but also emotional state, health factors, energy level, and external circumstances.

Arousal

As is the case with most natural body functions, the erection process appears simple and straightforward, but in reality, it is quite complex and susceptible to a wide variety of things that can go wrong.

There is a network of small, smooth muscles in the corporal bodies that, when the penis is soft, are in a natural state of contraction. Blood enters the corporal bodies through arteries running down the center of the tubes. The blood nourishes the penile tissue and flows back to the torso through a series of veins located just beneath the penile sheathing, the tunica albuginea.

When a man becomes sexually aroused, impulses are sent along *parasympathetic* nerve fibers in the penis that trigger the release of *cyclic GMP*, a chemical that relaxes the smooth muscles and blood vessels. As the arteries and muscles relax, blood quickly pours in. The spongy tissue expands as it fills with blood, and the tunica begins to stretch. When the corporal bodies expand and push out against the tunica, they pinch the outgoing veins. Pressure builds in the penis as blood pours in but can only trickle back out because the veins are pinched. As a result, the man has a rigid erection.

For this process to work, the blood vessels and nerve endings must perform flawlessly. If the arteries are blocked, blood will not flow in quickly enough to create the pressure necessary for an erection. If the veins have leaks in them, the penis will inflate initially but, like inflating a tire with a pinhole, will keep deflating. If injury, surgery, or illness damages the nerve fibers, the signal for the smooth muscles and arteries to relax will never arrive, and the penis will remain limp regardless of what kind of sexual activity is taking place. The signal to the smooth muscles and arteries can also be overridden by the effects of certain medications and by stress and distraction.

While the penis is becoming erect, a number of additional changes take place throughout the body. Breathing, heart rate, and blood pressure all increase. Blood flow to the skin may cause a rash-like appearance, called a sex flush, over various parts of the body. This blood flow also makes parts of the body, including the earlobes, lips, and nipples, more sensitive to stimulation. The testicles become engorged with blood and increase in size. The tunica dartos, the muscle lining the scrotal sack, thickens and contracts, drawing the testicles closer to the torso. A drop or two of a clear, slippery fluid from the Cowper's glands appears at the opening of the urethra.

Orgasm

People often use the words *ejaculation* and *orgasm* interchangeably, but this is not technically correct. When we talk about male orgasm, we are talking about a complex body response that may or may not include ejaculation. At the time of orgasm, intense muscular contractions will occur in the pelvis while a chemical reaction takes place in the brain, resulting in a release of tension and feelings of satisfaction and relaxation (Komisaruk et al., 2010).

Men can orgasm even if they do not ejaculate. For example, after the prostate gland is removed, it is physically impossible for a man to ejaculate, yet when sexually stimulated his body will still experience muscular contractions and brain-induced feelings of pleasure.

Men can also ejaculate without experiencing orgasm. For example, some men with severe cases of premature ejaculation can ejaculate not only before becoming erect, but before the brain can produce the pleasurable sensations associated with orgasm. Men with spinal cord injury can induce ejaculation even though no physical sensations register in the brain.

Ejaculation: Emission Phase

Male ejaculation occurs in two phases: emission followed by expulsion. The emission phase begins when sexual arousal reaches the necessary level of intensity. A series of contractions in the *vasa deferentia*, the seminal vesicles, and the prostate gland force sperm and ejaculatory fluid into the prostatic urethra. At the same time, the small circular band of muscles surrounding the urethra at the base of the prostate (external urethral sphincter) and at the opening of the bladder (internal urethral sphincter) contract, keeping the ejaculate inside the prostate. Once this emission phase occurs, ejaculation will occur, regardless of any distraction.

Ejaculation: Expulsion Phase

During the expulsion phase, the external urethral sphincter relaxes, opening up the passageway for ejaculation. At the same time, the urethra, prostate gland, and muscles at the base of the penis go into involuntary, rhythmic contractions spaced about 0.8 second apart. The timing of these contractions is similar to the timing of a woman's muscular contractions during orgasm. Because the external urethral sphincter relaxes, the ejaculate is expelled down the length of the penis and out the urethral opening.

Numerous factors can affect *ejaculatory latency*, which is the length of time between the start of stimulation and ejaculation. A man may take longer to ejaculate if he is fatigued, distracted, or lacks desire. Alcohol and some medications and other drugs can also delay or even prevent ejaculation. Anxiety, heightened sexual excitement, or a lack of recent sexual activity, on the other hand, can cause a man to ejaculate more rapidly than he is accustomed to.

Neurochemistry of Orgasm

At the moment of orgasm, it appears that the reward center of the brain (the *nucleus accumbens*) is briefly activated, resulting in a pleasurable sensation washing over the body. Heart rate, blood pressure, and respiration all increase, followed by a sense of release and relaxation. We still don't understand the chemistry very well, but it appears that the neurotransmitter dopamine plays a critical role, spiking right before orgasm and sensitizing the nucleus accumbens. Within seconds of orgasm, the hormone *prolactin* spikes and brings the person quickly "back to earth." Prolactin appears to be a sexual "wet blanket": when it is abnormally elevated in the brain, sometimes due to a medication side effect, a person will have considerable difficulty experiencing orgasm.

Postorgasm Changes

As noted, when a man becomes erect, impulses travel along nerve fibers (part of the parasympathetic nervous system) to relax the arteries and smooth muscles inside the penis. Shortly after orgasm, impulses are sent along a different set of nerve fibers (part of the sympathetic nervous system) to the same smooth muscles inside the penis. During a process called *detumescence*, the nerve impulses signal these muscles to contract. An enzyme, *phosphodiesterase-5* (PDE-5), is released to break down the cyclic GMP, the chemical that relaxed the arteries and smooth muscles in the first place. As a result, the muscles and arteries return to their normal state, and the pressure-squeeze on the outgoing veins is released. As the little muscles begin to contract, blood is literally wrung out of the corporal bodies into the veins and back out into the body cavity. The penis becomes flaccid again.

As the blood-flow pattern is reversed following orgasm, a man enters a refractory period, which is a period of time when the body is not capable of rearousal and orgasm. This refractory period can be very brief for young men—so brief that they may be ready to orgasm again before losing their original erection. The refractory period varies dramatically from man to man and often increases with age. As men approach their senior years, the refractory period can increase the downtime between orgasms to hours or even days.

AGING

A number of years ago, a man in his late 40s made an appointment with one of us because of an erection problem. He explained that he could get erect during only about half of his attempts at intercourse. This was particularly upsetting because he was in a new relationship, and he felt frustrated and embarrassed by his difficulty responding to his new partner. His partner was beginning to question whether she was doing something to turn him off or, worse yet, perhaps he didn't find her attractive. He was desperate.

We agreed that a 50% failure rate certainly suggested a problem, so we pressed for more details. The man explained that he had just ended a very bad 20-year marriage, the final years of which had been sexless. Now he was madly in love with his new partner. On the nights he and his partner got together, they would make love, and it would be wonderful—so wonderful that minutes later they would want to do it again. They were in the "honeymoon phase" of their relationship, and the novelty and excitement of a new relationship triggered a sexual appetite that the man had not experienced since he was in his 20s. But always during the second attempt, things wouldn't work—he couldn't get an erection. That's how he figured that he had an erection problem 50% of the time: the first attempt of each evening would be successful; the second attempt would not.

It never occurred to this man that the difficulty he was experiencing was perfectly normal for his age. When he was in his 20s, he could easily get an erection two, three, four, or even more times during the course of the evening. With the gradual deterioration of his marriage, however, it had been years since he last attempted to make love multiple times, so he was unaware of normal body changes that had occurred slowly over time. He had no idea that his refractory period had increased so that now it might take an hour or two after an orgasm before he would be able to become erect again. Had he known about this normal, age-related change in his sexual functioning, he and his partner could have been spared a great deal of worry and grief.

This example highlights the importance of awareness of the normal sexual changes that occur as men grow older. Many of these age-related changes can become evident as early as a man's 30s. These changes will continue slowly through each succeeding decade of life. In no way do these changes prevent men and their partners from enjoying sexual intimacy. Age alone will not eliminate sexual desire; it will not prevent a man from getting or staying erect; and it will not take away a man's ability to orgasm. Aging may slow down and modify how the body responds sexually, but it will not prevent a man from enjoying sexual activity. Men in their 80s can continue to have highly satisfying sexual experiences even though their bodies may no longer respond like the body of an 18-year-old. Knowledge of these changes prevents needless performance concerns that can easily distract and dismay both the man and his partner.

In this section we look at common changes that most men experience as part of the course of normal aging. When changes in sexual function are more dramatic or extreme than the changes described below, they may be due to more than aging: they may be the result of injury, disease, or psychological inhibition. Sexual dysfunctions, which are abnormal changes in sexual response, are discussed later in this chapter.

Decreased Sexual Drive

During their teens and early 20s men may feel like they're walking erections. It can seem like sex is always on their mind. If they're in a relationship, they'll tend to emphasize sexual frequency and initiate lovemaking every chance they get. As they move into their 30s, men still have strong sex drives, but the novelty of sex has begun to wear off, and job and family responsibilities compete for their energy and attention. By their late 40s and early 50s, many men find that their sex drives are beginning to decrease. A large part of this change is due to slowly decreasing levels of testosterone, the hormone essential for sexual appetite. Sexual desire, along with testosterone levels, continues to decline slowly as a man approaches his senior years. In later life, the man will respond with interest when presented with a sexual opportunity, but spontaneous thoughts about sex and an unrelenting drive to initiate sex will be much less common than during his younger years.

Psychological factors can inhibit sexual desire for men as they age. Men are not immune to vanity. As they grow older, many become distressed by graying hair, receding hairlines, protruding bellies, disappearing chins, drooping eyelids, and reading glasses. Gym memberships, hair coloring, and hair restoration products are part of a multimillion-dollar-a-year industry that caters to men trying to retain a youthful appearance. But changes in appearance don't seem to have a big impact on men's sexual desire. Whereas women often need to feel desirable to feel sexual desire, men apparently do not. Instead, men are highly concerned about sexual prowess. Some men, when they note subtle changes in their sexual response, feel threatened and pull back from sexual activity. Better not to be tested, they reason, than to be tested and fail. By avoiding sex, they avoid the potential humiliation of erectile failure. Unfortunately, in the process, they also miss out on opportunities to share physical and emotional intimacy with their partners.

Takes Longer to Get Hard

Whereas teens often fight to keep their erections down (outside the bedroom, of course), as men get older, it can feel like a fight to get and keep their erections. Accustomed to having instant erections in response to any sexual situation, middle-aged men may be threatened by finding that it takes longer to get an erection. This change is normal and should in no way interfere with lovemaking. Unfortunately, if the man begins to panic because he doesn't have an instant erection, he can worry himself out of responding.

Need for Fiction and Friction

Sex therapists like to say that an erection requires fiction and friction. The *fiction* refers to mental activity: think sexy thoughts and nature takes its course. *Friction* refers to the direct stimulation of the penis. When in his teens or early 20s, a man needs only one of these two ingredients. Either wearing jeans that are too tight or seeing a girl in a sweater that's too tight is often all that is needed to produce an erection. As he gets older, however, sexy thoughts or direct stimulation alone will usually not be enough. For a middle-aged man to become and stay erect, his mind will have to be focused on erotic thoughts, and his penis will require ongoing stimulation.

A common occurrence for a man as he gets older is to panic when his erection decreases during early sex play. When he was younger and became erect, it would seem that nothing short of an orgasm or an act of Congress would make the penis go down. Later in life, however, a disturbing change occurs. One night he goes to bed with his partner, and during the initial groping and caressing, an erection develops. Nothing out of the ordinary so far. Having learned to be a "good lover," the man focuses on pleasuring his partner further before attempting intercourse. He dutifully does all the things the sex manuals instructed him to do. He gently plays with her nipples, strokes her thighs, caresses her clitoris, maybe even tries to find and stimulate her G spot. Finally her quiet moans and pelvic rocking signal that she's ready for him. But, lo and behold, when he looks down, he finds that his erection has abandoned him. He panics and desperately struggles to regain the erection. Unfortunately, desperation is the slayer of erections, and he ends up having nothing to show for his efforts other than a cold sweat.

What is important for this man to realize is that as he gets older, his erections will require continued physical stimulation. Stop direct stimulation, and erections will likely go down. It's normal for an erection to go temporarily soft during love play. If the man doesn't panic, the erection will typically come back when the penis is directly stimulated again. It should take limited effort because he's not starting from scratch: the penile tissue is already stretched and additional blood has already collected in the pelvic area. The important thing is for the man not to fret.

Stress, fatigue, or distraction can occasionally cause difficulty in regaining or maintaining an erection. It's important for the couple to remain flexible. Contrary to the myth that good sex equals intercourse, partners can be highly sensual with each other without the presence of an erection.

Greater Variability in Erections

Most young men have two kinds of erections—rock-hard and harder than a rock. As men get older, however, erections become much more variable. A man in his late 30s or early 40s may find that on one day he has an erection reminiscent of his early youth, and on the next day an erection that's usable but pliable. Over time, rock-hard, rigid erections will appear less often, but the penis will still be able to become sufficiently erect for vaginal entry and thrusting. Sexual activity will continue to be highly pleasurable.

Another quite normal change in erections, but one that worries men, is the angle of their erection. Typically when standing, a young man will have an erection that points toward the ceiling, sometimes at a 50-degree angle away from the body. Young men often delight in the strength of their erections, taking pride in silly things like being able to hang a bath towel on an erect penis. Because of changes in penile blood flow and the elasticity of pelvic musculature as men grow older, the erect penis will eventually stop pointing to the ceiling, but instead to the wall, and in time, perhaps, even to the floor.

Takes Longer to Ejaculate

One often positive age-related change in a man's sexual response is the lengthening of the time it takes before ejaculation occurs. Age can be a surefire cure for rapid ejaculation. Young men tend to ejaculate very rapidly. With age and increased sexual experience, they develop the ability to last longer. As they enter their later years, however, some men find that it takes so long to ejaculate that, on occasion, they will end lovemaking before having an orgasm.

Although most women are quite accepting of the possibility that not every sexual encounter leads to orgasm, men have been conditioned to think differently. The lovemaking might be the most beautiful and exciting experience imaginable, but if they don't climax, men tend to write off the experience as a failure. Some men in later life even avoid lovemaking altogether rather than going through the frustration of not ejaculating.

It's important for men—and the women who love them—to realize that, as they get older, not only will it take longer to orgasm, but on occasion they might not be able to ejaculate. More important, older men need to discover what many women already know from experience—that lovemaking can be very satisfying even if there isn't an orgasm.

Ejaculation Changes

Even in his 30s a man will begin to notice changes in his ejaculation. It is very normal for the amount of ejaculate, the force of expulsion, and the number of muscular contractions to decrease with age. Young men can shoot a teaspoon of ejaculate a foot or more into the air. Older men may note that when they orgasm, perhaps less than a teaspoon of ejaculate will dribble, rather than spurt, from the urethral opening. These changes are normal and should not interfere with sexual satisfaction.

Detumescence Is Quicker

It takes a young man much longer for his erection to go down after ejaculation than it does for an older man. After an orgasm during intercourse, a young man may remain in his partner's vagina for minutes while enjoying the few additional moments of physical closeness in his postorgasmic glow. An older man may find his soft penis slipping out of the vagina almost immediately after ejaculation. All, however, is not lost. The older man also can enjoy physical closeness with his partner during his postcoital glow by cuddling with her. Like all the changes described above, quick detumescence is a change that should have no impact on sexual satisfaction, unless the man or woman is misguided by misinformation or unrealistic expectations.

Size: Everything Seems to Shrink with Age

An elderly patient complained, "Getting older, I can accept the aches and pains, thinning hair, poor hearing, and, thanks to Viagra, even the soft erections. But enough is enough—my !@#$%& penis is getting smaller!" Men do love their penises, no matter their age. And yes, many men will find that as they age, their penis will decrease in size. Part of the problem is the middle spread many men acquire as they get older—as we mentioned earlier, abdominal fat envelops part of the penile shaft, making it look shorter or nonexistent. This change is reversible—lose weight—but other changes occur that are irreversible (Freeman, 2009). Atherosclerotic changes in penile blood vessels and the buildup of inelastic collagen in penile tissue result in shrinkage of both the length and girth of the penis. A 30-year-old with a 6-inch erection may lose up to an inch by the time he is in his 60s. And while we're breaking the bad news, we should mention that the testicles shrink in size as a man grows older, perhaps in part due to age-related decreases in testosterone.

Thoughts on Sex and Aging

When looking at age-related changes in a man's sexual response, we might be tempted to conclude that aging has only negative effects: less desire, slower and less rigid erections, delays in ejaculation, even a smaller penis. As we've already said, however, these are normal changes and need not affect a couple's sexual pleasure and satisfaction. Nevertheless, these changes may make a man feel sad, helpless, or angry—all of which are part of grieving. It is important for him to recognize that his sexual response is different, that he will have feelings about this, and that he might need time to adjust. It is part of getting used to the "new normal" of being older. Grieving loss is a vital part of remaining open to passion and connection—and part of a life well lived.

Finally, it's important to realize that there are definite positives that emerge as men grow older. The sexual drive of an older man is often more closely attuned to his partner's drive than when he and his partner were younger. Many men in long-term relationships become more comfortable with physical and emotional intimacy. They have learned to feel more secure about their manhood and sexuality and, as a result, become far more sensitive lovers. We have often seen older men who have become much more responsive to touch. When we work with older couples, we're impressed hearing them talk about how much they enjoy the eroticism of touch—massaging, holding, and caressing each other. Sometimes women muse about how much their physical relationship has changed from the early years when sex involved "copping a feel, having a quickie, and falling asleep." They describe how genital sex has become only one portion of an extended, loving, physical connectedness between the two partners.

SEXUAL DYSFUNCTIONS

Slight alterations in the phases of sexual response are perfectly normal with aging. Sometimes, however, the phases of sexual response can be totally disrupted or shut down by psychological or medical factors. These sexual dysfunctions can be very alarming, both to the men who experience them and to the women who are their sexual partners. Understanding why they occur can ease the minds of couples and steer them in the right direction for help.

Loss of Desire

According to social stereotypes, real men want sex, and lots of it. It's women, not men, who get headaches and try to avoid sex. But it's just not true. Loss of sexual desire is a common problem for both men and women. In a 1994 U.S. study of more than 1,300 men aged 18 to 59, almost 16% acknowledged lacking interest in sex

(Laumann et al., 1994). In a 29-nation study of 13,618 men between the ages of 40 and 80, the incidence of low sexual interest ranged from 12.5% to 28%, depending on the geographic region (Laumann et al., 2005). Causes of this problem can include medical illness, testosterone deficiencies, adverse reactions to medication, depression, relationship problems, sexual conflict, reaction to erection problems, and stress.

It's very difficult for men to admit to others, or even to themselves, that they have lost their interest in sex. They will deny it, bury themselves in their work, and, when pressed, make excuses to avoid sexual intimacy. If confronted directly about his avoidance of sex, a man may try blaming his partner, suggesting that her weight gain, past history of sexual indifference, or unwillingness to experiment has finally beaten down his interest in sex.

If a man loses his sexual desire, a physical examination should be the first step in trying to understand and resolve the problem. A healthcare provider can make sure that there are no medical problems affecting the man's sex drive. If a medical problem is discovered, the healthcare provider can prescribe appropriate treatment.

For example, when hormone levels are abnormally low, testosterone can be administered in a number of ways: an injection, a gel applied on the skin, pellets inserted beneath the skin, or a mouth patch placed on the upper gum and absorbed through the mucous membrane in the mouth. In appropriately screened cases, testosterone augmentation can help to restore sexual desire as well as improve erectile response. Oral testosterone supplements are ineffective and can have undesirable liver complications. Despite claims often made in the popular press, however, testosterone is not a miracle drug and offers no advantage when hormone levels are already normal.

Sexual desire for men, whether acted upon or not, can be active and vital even in the face of chronic illness and treatments that eliminate testosterone altogether. As with women, the quality of their relationship and history may, in some cases, trump even the most daunting of challenges.

It appears that dopamine *agonists* (medications that increase dopamine activity) may have a positive impact on sexual desire. Although as of early 2011 no dopamine agonist is currently approved in the United States for the treatment of low sexual desire, experimental drugs are undergoing clinical trials and show promise as a new approach for addressing this problem.

If a man experiencing low sexual desire gets a clean bill of health, consulting a sex therapist may be a helpful next step. For more information on sex therapy, see Chapter 16.

Erection Problems

The sexual problem that strikes the greatest fear in the hearts of men is not being able to "get it up." Potency and manhood are immutably connected in the male psyche. Many men cannot escape the belief that to be impotent is to be less of a man. As a result, erection difficulty can lead to significant personal and relationship problems.

Unless there is an injury or a psychological trauma, erection problems usually don't happen suddenly. More often, over a period of months the man notices that it is more and more difficult to get and stay erect. Noticing the dramatic decline, the man will often say nothing to his partner. Instead, he begins to pull back sexually, often as a form of denial or self-protection. The man may rationalize that avoiding sex spares his partner the frustration of "being left high and dry." All this often goes on without a single word being spoken between the partners.

Meanwhile, the man's partner notices his withdrawal. How can she miss it? A man who for years has had a robust interest in sex is suddenly asexual. In time, it's not uncommon for the partner to start worrying. *Is it something about me?* she wonders. *Or is he seeing someone else?* Frightened, hurt, and concerned, she may withdraw, become irritable, or turn to a Victoria's Secret catalog in hopes of reigniting his interest. And still, often all this goes on without a single word spoken between the partners.

Erection problems are common. In a study of men between the ages of 18 and 59, 10% were unable to achieve or maintain an erection (Laumann et al., 1994). In the 29-nation study of men between the ages of 40 and 80, complaints of erectile problems ranged between 13 and 28%, depending on the geographic region (Laumann et al., 2005). Difficulty increases with age, so that in a study of a cross-sectional sample of men between the ages of 40 and 70, 52% reported some form of erection difficulty (Feldman et al., 1994). In a study of almost 32,000 health professionals, less than 2% had erectile problems before the age of 40, 4% between 40 and 49, 26% between 50 and 59, 40% between 60 and 69, and 61% over the age of 70 (Bacon et al., 2003).

Not all that many years ago, practitioners assumed that the majority of erection problems were due to psychological factors. Performance anxiety was seen as the main culprit. We assumed that most men with this problem were so worried about performing well that the pressure and anxiety actually overrode the body's signals to respond sexually. Thanks to new diagnostic technology and increased understanding of how erections occur, we've come to realize that the majority of erection problems are due to medical problems. Medication can interfere with erections. The penis may have damaged blood vessels due to poor diet, smoking, or high blood pressure. Injuries, surgery, or diseases that impact the nerve fibers controlling erection can also lead to erectile dysfunction. There are still many bona fide cases of erectile failure caused by psychological issues, but a medical evaluation should always be the first step when addressing an erection problem.

How can doctors determine whether the erection problem is medical or psychological? Tests can measure blood flow in the penis, check for leaking veins, and determine whether the nervous system is working properly. One particularly helpful and easy diagnostic procedure is monitoring to see if a man gets an erection when he's sleeping. Most every man is familiar with what is called, in the vernacular, a "piss hard-on." Every few mornings, a man will wake with an erection. He gets up, urinates, and the erection goes away. He assumes that the erection was the result of a full bladder; thus the term "piss hard-on." The penis, however, is not a water balloon, and the erection has nothing to do with the condition of the bladder. Normal sleep consists of 90-minute cycles, and one of the stages of these cycles is called the REM, or rapid-eye-movement, stage. During the REM stage, the body goes through a number of physiological changes, including the pooling of blood in the pelvis. As a result, every 90 minutes during sleep men generally get an erection lasting 10 to 15 minutes. Likewise, women lubricate every 90 minutes during their sleep. Morning erections occur only on those mornings when the man happens to wake up during the REM stage of sleep. On other mornings, when he awakes during other stages of the sleep cycle, he won't have an erection—but he'll probably still have a full bladder.

We have been able to capitalize on this phenomenon to help assess the cause of erection problems. By simply asking the man about his morning erections, we can get a good idea about whether his penis is still capable of functioning normally. If the man is in doubt, we can send him home with a special monitoring device. If the man's erection difficulty is due to psychological problems, he should still get erections when he's asleep. The reasoning is that when he's sleeping, performance concerns and sexual inhibitions shouldn't come into play. Without the negative influence of the mind, the body is free to respond normally to physical cues. If, on the other hand, he can't get erections when he's awake or asleep, chances are there's a medical reason.

In recent years there have been a number of exciting advances in the treatment of erection problems. Let's take a look at some of these treatment options.

Hormones

Although testosterone primarily affects sexual desire, it also appears to influence genital sensitivity. When a man has an erection problem and his testosterone level is abnormally low, testosterone augmentation (see above) may improve erectile functioning. This is particularly likely if the erection problem is caused or complicated by low sexual desire.

Corrective Surgery

Vascular surgery performed to repair or bypass blocked or damaged arteries supplying blood to the corporal bodies in the penis is rarely performed because of a low success rate (perhaps 5%). In carefully screened cases, however, such as younger men with a single damaged artery resulting from a pelvic injury, vascular reconstructive surgery has had a 50–75% success rate in improving erectile functioning.

Years ago, surgery was a common intervention for a condition called *venous leak*. Some men develop small leaks in the veins leading away from the penis. Every time there's an erection, the penis can't maintain the internal pressure necessary to sustain it because blood keeps leaking back into the torso. In efforts to restore potency, surgeons would *ligate* ("tie off") the damaged veins, but follow-up research has demonstrated that the effects usually were not permanent. Today, when a man has a venous leak, in most cases the use of a vacuum constriction device (see below) or a constriction band produces good results.

Sometimes the erection problem is due to a condition called *Peyronie's disease*. In this condition, the sheathing surrounding the corpora cavernosa develops a fibrous plaque or scar, often due to vascular trauma or penile injury. As a result, when the penis starts to expand, the sheathing can't stretch uniformly, which causes the shaft to curve. It's similar to pinching a balloon when inflating it: the balloon will curve around the point where it can't expand. In cases of Peyronie's disease, the curvature can be so severe that the penis is unable to become sufficiently erect for intercourse. Oral medication may be used initially in efforts to decrease inflammation and possibly dissolve the plaque. Injections of enzymes directly into the plaque have limited success. In extreme cases, various surgical procedures, including removing and patching the affected sheathing, have been successful. As a last resort, penile implants (see below) are sometimes used.

Vasoactive Medications

In 1998, a little blue pill revolutionized not only how we treat erection problems, but also how mainstream media acknowledged sexual problems. Shortly after Viagra was introduced on the market, decorated war hero, distinguished member of the U.S. Senate, and former presidential candidate Bob Dole announced in a nationally televised commercial that he had "ED," erectile dysfunction, and told men to have a talk with their doctors because something could be done about this problem. And more than 30 million men have indeed had that talk.

The sponsor of that commercial was the manufacturer of Viagra. Viagra is a *vasoactive medication*—that is, a medication that increases blood flow. Since 1998, two additional vasoactive medications have been introduced, Levitra and Cialis. Despite minor differences among these three medications, all three essentially do the same thing—they specifically target penile blood flow. As you read earlier in this chapter, erections occur when cyclic GMP is available to relax smooth muscles and arteries in the penis. Many erection problems are due to impaired blood flow or damaged nerve fibers. Because of these problems, the penis requires more cyclic GMP than is available for producing an erection. Viagra, Levitra, and Cialis all inhibit PDE-5, the enzyme that breaks down cyclic GMP. While the PDE-5 enzyme is inhibited, even a limited amount of cyclic GMP can have a maximum effect.

The most common question we are asked about *PDE-5 inhibitors* is "Which one should I take?" In our experience, none of the three stands out as superior. Viagra has been on the market the longest, and practitioners have far more clinical experience with this medication than the two newer medications. Levitra may act a little faster (15 vs. 20 minutes) and last a little longer than Viagra (5 vs. 4 hours). Cialis is referred to as the "weekend drug" because its vasoactive action continues for up to 36 hours. A second version of Cialis was released in 2009, a daily dosage version that allows men to feel "ready to roll" 24/7. The bottom line is that all three medications are highly effective (70–80% of men report improved satisfaction with erectile response), and the final selection is usually based on physician recommendation or the best results and least side effects experienced during trial and error.

There are common misunderstandings about PDE-5 inhibitors. For example, contrary to popular belief, they do not create automatic erections. One can't simply take a pill and sit back and wait expectantly for an erection to appear over the next 20 to 30 minutes—sexual stimulation is required for these pills to work their magic. Erections aren't guaranteed, even if the pill worked previously. As helpful as these medications can be, they can still be neutralized by psychological factors. If a man is overly distracted by performance concerns, sexual stimulation can be sufficiently compromised to override the vasoactive effect of the medication. PDE-5 inhibitors are not aphrodisiacs. They do not chemically create increased desire, although restored potency can boost a man's confidence and satisfaction, making him more receptive to more frequent sexual activity.

Restored potency can create new challenges in a relationship. After years of erection problems, a guy suddenly experiencing adolescent-like erections can feel like a kid in a candy shop. After a while, his partner can become so exasperated by the nonstop sexual overtures that she finds herself yearning for the more languid times before Viagra. Some couples report that chemically assisted erections tend to shift the focus of their lovemaking from a sensual, intimate interaction that did not necessarily rely on intercourse to a frantic, phallocentric (centering on the erect penis) attempt to exhibit sexual prowess.

Another common challenge encountered by many couples using PDE-5 inhibitors is establishing a comfortable sexual rhythm. If the man takes a pill, he may end up feeling doubly frustrated if an hour later his partner declines his invitation to make love. Not only does he feel disappointed sexually, but he may resent that he just wasted $10, the average cost of a single dose of a PDE-5 inhibitor. Likewise his partner may resent the implied expectation to "stay up" for sex if he has already taken a pill, even if the mood had passed while waiting for the medication to kick in.

Couples struggle with how to be spontaneous when intercourse is going to depend on chemical assistance. "Would you like me to take my pill?" is hardly a romantic or sexy invitation. A scene of spontaneous passionate kissing and caressing, interrupted by the guy saying, "Hold that thought for 20 or 30 minutes while I go take my pill," will never be found in a Harlequin romance novel.

Although there is no single, simple solution to the challenges described above, a few principles can help. Restored potency is wonderful, but a broader focus on emotional connection and sensual touch that extends beyond the genitals is far more critical for satisfying lovemaking. On some occasions it can be better to skip the pill and make love anyway—spontaneous, passionate, and erotic lovemaking, even if intercourse isn't included. On other occasions, plan. Discuss, tease, joke about making love later that day, that night, the coming weekend, without necessarily making reference to any medication. And when medication is used, avoid the mindset that we must get our money's worth from this outrageously expensive little pill. A pill taken needlessly is not a big deal—but making it a big deal can create needless pressure and resentment for both parties. Men need to look at taking a PDE-5 inhibitor before sex like packing a condom just before a date—they may or may not get lucky, but at least they will be prepared. And, of course, as we have recommended continually throughout this book, talk openly with each other about these challenges and how to overcome them. Often these little pills remain in the medicine cabinet or prescriptions go unfilled just because people haven't figured out how to preface their lovemaking with a discussion that should occur well before the anticipated event. Really before—perhaps the day the prescription arrives home in his jacket pocket.

Side effects from these PDE-5 inhibitors are rare and usually mild and reversible when they occur. They can include headaches, facial flushing, nasal congestion, stomach irritation, muscle cramping, backache, rashes, difficulty differentiating the colors blue and green, and shortness of breath. A number of highly publicized deaths attributed to PDE-5 inhibitors have, however, alarmed the public. Most of these deaths have been due to a lethal drug interaction. Men taking nitrates should not use a PDE-5 inhibitor. Nitrates dilate blood vessels and are often prescribed for angina, which is chest pain caused by constricted blood vessels. Because PDE-5 inhibitors also dilate blood vessels, the double impact of the combined medications can relax the blood vessels so much that blood pressure drops too low, triggering a fatal heart attack.

You may recall when watching a television commercial for a PDE-5 inhibitor a narrator at the end rattling off in a rapid-fire monotone a series of warnings and disclaimers, including "In the unlikely event that an erection lasts more than 4 hours, seek medical help immediately." Most guys when hearing this think, "If I had an erection that lasted 4 hours, I'd throw a party." But a 4-hour erection, a rare side effect called *priapism*, truly is a medical emergency. Blood flow to the penis is partially restricted during an erection, and if over time there is not an ample supply of fresh blood, penile tissue will be deprived of oxygen. Without oxygenated blood, penile tissue becomes necrotic—it dies. In an emergency room, physicians will treat the priapism with adrenaline to reverse the erection or, if necessary, perform a surgical procedure to remove blood from the penis, allowing fresh blood to flow in and replace the aspirated blood.

Two other possible serious side effects have recently been reported in a small number of men taking a PDE-5 inhibitor—gradual hearing loss and a sudden onset of a rare form of blindness. Initially experts suspected that the vision loss occurred as a result of the medication impacting blood flow to the optic nerve. But further investigation has not supported a direct link between PDE-5 inhibitors and blindness. This rare form of blindness typically occurs in older men with a history of hypertension, diabetes, and heart disease—the same characteristics of men most likely seeking medical treatment for erection problems. In the case of hearing loss, increased blood flow to sensitive tissue in the ear is a suspected cause. Whether a direct link exists between the use of a PDE-5 inhibitor and hearing loss continues to be studied carefully.

For the sake of safety, especially in light of the potential side effects described above, PDE-5 inhibitors should be taken only under a physician's supervision. Ordering this medication on the Internet or buying it on the black market can be dangerous. Working with a physician not only ensures safe and effective use of the medication but can also uncover medical causes for the erection problem. Many men now taking a PDE-5 inhibitor were unaware of cardiovascular problems until they were screened for their erectile dysfunction. In some instances, this discovery was lifesaving.

In recent years, oral vasoactive medications have gotten most of the press, but they are definitely not the only game in town. Before Viagra's introduction in 1998, vasoactive medications were being used, not through oral administration, but by means of injection or insertion. Alprostadil (Caverject, Edex), papaverine, and phentolamine, either alone or in combination, can be injected directly into the corpora cavernosa. Their chemical actions differ from PDE-5 inhibitors but produce the same result—dilation of blood vessels in the penis. As an alternative to injection, alprostadil can be inserted as a gel-like suppository (*medicated urethral suppository for erection*—MUSE) into the urethra of the penis, bypassing the hassle and anxiety associated with needles and shots. These substances begin to act within 5–10 minutes of administration, with the full effect taking place within 20 minutes. Injections make erections possible for a 1- to 3-hour time period; the suppository works for 30–60 minutes. Pain is the most common side effect—pain from the injection, pain during the erection, or pain after the erection. Side effects that are rare but of concern include priapism, Peyronie's disease, and penile fibrosis (irreversible damage to penile tissue).

While oral medications are the first line of treatment for erectile dysfunction, the use of injectable or suppository vasodilators offers a viable alternative when PDE-5 inhibitors can't be used due to medication interactions (e.g., the simultaneous use of nitrates) or when the oral medications failed to produce satisfactory results. In the latter case, injections or MUSE can be substituted for the PDE-5 inhibitor or MUSE can be combined with the ineffective PDE-5 inhibitor.

Penile Implants

When damage to the blood vessels, nerve fibers, or structure of the penis is irreparable, penile implants may be a treatment option. A surgeon will implant cylinders into the corpora cavernosa, the top two spongy tubes in the penis. The cylinders may be either malleable (bendable) rods encased in silicone or inflatable tubes. With the malleable implants, the penis is permanently enlarged. During nonsexual situations, the man bends the penis downward to remain inconspicuous. When the man wants to make love, he bends the penis upward to position it for intercourse. This style of implant is particularly popular with older men who prefer something simple and who are less likely to spend time in gym locker rooms. Walking around in a locker room or shower area with an erection doesn't help to make new friends.

Men not wanting to contend with a permanently enlarged penis often prefer inflatable implants, because the penis appears flaccid during nonsexual situations. During sexual situations, the man squeezes a small pump in the tip of the implant or in the scrotal sac, which transfers saline solution from the back of the implant or from a reservoir placed in the abdominal cavity. As the fluid fills the tubes, the penis becomes rigid. When the man releases a seal in the pump, the fluid recedes to its reservoir, and the penis becomes flaccid. For diabetic patients, inflatable implants are usually preferred—they are less likely to damage internal tissue because, unlike the malleable implant, they are not always rigid and thus less likely to create injuries that can overwhelm a diabetic patient's compromised capacity to heal.

After surgery, the size of the erect penis is decreased slightly, but this change should have no effect on either the man or woman's sexual pleasure and satisfaction. Because the corpus spongiosum, the corporal body surrounding the urethra, is not affected by this surgery, a man's ability to urinate and ejaculate remains intact. The man usually retains normal sensations in his penis, unless sensation had already been lost due to injury or disease. The erect penis should feel normal to the woman; it will not feel like a foreign object poking at her.

Inserting the implants will damage delicate tissue in the corpora cavernosa and destroy any remaining ability the penis might have to become erect naturally. Implant surgery, therefore, should be considered a last-resort treatment. In cases where there were no other viable options, penile implants have allowed men to resume a full, active, and satisfying sex life.

Vacuum Constriction Device

A treatment option called a *vacuum constriction device*, or VCD, is a large plastic tube with a pump on the end of it (the device resembles a breast pump). When the man places the tube over his penis and flush against his torso, he creates a vacuum by pumping air out of the tube. The vacuum draws blood into the penis, causing it to expand and become erect. The vacuum is usually powerful enough to overcome even severe blood-flow problems. Once the penis is erect, the man slips a specially designed rubber band off the tube and onto the base of the penis. The constriction band traps the blood in the penis, which keeps it erect after the vacuum tube is removed. The band can remain on the penis for up to 30 minutes without risk of the restricted blood flow causing tissue damage.

The VCD is a safe alternative for men who do not want to deal with medication or surgery. Many men with erectile problems prefer this surefire mechanical approach to making the penis erect. The resulting erection can be a source of pleasure for both the man and his partner. This device does not interfere with orgasm, although ejaculation may be difficult. Because the band exerts pressure around the base of the penis, semen can be blocked. This is not a birth control device, however. If ejaculation is forceful enough, the semen can still be discharged.

The VCD does have some potential drawbacks. Some couples complain that the process of using the equipment to inflate the penis deflates the romantic ambience. Many couples have worked around this complaint by having the man generate the erection before he joins the partner to begin their love play. Some men don't like the VCD because of the subtle differences between normal erections and erections created with it. VCD-assisted erections tend to "hinge" or bend at the point where the band is located. (Remember that the penis continues past the abdominal wall and is anchored to the pubic bone.) With a VCD, the corporal bodies are engorged only from the constriction band forward. Behind the band, the penis is flaccid. As a result, it can be more difficult to align the penis with the vagina for entry and thrusting. Some men are distracted by subtle changes in skin coloration and temperature when the penis is erect. Because normal blood flow is greatly restricted, the penis may have a slightly blue or grayish hue and may be cool to the touch. None of these changes—hinging, color, or temperature—should prevent a couple from enjoying intercourse. Some men or their partners, however, are turned off by these changes and opt for another solution.

Despite the drawbacks, tens of thousands of men and their partners have been happy with this inexpensive, safe, and effective device. Men who take blood thinners or who are at risk for internal bleeding may not be good candidates for this treatment option, however.

Sex Therapy

For erection problems largely attributable to psychological causes, sex therapy (see Chapter 16) can be very helpful. Even when the erection problem has a physical cause and responds to medical treatment, counseling can help the man adjust to changes in his erectile functioning and their effects on his self-esteem. Counseling can also help the couple overcome the aftermath of the blame, embarrassment, or self-doubt that they may have experienced before the erection problem was diagnosed and treated.

What's New on the Horizon

Because of the significant number of men with erection problems—perhaps 150 million worldwide (McKinlay, 2000), and with the baby boomers quickly approaching their senior years—we anticipate a continued flurry of research and development to produce new and better treatments for erectile dysfunction. New oral drugs that use slightly different mechanisms of action to speed up and prolong erectile responsivity are in development. New means for delivering vasodilators are also being examined. Earlier we discussed how Alprostadil, a *prostaglandin* (a type of hormone that dilates blood vessels), is currently introduced into the penis by injection or urethral suppository. A new means of administering Alprostadil, as a cream applied directly to the penis, is available in Asian markets. Regulatory approval is currently being sought in the United States, Canada, and Europe. A novel approach for improving erections focuses on the brain rather than the penis. A synthetic peptide (a chain of amino acids that can activate select cells), currently referred to as *bremelanotide* (PT-141), activates a part of the brain that stimulates erections. Originally designed to be delivered as a nasal spray, bremelanotide is now being tested as a subcutaneous (under the skin) injection. The good news for men is that "subcutaneous injection" means the injection doesn't have to be made directly into the penis. Perhaps the most radical and potentially exciting approach to treating erectile dysfunction is gene therapy, which would replace proteins in the penis that are malfunctioning and interfering with the normal erectile response.

Rapid Ejaculation

As common as this problem is—28% of a U.S. sample of 18- to 59-year-old men and between 12.4% and 30.5% of 40- to 80-year-old men from 29 nations complained that they climax too quickly (Laumann et al., 1994; Laumann et al., 2005)—rapid ejaculation is very difficult to define. How quick is too quick? Experts have disagreed for years. In the past, many doctors and therapists would use length of time prior to ejaculation or the number of thrusts as the criterion. For example, if a man ejaculated within 2 minutes of entering the vagina or before completing 100 thrusts during intercourse, he would be diagnosed as a rapid ejaculator. But something was missing with this approach. Not only did it encourage people to take a stopwatch into the bedroom, it also failed to take into account other important factors such as the duration and quality of the overall lovemaking experience. According to this definition, a man could last 3 minutes, skip additional sex play, and still feel reassured that everything was normal. We don't think so.

Some experts have suggested that a man is a rapid ejaculator if his partner fails to orgasm at least 50% of the time. The problem with this definition is that we have learned that more than half of all women have difficulty experiencing orgasm from intercourse alone, regardless of how long it lasts. Other experts have defined rapid ejaculation as occurring when a man does not have control over his ejaculatory response. But as most men will attest, a man at best may have partial control over when he is going to ejaculate, but certainly not total control.

Again, how quick is too quick? Certainly when a man ejaculates before getting out of his clothes, or before he enters his partner's vagina, or within seconds of entry—that's a problem that should be addressed. But beyond these extreme cases, a more general factor should be taken into account. How satisfying is the lovemaking experience for both partners? If lovemaking is reduced merely to the time the penis is in the vagina, satisfaction may be unlikely. Some writers make the distinction between *intercourse* and *outercourse*. Lovemaking should typically involve talking, holding, caressing, and stroking both before and after intercourse. When this is the case, the length of time that intercourse takes place becomes far less significant; satisfaction will come from the whole experience, not just part of it.

Rapid ejaculation rarely has a medical cause. Some have actually argued that rapid ejaculation was bred into the human species during the early millennia of evolution. The theory goes that the individual who could quickly impregnate his mate before having to fight off competing males was more likely to contribute to the species' gene pool. Consistent with this line of thinking, copulation for virtually every animal species is very brief. Others, however, argue that unlike other living species, rapid ejaculation is not very adaptive for humans. Because humans are social and capable of emotional bonding, making babies is not the only function of sex. For humans alone, mutually satisfying and enjoyable sex facilitates an emotional bond between the two partners.

As for why some men tend to ejaculate much more rapidly than others, there is no agreed-upon answer. Some people suggest that rapid ejaculation is a learned response going back to adolescence, when a male would masturbate quickly to lessen chances of being caught. It's clear that experience and frequency also influence ejaculatory control. Most young men ejaculate very quickly, but with experience their ejaculatory latency—the time it takes to ejaculate—increases. Likewise, the frequency of sex influences ejaculatory latency. If a man goes without sex for an extended period of time, he will ejaculate much more rapidly than if he has sex two, three, or four times a week.

Anxiety may be another possible factor contributing to rapid ejaculation. We know that the ejaculatory response is partially controlled by the sympathetic nervous system. Men who are very sensitive to the physical effects of anxiety, which are mediated by the sympathetic nervous system, appear to be susceptible to rapid ejaculation. In our clinical practice, we have noted an increased incidence of rapid ejaculation in patients with anxiety disorders, phobias, and obsessive-compulsive disorders.

Rapid ejaculation can affect not only the man but also his partner and their relationship. Unless he is so self-centered that his partner's satisfaction is of no consequence, a man who ejaculates too rapidly will often feel embarrassed and humiliated. The partner, too, may struggle with a variety of possible reactions. Some women blame themselves, assuming that they must have done something wrong to make the man ejaculate so rapidly. Many women feel cheated when the pleasure of being physically connected is cut so short. Some of these women resent repeatedly having to hide their disappointment and feeling obligated to comfort and reassure their partner. Others can't accept normal feelings of disappointment but instead feel guilty over what they inaccurately label in themselves as insensitivity. Any of these responses—embarrassment, humiliation, guilt, disappointment, or resentment—can lead to stress and strain in even the best of relationships.

Sex therapists have found a number of behavior-therapy techniques to be helpful in extending ejaculatory latency for the majority of men experiencing rapid ejaculation. The success rate for treating this problem has been encouraging. When premature ejaculation is the result of a hypersensitive penis, a numbing cream or spray containing lidocaine can be helpful. For the really difficult cases, we have found that small doses of select antidepressants (Paxil or Zoloft) can also increase ejaculatory latency. Dapoxetine (Priligy), an SSRI (selective serotonin reuptake inhibitor) similar to Paxil and Zoloft, is still undergoing clinical trials but appears quite promising and will likely be the first FDA-approved treatment for premature ejaculation.

One final word about length of time. As you've read above, we've tried to discount the significance of actual seconds or minutes that intercourse lasts. We also want to dismiss a fallacy that is perpetuated by porno films and locker-room bravado. When we ask men how long they think most other men can go during intercourse, it's not uncommon to get answers like 20 minutes, 30 minutes, or more. Believing that to be true, even when sex is good, many men still feel inferior, thinking they have far less ejaculatory control than normal men do. In reality, however, based on survey data, it appears that the average length of time between entry and ejaculation is somewhere between 4 and 7 minutes.

Now if lovemaking in total lasts only 4 to 7 minutes, the likelihood of sexual dissatisfaction is quite high. As we described earlier, however, lovemaking should be much, much more than merely intercourse. The likelihood of sexual satisfaction will be far greater if the entire lovemaking experience includes extended touching, caressing, and sex play, of which 4, 5, 6 minutes or more of intercourse is only one component.

TWELVE

Relationship Matters in Satisfying Sex

This chapter is meant for you if you are in a committed relationship: the *strength* of your relationship, not technique, is the most significant factor in predicting sexual satisfaction. This fact is borne out over and over by research and the work of professionals from various disciplines. Whether you were married in a castle or have tentatively and hopefully moved in together with a ceremony consisting of sharing a pizza, your relationship is no fairy tale. Fairy tales end at "ever after," but when you join with a partner, "ever after" is actually the *beginning*.

Your relationship will not be free of conflicts and stress, but with proper care it can endure and adapt without allowing a stockpile of resentments to obscure your course. Think of you and your partner in a small boat (a metaphor for your relationship) together. If your relationship gets mired in disappointment and resentment, it is like putting down a heavily chained anchor: you go nowhere. A strong relationship doesn't sustain you intimately and sexually just when you're sailing along, but also when life is very challenging.

This chapter will explore what factors are most influential in building and maintaining a strong relationship and how your relationship is mirrored in your sexual experience. But first we'll cover some fundamentals and describe how we are almost *designed* to experience serious disappointment in our relationships, necessitating us to forge new awareness and self-responsibility. We'll move first into couple patterns and behaviors that are distressing at best and destructive at their worst, and then into what to do about these behaviors and how to build a skill set as a couple and individually. We include information about the unique challenges of being in a lesbian relationship. Chapters 13 and 14 will discuss ways to manage sexual challenges and ways to care for sexual aspects of your relationship. For all of you, our commitment is to help you gain new ways to communicate and address problems, freeing your relationship and you.

THE VERY BEGINNING: YOUR BRAIN

Every morning Regina, who lives on the outskirts of Chicago, hops on the elevated train for a 40-minute ride into the city for a three-block walk and elevator ride to the 27th floor of the office building that houses her small work cubicle. "What a city!" she thinks as she glimpses the skyline, juggling her coffee on her way. The city includes skyscrapers, a rail system that runs in an efficient loop, dropping and picking up passengers to innumerable destinations, bridges crossing the Chicago River, power lines, wireless connectors, telephone lines, cell towers, electricity that lights the night, and underground connecting systems. The intercommunication systems and transportation control and maintain order. But what's in Regina's head, her brain, the control center for every action, thought, and memory throughout her body (Siegel, 2007), is actually more intricate than the city surrounding her. "It has been called the last and the greatest biological frontier, more complex and more challenging than anything else in the entire universe" (Hales & Hales, 1996). The "universe" of your brain is like our Milky Way: continually under exploration with astonishing discoveries revealed. Until very recently, scientists and doctors couldn't *see* how the brain worked. (It is entirely covered by bone, after all. You can research for yourself the successful and less productive methods employed in the quest for understanding how this organ works.) Scientific curiosity in the 19th century was, of course, limited by the technology of the times. At one time scientists attempted conclusions about the brain by measuring and making inferences about the skull and its bumps and shape. Studying behavior changes in patients who had experienced a head injury was a significant advance, moving the view of aberrant behaviors away from simple willfulness on the part of the patient. Electroencephalography, a means of gathering electrical information nonintrusively from the brain itself, has evolved as a useful technology (Hockenbury & Hockenbury, 2003). Most recently brain-imaging technologies are providing a powerful, breathtaking "telescope" into the brain.

Our most current understanding is that the brain has evolved to accommodate new demands, thus changing in size, shape, and character, and that it is composed of three specific brain sections, each one having its unique functions. Your brain is the operating system, of course, with neurons and neurotransmitters, and interconnections with each portion of the brain controlling all the body's actions. Using a very limited example, your brain is like your hand inside the Sponge Bob sock hand-puppet that makes your toddler nephew peal with laughter at the antics you produce. Now, describing the complexity of the brain in an abbreviated manner is as absurd as comparing it to a sock puppet, but our description here is, of necessity, brief.

Three Brains in One

- The *cerebrum*, also called the *neocortex*, also called the *forebrain*. By far the largest portion of the brain, among other functions, this area provides the wonderful gifts of critical thinking, speech, language, expression in the form of writing, and, for our purposes, the essential function of *appropriate* inhibition of one's impulses.

- The *limbic system*, also called the *midbrain*. Among other critical functions, this control center regulates body temperature and helps us interpret many body sensations. For our purposes, this brain area is the center of emotion and associating emotion with events. Bonding, attachment, love, and sex blossom from this system, intersecting with the neocortex.

- The *brainstem*, also referred to as the *reptilian complex*, also called the *hindbrain*. This most primitive brain section, and the oldest in human evolution, is literally life-sustaining. Among other autonomic (involuntary) functions, we breathe because of our brainstem. For our purposes, sex drive and reproduction are located on the brainstem, the most intractable of all of the brain areas. The *fight-or-flight* response, originally a self-preserving function, is now frequently evoked during the intensity of a conflict (most often with impotent results). The brainstem functions are very resistant to change. This means that the fight-or-flight response can bulldoze the neocortex's modulating influence of appropriate inhibition, although very often the more sophisticated brain function takes the "high ground" and quells the potentially damaging impulses.

"BUT EMOTIONS TELL ME I'M ON THE RIGHT TRACK, RIGHT?"

What does this have to do with you in your relationship and how you interpret feelings and negotiate with your partner?

> Carly was into it. She could feel her body urging toward Dan's, their responses in tune. Dan pulled back from Carly and positioned himself so that his mouth was on her belly, tickling and kissing her first gently and then with more force. His hands moved to her thighs and spread her legs apart, his mouth moved downward. Both of them felt the moment: Carly shifted her bottom and moved her legs so that Dan's hands could remain, but it was clear his mouth was not welcome near her vulva. Dan raised himself up and both of them disengaged their bodies. "Carly," Dan snapped. "We've been over this so many times! Why can't you loosen up just a little? Do you want sex to be the exact same way until we die—or die of boredom?" Carly's face contorted. "You always ruin things, Dan! Why do you always push me to do what I am uncomfortable with?" The familiar argument ensued, rising in intensity.

Even though individual responses are so automatic that neither Carly nor Dan could delineate what *really, underneath*, prompted their reactions, both were "stuck" with their intense perceptions that their response was justified, and, conversely, the other's response was way off base. After all, both of their central nervous systems were giving each of them all the clues they needed: "I'm feeling it intensely; therefore my reality is accurate." So, being rational adults, do Carly and Dan calm down and discuss the situation rationally, using "I" statements?

No. Escalated emotions also excite body responses: hearts race, breathing is rapid and shallow, and adrenaline is almost palpable. Good luck to any of us on getting something substantial accomplished in such a state. And yet all this physical evidence convinces us that we are on the moral high ground. Perhaps for self-preservation or intense need for affirmation we persevere with what isn't working. Even though they've been down this path before, Dan and Carly continue their fruitless arguments. Is there a way to release a couple from this futile cycle?

"If I Stumble, I Can Count on You to Catch Me Every Time"

Harville Hendrix is a prominent therapist and author. In his work he starts at the beginning—the very beginning—before we are even born. He postulates that all of us (hopefully) begin in an environment where our needs are met and we experience a never-again-achieved security. Furthermore, we all have a deep desire to replicate this sublime existence and pursue it with our own form of "magical thinking" (Hendrix, 1988, p. 17). Our adored partner will re-create this supposedly pure Eden, and when this person can't or won't do that or expresses needs of his or her own, we temporarily dissolve into an abandoned, misunderstood puddle of feeling. Helen Fisher's work emphasizes how our chemical composition contributes to all of this (Fisher, 2004). The powerful hormones generated by romantic love which we discussed in Chapters 3 and 4 tune out flaws of the beloved, prompt us to take more risks, idolize, and perceive that all needs will be met.

When the idealization collapses, love often degenerates into either a cold war or an easily ignited fury. What's interesting is that both are sides of the same coin! Either way, raging love or icy fury, we are clinging to the fantasy that our partners make us complete, and they can bestow or withhold that power (Hendrix, 1988, p. 8). But this is not a life sentence. With increased understanding, self-awareness, and a foundation of friendship, couples can and do struggle through this challenge, emerging with new strengths.

What's in Your Luggage on This Relationship Journey?

We've all heard it: *emotional baggage. That's not me*, we each think, as we calmly contemplate the history we carry inside ourselves. Couples, as they begin life together, believe their good intentions will free them of any negative history they might have brought into the relationship. But our emotional baggage cannot be tossed overboard.

It is intricately entwined with all of our development and encoded every bit as much as our reach and grasp of objects.

React first, think later—that's us. As infants the part of the brain that records emotions, the amygdala, is busy firing away, making emotional associations and hard-wiring those connections for future reference. Meanwhile, the hippocampus, the part of the brain that actually makes *sense* of these emotions, lags far behind. So Baby is frightened by a loud noise, but it will be some time before she can interpret this as a banging door, disruptive but not threatening. Furthermore, the emotional connections we make very early in our development stay put and partially determine our emotional response patterns throughout our lives. "Adults, then, can be plagued by chronic, debilitating emotional outbursts linked to past events that they neither remember nor have any way of recovering . . . " (Atkinson, 2005, p. 26).

What does this have to do with couples? Well, if we don't have any recorded memory of what started the whole emotional response in the first place, we are in a perfect position to categorically place the response squarely and resolutely on the "behavior"—or lack thereof—of our partner. And it's hard to talk us out of that.

Of course this isn't the end of our emotional stories. Our emotional response system doesn't stop developing when we've graduated from wearing diapers. We're influenced and shaped by many factors, such as inherited traits and family interactions—one family may be robust, raucous, and another may be intellectual, analytic, and in general quieter. Chapter 10 describes how specific experiences can shape or alter our emotional responses. The intention here is to emphasize that (1) we are wired to react very quickly emotionally, (2) our emotions frequently misinform us, and (3) our feelings tend to cement our convictions that our position is right. However, we can and do learn to modulate our responses, calm ourselves, and learn and exhibit empathy.

How to Avoid Sinking Sex and Flooding Your Relationship

In this section we will discuss common ways we sabotage our relationships. Too often we operate from an "If he/she would only . . . " narrow lens. We all need to regulate our togetherness with our partner, along with our need to be independent individuals. When the patterns we present here become habitual, they are difficult to break. (With commitment, we can break patterns, incorporate new skills, and rewire some of that brain reactivity. Later in the chapter we discuss the strategies and tools that work to move from negative to positive interactions and how to move from futility to confidence.)

Could You Be "Setting Up" Your Partner to Fail?

Are you prone to keeping mental track of how many times your partner doesn't reciprocate, forgets to do something you asked, or doesn't respond to your overtures?

If you are vigilant about collecting grievances, eventually you will have a great tally in your favor. The companion "setup" is that you keep a mental tally of all the exceptionally good things you've been doing that your partner doesn't even acknowledge, like driving his mother to her radiation treatment every day last week. What happens to grievance collections? They pile up like poker chips and are often cashed in in the bedroom: if your partner withholds from you, you can withhold just as powerfully (Berne, 1964). It's important to note that both you and your partner might be participating in this no-win situation. In this kind of game, no one can win, and the payoff is always painful. If this seems to apply to you, talk to your partner about starting fresh and without the score card.

Do You Just "Check Out"?

Checking out is different from the healthy balance of closeness and autonomy, which we'll discuss later. Dr. John Gottman, an educator, author, and scientist, calls this "stonewalling" (Gottman, 1999, p. 33) If you find you (or your partner) are frequently disengaging, becoming stony or mute, you could be moving into a pattern that is actually one of the most destructive to a relationship. There are many variations: you don't want to attend an event, but you go. Then you isolate yourself in ways that make it explicitly clear that you don't want to be there. This pattern may begin because the assertive partner mows down the other with relentless persuasion or criticism. Earlier we talked about Dan and Carly. When Carly couldn't respond to Dan's advances outside of her sexual comfort zone, Dan responded strongly, and Carly responded in turn but in an ineffective (although engaged) way. If this pattern continues, one of Carly's defenses might be to roll over and avoid not only the conflict but the relationship too, not to mention sexual overtures when they are offered. Stonewalling is dangerous to a relationship. It can escalate to the point where the stonewaller acts like a single person alone in the house or apartment. The tuning out and indifference are very problematic in a relationship. Stonewalling does just that—builds a wall that treats the partner and the relationship as if they don't exist.

"But I've Been Saying This Forever!"

Couples don't always see eye to eye, and most major conflicts in couples remain unresolved. This does not spell the death of the couple. Although there may be some fundamental "deal breakers" that are so critical that they can't be negotiated, most couples learn where the potholes are and slow down and steer around them. For example, one partner may yearn to be a parent, while the other partner adamantly wants to remain unfettered by parenthood. Perhaps they both thought they could change the other's mind.

Most conflicts aren't so extreme that couples separate. Conflicts aren't awful: every close relationship has them. Conflicts come from wishes, hopes, values, traditions, work overload, and so many other factors. Small conflicts dissolve; major conflicts stick around. It's when an individual holds on to a fantasy of fusion—perfect agreement, where if you love me you will give all—that the trouble begins. Resolution of conflict by one partner continually giving in to the other doesn't lead to perfection; it leads to weariness and a lack of distinct viewpoints. In these partnerships there is little tolerance for differences of opinion.

Are You Way Overactive—or Underactive—in Your Relationship?

Mary Lou sat on the couch, huddled in a blanket, shivering, waiting for Jill to fix the situation. It was dark and cold; the power was out because of an ice storm that made even stepping outside the front door treacherous. At the same time Jill, using their Coleman lantern, was gathering candles and matches. She pondered over which boots she owned that would give her the best traction outside, considering everything was covered with half an inch of ice. Outside she used a sledgehammer to break free some firewood that she then gingerly carried into the house. A few blocks away, Keisha and Will kept a running dialogue. "You take the Coleman. Darn! Where did I put those batteries!" Keisha, from the other room: "In the laundry room, second shelf." Will: "I'm gonna try to get outside for some firewood for the fireplace. Can't believe how cold it is!" Keisha called from the living room where she was gathering candles, "I think your lace-up boots will give you more traction. And use that walking stick thingy that's in the garage somewhere."

In one scenario we have what we call an overactive/underactive couple. We can extrapolate that Mary Lou's passivity and Jill's take-charge patterns permeate their relationship. Mary Lou is dependent to the point where she has little self-sufficiency, problem-solving skills, or power. Jill, on the other hand, has overresponsibility, a feeling of needing to keep everything in manageable order, including major decisions, finances, and sex. Let's assume that Keisha and Will have a more equal relationship. They talk over decisions, perhaps heatedly at times. Their conversation conveys that they speak frequently and they work collaboratively and efficiently when faced with a big challenge, like prioritizing and creating a safe environment as best they can during a major ice storm. The couple relationship that Mary Lou and Jill display is *not* dependence/independence. It is dependence/dominance. In such a dyad, the overly dependent partner not only displays less assertiveness but also has fewer problem-solving abilities to draw from. Because they have less input in the running of the household and finances, they can resort to "barter sex" to get what they want. Dependency can also breed resentment, experiencing the partner as controlling or withholding. Interestingly, African American women are much more likely to describe themselves as dominant. This may be explained as a cultural difference, where African American women are *expected* to be more assertive and active about when, where, how, and what occurs (Soet et al., 1999).

When it comes to sexual activity, women who feel they are dominant in a relationship appear to have no difficulty contributing—or even determining—the frequency, type, and location of sex, as well as safer-sex practices. Women who are passive or dependent in a relationship acquiesce to their partner's wishes, including time, place, frequency, and yes or no to safer-sex practices.

Are You "Just Offering Constructive Criticism?"

We might rename this *destructive* criticism. This by no means indicates that couples who have chosen each other as partners either don't have complaints or will ignore them until one of them develops an ulcer. Gottman describes a world of difference between complaints and criticism (Gottman, 1999, pp. 24–25). Criticism incorporates the *always/never* accusation. "You *never* put gas in the car," "You *always* have a headache or something when I want sex." Even more toxic is when criticism undermines the very integrity of the partner. Instead of addressing the issue, even with frustration, a partner who attacks the character of the other ("I guess you're just too stupid to remember . . . ") is left with very undesirable responses. The most common would be defensiveness (discussed next), either pleading or raging to reestablish integrity. Criticism often begins with intensity far beyond what the circumstances indicate (Gottman, 1999, p. 24).

Respect generates cooperation. Criticism that attacks may offer temporary superiority to the attacker but diminishes the person attacked and cumulatively erodes self-esteem. Sex in these circumstances can become perfunctory, with the diminished partner acquiescing for fear of further retribution. This situation isn't gratifying for either partner and can lead to even more devastating relational or personal outcomes.

"No, Wait . . . but I . . . "

The inevitable companion of attack is defensiveness. In some cases this is the only mode of communication a couple has, outside of superficial conversation. Otherwise, the couple's world silently and separately revolves around the next go-around. The household seethes with tension in this environment. Communication withers to a debate, albeit a highly charged one, where each participant prepares a rebuttal even as the other is making his or her own point. Gottman says that "research shows that this approach rarely has the desired effect" (Gottman, 1999, p. 31). He also incorporated this as one of the "Apocalyptic Horsemen" that can—and may well—lead to divorce or separation. As therapists, the three of us have yet to see a couple where this particular interaction leads to a satisfactory outcome. It would be a rare occurrence indeed to hear an outright attack followed by "You know, you're right. Now I get it; I'm so sorry." The only way for this to dissipate is for it to fizzle out. The problem is, the attack/defend mode isn't the only thing that fizzles out. Continual experience with this futile attempt at solving problems has the result of avoidance, with little hope of intimacy, sexual or otherwise.

"We Have a Dog?"

> Allesia was astonished to see a four-legged creature in the laundry room. "Uh . . . Danelle, where did this come from?" Danelle looked up from the floor where she was lacing her running shoes. "That's Magic. He's a rescue dog, and I brought him from the Humane Society a week ago." "Hmm . . . " Allesia responded. "It might have been nice to know," she said as she moved toward the stairway, with the project report that was due on her mind.
>
> Allesia and Danelle tried couple counseling for their waning to nonexistent sex life. When the therapist asked them to visualize time for intimacy, even 15 minutes twice a week, at first they were defensive about their varied activities, and then they were mutually mute. That interaction was an exact replica of their relationship. Their therapy lasted for three sessions because they could not coordinate their schedules.

Most couples experience demanding schedules, juggling not only their individual commitments but their family's and partner's as well. Much of the time "balance" is just a word, and "juggling" is more descriptive of their lives. But there is a subtle line that, when crossed, results in parallel lives with little to no connection between the two partners. Sometimes one partner "exits," working unpredictable hours, holing up for hours with the computer or other "loner," excluding activities. In this case the frustrated partner pursues, while the disengaged partner retreats. The further the retreating partner goes, the more persistent the pursuer becomes.

Eventually one says "You're ALWAYS nagging me about something! I can't stand it!" The retort, predictably, is "I can NEVER reach you!" There's no comfort here. There is little or no sharing, cuddling, or gratifying intimacy.

Could Contempt Be Creeping into Your Relationship?

Again borrowing from Dr. Gottman, contempt is poisonous to a relationship. The keys to this downhill slide are sarcasm, cynicism, name-calling, eye-rolling, sneering, mockery, and hostility (Gottman, 1999, p. 29). How does a couple recover in this situation? It is a minefield of threats, implicit and explicit. Attempts at reconciliation from either partner would most likely be met with distrust at best. The contemptuous partner (or eventually both partners) gives no quarter. Here are the most likely outcomes for this relationship problem: divorce, affairs, major illness, escalation to physical violence, escapism so that neither is in the same space as the other except rarely, and spillover so that friends, relatives, or coworkers get the lowdown on how bad things are. There is no room in this scenario for intimacy in any form. The hope would be for self-reflection, self-awareness, and self-responsibility before any repara-tive couple-work would begin. If the couple end the relationship and do not engage in self-reflection about the relationship, the likelihood is high that they could find themselves in a new relationship that reflects the old.

CYBERSEX

Cybersex, at least in common use, is about as old as the average college student is today. This means that our dominant culture has about that much experience and wisdom in incorporating it into daily life. In the 1950s television programming became available on a few channels for most daytime and evening hours. The explo-sion of available options—on TV and the Internet—is new territory for couples and families.

Cybersex, for our purposes, is defined as the vast, burgeoning field of Internet sex. It may involve everything from seeking and viewing "soft" porn to using web-cams to expose oneself explicitly to another and masturbate in that person's "pres-ence." In fact, there are so many forms of cybersex that we could bury this chapter in their descriptions. It is virtual connection with another for the purpose of a sexual connection. It can be interactive or just involve viewing with no direct or indirect contact with another person.

Does cybersex impact committed relationships, and if so, how? For many cou-ples, exploring online sexual content is titillating and fun, and stimulates their own sexual interaction. Men are verifiably more aroused by visual images than women. If a woman is in a heterosexual relationship, and she is open to and accepting of his interest in cybersex, this agreement may cause no problems. It is certainly some-thing to discuss carefully.

Problems, and serious problems with serious consequences, can and do arise from cybersex. At the mild end of the continuum, a woman may be distressed by the increasing time her partner spends alone, closing himself off in another room, minimizing or rationalizing his absence. At the other end, "real-world" life may be imperiled by cybersex in terms of increasingly risky behaviors, too much time spent on the Internet, and avoidance of sexual contact with the partner.

Cybersex is seductive in more ways than one. It suggests that gratification is quick and entirely under one's control. There is no real reciprocal responsibility, such as opening oneself to vulnerability, or facing the inevitable ambiguity of face-to-face sexual intimacy; for example, tolerating one's own anxiousness about whether what is happening is gratifying to the partner. Just like sex portrayed in the movies, most cybersex seems to be without consequences and, in fact, is relatively effort-less. Cybersex may be the ultimate in objectification. There is no reciprocity, and the participant responds powerfully to this one-dimensional sexual experience. The viewer's fantasies are the stand-in for love, intimacy, and affection. Furthermore, if the participant is displeased with any aspect of the scenario, it can be altered with a few clicks of the mouse. Interpersonal relationships are not quite so simple.

A couple's intimacy can quickly degrade under these pressures. In a hetero-sexual couple, for example, the man may lose interest in the trials of intimacy and the challenges of sex with his partner. Perhaps "partner sex" had become routine, or the man had become accustomed from an early age to becoming quickly aroused by an ever-changing supply of erotic material. Cybersex problems can mimic alcohol or drug abuse. Here, the woman attempts to "catch" her "offending" partner in the act. This is a perfect setup for failure, because she will sag under the futility of her attempts, and her partner might well feel justified in continuing or possibly acceler-ating the behavior because of his "overcontrolling" partner. Moreover, cybersex can, for him, become a haven away from the increasing tension and conflict and thereby be even more seductive.

If cybersex problems are affecting your relationship, this is no time for self-help books. Competent, expert outside help is indicated. Not all therapists—even sex therapists—are prepared to assist a couple through the process of managing the treatment interventions indicated when Internet sex becomes a problem for a couple. One crucial variable is that the persons *themselves* must be motivated and committed to change. Whether the programs being considered are residential treatment centers, outpatient hospital or agency based, independent couple or individual treatment, all possibilities should be explored as to the staff's qualifications and training, the phi-losophy and approach of the program, and the interventions and methods employed. If independent treatment, such as a therapist not affiliated with a program, is sought, the experience, training, and efficacy of that therapist should be explored.

WOMEN WITH WOMEN: BEING LESBIAN

Chances are you grew up with heterosexuality all around you and the expectation that someday you would be part of the "husband and wife" couples you saw in books, on television, in your family, and in your neighborhood. Despite this, same-sex attraction and pairing has existed and "survived" religious, cultural, legal, medical, political, and community persecution throughout history. We want to stress here that all of the issues throughout this chapter apply to you. It would seem fair to be exempt from all of the couple pitfalls and be able to avoid all of the self-examination it takes to maintain a healthy relationship since you have enough to deal with with-out having those concerns. But no—no free passes. We all are prone to the same reactions and have the same personal patterns of responses.

Even if you are an Olympic medal winner, a famous golfer, or the mayor of your city, as a lesbian, you know that labeling and categorizing often go hand in hand with discrimination. The simplest of acts for a straight couple—holding hands in public—must be negotiated carefully by a lesbian couple. Stigma and discrimination actually affect a lesbian couple's sense of safety and happiness in the world. Research indicates that "the marriage benefit" that straight couples enjoy gives them a greater sense of well-being, as well as more respect and stature in their communities, than that of straight or gay cohabiting couples or single people. Lesbian couples are denied this well-being and respect that comes with social acceptance (Wienke & Hill, 2000). This "invisibility" can lead to isolation and create a strain on a relationship. If possible, seek out other lesbian couples and queer-friendly social groups. This may be easier in urban than rural areas, but lesbian women and couples are part of the fabric of almost every community.

Being a Couple: Under the Covers and in the Grocery Store

One of the first challenges you will face in your relationship is that those husband/wife roles that were likely modeled for you as a child just don't transfer. All couples have to negotiate: you just have to negotiate a lot more. Lesbian and gay couples have neither the social support of marriage nor the assumptions. So same-sex couples learn early to communicate and discuss candidly many aspects of being in a partnership, such as financial arrangements, chores, purchases, and so on (Rostosky et al., 2006). This can have a positive effect in the bedroom. Sex therapist and researcher Margaret Nichols reports that lesbian sexual functioning and satisfaction emphasizes each woman taking responsibility for her own orgasm and openly communicating with her partner about how she wants to be touched sexually (Nichols, 2000). Compared with straight couples, lesbians tend to have more varied sexual activity during sexual play, to include masturbation in sex play, to be more experimental, and to achieve orgasm more frequently in their sexual play (Leiblum & Rosen, 2000). Lesbians enjoy oral sex, vaginal penetration with fingers, hand, or objects, and touching and rubbing skin and genitals. If you are in a relationship with a woman, you are likely to see your relationship as positive and committed and as functional as the heterosexual relationships in your circle. But there are no commonly accepted definitions and guidelines for being a lesbian couple. You'll need to figure out what being a lesbian means to each of you and to your relationship.

Throughout this book you've seen that the emotional intimacy and quality of the relationship that you are in trumps the sexual aspect, but sex is important. No surprise that women and women couples predominantly express the same values. Your relationship is vulnerable to the same sexual problems as any: sexual desire problems, problems with making sex a priority, your personal history, fertility concerns and conflicts, and all the rest. And no, just because you are partnered with a woman does *not* mean that she will understand and intuit what you want and need sexually.

Some Last Concerns

Safer sex is as important in same-sex relationships as in straight ones (see Chapter 9). In addition, whether lesbian, bisexual, or straight, alcohol and safer sex don't mix well. You'll make your best decisions when you are sober.

Finally, find healthcare providers you can trust and rely on. You need good gynecological care just like straight women. We wish that finding a healthcare provider was easy, but it is not. You may have to interview several before finding someone who is queer friendly. It is worth the search for the sake of your health and that of your partner.

NECESSARY TOOLS TO STOW ON THAT BOAT YOU'RE BOTH IN

This section will give you a chance to acquire some valuable tools, forged from the best material, that will make not only your love relationship but *all* of your relationships function better. The term *tools* is strong and brings to mind an array of tangible items we keep accessible in our houses or apartments. We want the tools that we accumulate to help repair, strengthen, or facilitate the project that needs help, whether it is to fix the cupboard doors that don't align properly or precisely cut the material for the quilt that is painstakingly being constructed. We also want the tools to be reliable and strong enough to do the job. We need tools in interpersonal relationships too: they must be tools we can rely on to manage major conflicts and to take preventive measures. If the steps leading to our front door were sagging and cracked, we would be wise to repair them before someone gets injured. And, for example, if we recognize that we are being overly critical and even contemptuous of our partner, there are tools we can use to mend this problem.

It may surprise you to know that the tools we rely on most as therapists are tools that are focused on YOU. We'll leave the negotiating, the "I" statements ("I hear that you think I am controlling"), the mirroring ("Here's what I heard you say"), and the conflict resolution to you.

Earlier in this chapter we described a number of ways you—all of us—can "sink sex and flood your relationship." We will *not* in this section revisit each of these and offer tailored solutions. The answers will come from within you as you learn to be less reactive, more self-assured, and more empathic to your partner. Also, as has been true of most of this chapter, these tools will not be designed primarily around sex matters. Some specific suggestions and correlations will, of course, be incorporated. But, to repeat what we said earlier, the more science and sexologists learn about sex and relationships, the clearer it becomes that in the short *and* long run the strength and satisfaction of your relationship is the strongest, although not the only, factor in how gratifying your sexual experience remains over time.

"We Truly Meant to Take TIME Just for Us This Week, but . . . "

I had a deadline to meet on a major project. . . . My social outreach committee at the church/mosque/synagogue had me on the phone every minute. . . . It was my turn to carpool all week . . . I get up at 4:30 so I can work out before I go to work . . . I'm in bed 10 minutes after dinner, it seems. How long could we make this list? Single, newly in a committed relationship, married with children and their demands, partnered and dealing with aging parents, or retired, every single individual has such a list. An exception is a couple in that "romantic" phase of love we discussed earlier, propelled by attraction and hormones that create the most powerful drive we have. In that case time is no problem. When is the last time YOU thought and said out loud some version of "I'll have much more time when the kitchen renovation is done"?

If you can't visualize it, you can't achieve it. The calendar on the refrigerator is daunting with all its notations about doctor appointments, soccer practices, business trips and the like. When we ask couples where intimate time exists in their schedules, most stare blankly, or offer "When [this] is done, we'll have time." There is no place on the calendar, concretely or mentally, for time together. If you wanted a special dinner, you would have to decide on the menu, list ingredients you needed, shop, cook, and so on. At every level you know that, even if you got the ingredients and set them all carefully on the kitchen counter, they would not compile themselves into the dinner you envision. Our primary sex-and-relationship educators, television and movies, show us that sex is "spontaneous" and is fueled by an electric desire between the two of you. Sexual intimacy needs its space and planning too. When couples in therapy are confronted with the notion that their intimate lives might need attention, we've seen them roll their eyes and say "Oh, *please* don't suggest 'date night.'" We didn't, but it is interesting how defensive people become about their inflexible schedules. Our message: Review how you visualize time for intimacy together. Set a ground rule about becoming defensive about your own activities. Defending will close communication and create inflexibility. If you can, for a predetermined amount of time, perhaps an hour, sweep away the "noise" of all the competing demands so you can have this discussion without distraction. Set the stage for developing a plan about time together and follow through on the next stages.

Speaking of Tools, Avoid Becoming a Sledgehammer

Reflect on this statement for a moment: "So, are we *ever* going to have sex again?" What responses are available to the partner? The question was accusing, diminishing, and self-righteous. "I'm concerned about why our sex life has dwindled so much" is a whole different ballgame. Stockpiling the hurts until you explode in anger is unfair—and, furthermore, impotent. Speak up and avoid collecting those useless poker chips. Accelerating from 0 to 60 in seconds is for race cars, not for people. Blowing up over a partner's perceived neglect or misdeed does not justify raging about it. Rage creates fear, withdrawal, and sometimes activates responsive rage in the partner. It is bullying and unfair. Take responsibility for what Gottman calls "softer startup" (Gottman, 1999, p. 158). If there is a problem, approach it as you would want to be approached. That would likely be respectful and not explosive. Do a personal inventory about how you have approached your partner with complaints in the past month. Completely avoid the "but she/he. . . . " This is about your personal approach to addressing and bringing up problems.

Stand on Your Own Two Feet

We've said it many ways: you are *you*, and having a partner can't make you "complete." To be an intimate partner, you have to be able to *differentiate* yourself from your partner. This means you are distinctly you, separate from your partner. If you are thoughtful, you will not interpret this as *so I can do what I want, spend what I want, and not be accountable.* That kind of behavior is anything BUT differentiated: it is immature and inconsiderate and exploitative. Differentiation is difficult to describe and to understand beyond the basics: "I like coffee; you like tea." Simply stated, *low* differentiation means you rely much more on your partner's reaction and response to you than you do on your own internal security and self-validation (Schnarch, 2000). This does not mean that you smugly hold on to your position and reaction in an argument with your partner. In fact, the more differentiated you are, the more likely you are to be open and empathic with your partner's expressions and more open to his or her feedback to you. It's called growth. When it comes to sexual intimacy, if you are poorly differentiated, your entire sexual *adequacy* is determined by how much you perceive your partner is satisfied. Now of *course* we want to please our partners intimately. However, relying solely on validation from your partner, all the while being anxious about whether what you are doing is "working," looks a bit like you are trying to Velcro to your partner, to merge into some kind of sexual perfection. Maintaining a separate self, less reactive to your partner as the primary barometer of your self-esteem, is crucial to a strong relationship. As difficult as it might be, give up the futile struggle to merge with your partner. Take steps, whatever it takes, to manage your anxieties yourself. Expect a counterreaction from your partner if this pattern is changed. If you have taken steps to be more independent from your partner's reactions, you will be better equipped to manage the discomfort of changing established patterns and interrupting the inherent disappointments in those patterns.

Wise Up

Marisa and Sandra saved money for 2 years, first putting the day's spare change into a jar and then saving discretionary money every chance they had. Their dream was a vacation—an Alaskan inland cruise that they planned carefully. The first day on board Sandra got seasick, dizzy and nauseated, and she had to skip exploring the ship with Marisa. At Sitka they realized their planned day trip didn't fit for them, so they scrambled to make other plans. The trip turned out to be a wonderful memory, but it had not gone as they had planned.

Your relationship will inevitably unfold the same way and predictably with greater challenges than seasickness on a vacation. The dreamy and enlivened countenance of bridal couples at their weddings often makes us smile and bask in their aura, perhaps reviving in us memories of our own uncomplicated expectations. Yes, we all know the next part of the story. But often we hold on to blaming the other for our own distress that life did not turn out the way we had hoped. Eventually each one of us has to learn to work on our own internal skills for managing disappointment and loss (Hendrix, 1988, p. 168).

Wisdom has been described as the capacity to cope in the real world, caring about others, avoiding being self-centered or self-absorbed. This capacity for wisdom is deep in the brain's working and becomes more prominent in middle age. As we age, we are more capable of seeing the bigger picture and not making instant judgments. Yes, young people can be capable of wisdom. Still, "middle-aged" persons learn, express, and experience stimuli differently. When presented with a task while undergoing an fMRI, "younger brains, as expected, used only the left side of their frontal lobes to first learn the words—called encoding—and switched to the right side of their frontal lobes to retrieve the memory . . . older adults . . . not only engaged less of their frontal lobes' left side to form the word memory initially, but they then proceeded to use both sides, right and left, to do the harder job of recalling words" (Strauch, 2010, p. 94). The results of this are that as we get older, we are more capable of viewing problems in their larger context; we're calmer and, in fact, happier.

Wisdom has also been described as *"thinking and curiosity"*—managing decisions in an environment that is unpredictable, examining issues carefully, and avoiding black and white thinking. Wisdom is *reflective*—seeing and respecting different perspectives and caring *empathically* for others (Strauch, 2010, p. 45). Self-centeredness is the opposite of wisdom. Take your own inventory. Open yourself to hear your partner's perspective. Together you may do a much better job of problem solving. Exhibit empathy and respect for your partner.

Calm Down

Amal listened with one ear, bored to the point of dozing, while the airline steward recited, "If the oxygen masks drop from overhead, put your own mask on before helping your child." Amal didn't have a child, but she understood that if she had, she would be getting sufficient oxygen to allow her to be alert and calm enough to do her part to help the child in what could be a dangerous situation. Perhaps outbursts from your partner or you won't lead to calamity, but the distress can send your adrenaline soaring, allowing your reactive self to rule: sky-high heart rate, rapid breathing, gastrointestinal processes slowing or shutting down, altered sense of time, high alert, and a fight-or-flight condition for how you will react. At this point it seems ludicrous to imagine that you would have any real control over your physical or emotional responses. Furthermore, it seems irrefutable that your response is appropriate. You are temporarily overwhelmed, flooded with emotions. Your partner may be experiencing exactly what you are. Your alert system might be keen, but your vocabulary seems to have been reduced to a dozen words, all in high volume.

Let us *assure* you that nothing of value will or can be accomplished in this hyper state. The only way to stop this flailing is to stand, stop, move away, and take control of yourself. Also, at a calm later time between you and your partner, tell him or her how you plan to work on your part of the ineffective arguments that recur between you. We recommend that you avoid overexplaining or apologizing for your plan. These concepts are not meant to be punitive and withholding to your partner, but to be an effective tool to move you out of an unproductive and highly distressing pattern. Even before you need it, long before this hypothetical fight, spend some time building yourself an imaginary safe and wonderful place. A sunny beach you've visited often, a rain forest you've never seen, a softly lighted room loaded with down pillows—your own creation in your mind. You'll need it. At the time when you are flooded, move to another place. You've already prepared your partner that this is your plan.

Sit in a comfortable chair with arms. Become aware of your body sinking into the chair. How you control your breathing is essential: breathe in slowly and deeply through your nose and exhale just as slowly through your mouth, forming your lips as if you are gently blowing out a candle. If you are tempted to gnaw on grievances from the argument, remember, you'll get nothing of value from this. Retreat to your own mental place. Concentrate on bringing your heart rate down (adapted from Gottman, 1999, pp. 178–179). Don't rush this process; you'll actually save time in the long run, and you'll be less exhausted.

These strategies work.

1. Said again, only YOU can calm yourself and reduce your tension.
2. Take the breathing, relaxing, and imaging exercises seriously. They work.
3. Letting go of your feelings of being a victim to your partner's presumed insensitivity requires practicing, and then practicing again so you don't tie your own shoelaces together as you're working hard to break away from the damaging "defaults" that keep automatically reappearing.

Be Positive! Now *That's* Easy to Say

Love is a decision, not a feeling. We can't trace the origins of this often-repeated statement, but we can affirm its wisdom. In fact, love isn't a decision—it's a continual set of decisions focused on the positive. Or, as the American philosopher William James said, "Wisdom is the art of knowing what to overlook." When it comes to your relationship, there's a bit more to the story: you have the ability to experience interactions through the lens of the most charitable interpretations. Was there malicious intent in your partner's misstep? If yes, address it. More often issues between couples move from frustration to anger because of stress, external factors, mis- or overinterpretation, or exaggerated expectations. Of *course* we don't mean that you smile beatifically and accept anything that comes your way. Just work on being discriminating, and as we've been saying throughout, not immediately and defensively reactive.

A balance between positive and negative statements to our partners is essential. This is *not* a one-to-one ratio. Negative experiences or feedback are much, much more potent than positive. We remember them more vividly and longer and place much more weight on the negative. Imagine this: you are asked, and you prepare to present a half-day seminar at your synagogue. Of the 12 participants, 11 give you good to excellent evaluations, but one person was dissatisfied and liberal in expressing this. What impression stays with you? Gottman's research has shown that the ratio of positive and negative interactions between couples needs to be 5 positive to 1 negative for the couple to be stable (Gottman, 1994, pp. 56–57). To stress how influential this is in the well-being of couples, what might seem a rational ratio would be, say, two to one. But this doesn't work because of the much greater power of the negative and, in fact, has the exasperating effect of erasing the positives. But it is not realistic or desirable to set a goal to do away with negative interactions altogether. They are a part of the pattern of pair bonding. As therapists, at times we'll see couples who, when asked directly, cannot come up with one positive reflection about their partner. We assume those couples are hoping we'll produce our magic wands to take the place of their doing their own work on their own relationships. Instead, our experience informs us that this couple very well might not stay together.

If this ratio of 5 positive to 1 negative does not exist in your relationship, discuss this with your partner and pay serious attention to your own contribution to why this isn't happening. Recognize that we are all attuned to react to negatives and that it takes motivation and persistence to be alert to positives.

Talk about Sex—You Can Do It!

We are truly fortunate if we have eyesight, hearing, and the ability to use our voice. We also have language, something we can use in remarkable ways. But the closer we get to our most intimate issues, the fewer words we seem to be able to find, particularly with our partners, and most particularly if things aren't going all that well. We have wonderful, well-practiced ways of avoiding. The sexual issue may be that one or both of you wants to expand your sexual repertoire or explore inhibitions or discuss frequency concerns. If there is sexual dysfunction, whether it has recently occurred, been of long standing, is health related, trauma related, or other related, avoiding talking can have as many ramifications as risking the discomfort of tackling the issue. Some issues resolve spontaneously, but that often isn't the likely outcome. Avoidance can expand way beyond the talk thing. It can and often does happen in the bedroom (we should say *doesn't* happen in the bedroom). As therapists we know that avoidance can extend into days, months, and sadly even years. You're reading this, so if it applies to you, get started. Chapter 14 will challenge you to go much further with discussion and exercises designed to enhance your sexual experience and pleasure. The following points can function as preliminary considerations that can ensure your success with the discussions and exercises you plan together.

- *Do the preparation to have a discussion.* This will take the two of you, so plan ahead. Don't bring up a sexual conflict between you while you're driving to your brother's wedding. Agree in advance about a time and place where you want to talk. If you are the initiator and your partner balks at the whole idea, as calmly as possible state how important this is to you—and to you as a couple—and that you will be making the request again fairly soon. And do it. Take into account each other's traits. We're often less tolerant of the partner's traits than other features about him or her. For example, women tend to use many more words to communicate than men do. Avoid mentally drumming your fingers in frustration; calm your own impatience. Ground rules are always important. Discuss these. Possibilities: one talks and the other respectfully listens. Ideas that are expressed might be written down so they aren't forgotten, not criticized by the other, but discussed later. If your partner suggests installing a trapeze in the bedroom, maintain eye contact and write the idea down. Time later for keeping or tossing out ideas. Reassurance that both of you want a change and that you care for each other could be repeated often. Of course there will be other ground rules that are unique to your circumstances. When you set a time for a discussion, follow through. Many find, especially if there are children at home, that a neutral place away from home is best.

- *Reminisce about good sexual experiences.* A way to relax into the process of discussing current problems is to reminisce about positive sexual experiences together. Discuss details and what you especially loved (Zoldbrod & Dockett, 2002). If good sexual experiences are either obscure or nonexistent, try referencing some romantic or sexual content you were drawn to in the media. Caution: there is a real risk here of overidealizing the dramatized "intimacy" portrayed in movies or on TV. Talk about the possibility, even likelihood, of this idealization and how that could inadvertently contribute to the problems you're experiencing.

- *If you have pain with sex, talk about it right away!* Do not override your experience of pain, ever. You won't be doing yourself or your partner any favors by doing so. Chapter 8 thoroughly discusses pain with sex. Talk to your partner right away about pain and seek medical evaluation. In many cases, pain problems are much

more responsive to treatment earlier than later. Recall that we said earlier that negatives are much more potent than positives. If you have even a couple of painful
experiences with sex, your mind and body can quickly learn to anticipate pain and
so avoid it.

   • *Avoid comparing your "perfect" sex with a former partner.* What could possibly
be gained from this approach? It isn't going to be met with "Oh, that's interesting.
I wonder what I could do to help you have that experience again?" More likely, the
hoped-for discussion will be derailed. If your partner promotes this by asking about
your previous sexual experiences, address how this can't be helpful to the two of you
and is only really diverting you two from your own issues.

   • *A sexual discussion requires empathy.* Any charged discussion has the potential
to make us anxious about what we're about to say and vigilant about how the other
person may respond. Openness and heartfelt concern about what your partner is
feeling and expressing is empathy. Truly listen and observe. Ask questions for further clarification, not to challenge your partner.

   • *Is a sexual dysfunction involved?* Possible underlying medical causes are discussed throughout this book. When it comes to talking, there are several things that
seal most couples' lips. One is fear of hurting the other's feelings. A sense of despair
may prevail. Take the leap and suggest, "Let's set a time and discuss this lack of
sexual interest, when it began, and see if we can put the pieces of this puzzle together
the best we can." As you are deciphering a problem in discrete parts, you may come
to a brick wall of communication. Take a break. When you resume, acknowledge
that you've come to a sore spot, a place where you're stuck. Using your wisest brain,
the part that can see the big picture, tenderly recognize the vulnerability of both of
you and talk about the feelings that this evokes. First consider one thing that you can
do concretely about the problem and follow through with that. You've then taken the
first step of taking control of the problem rather than having it control you.

   • *If you want a more adventurous sex life, start kissing.* Yes, that's what we're recommending. Don't skip the "setup" and do arrange a time for discussions, but just
before your discussion, spend 15 to 20 minutes exclusively devoted to kissing and
holding each other. Kissing gets short shrift in many couples' intimacy. The following lesser-known facts about kissing come from Helen Fisher's book *Why Him? Why
Her?* Kissing sets off more brilliant fireworks in the brain than you've ever seen. All
of the senses are involved in kissing. Your lips, tongue, and mouth are exquisitely
sensitive, packed with neurons that are responsive to the most subtle sensations.
The hormones associated with attachment are elevated, and stress hormones are
reduced. Male saliva contains an abundance of testosterone that can prompt sexual
desire (Fisher, 2009). Now that you have relaxed into each other with the intimacy
that comes from kissing, talk about what you would or wouldn't like to see happen with sex. Begin with the things that you like very much and express how you

would like to see these expand. Move into steamier water: what would be exciting? Many ideas can be found in Chapter 14. Look that baggage of inhibitions you carry around right in the face. With *attitude*. For instance, exposure to some erotic material might expand your comfort zone (it often does) and might be fun to do together. The discussion of erotica in Chapter 14 is respectful of your personal boundaries and at the same time suggests ways to explore this further. Finally, if you make a commitment to do something specific to increase your openness, *don't procrastinate: follow through.*

Your relationship is, or may become, the most cherished and valuable thing in your life. Children grow and go, and we celebrate as they forge their own relationships and lives. Jobs end. Citations and awards end up hanging on a wall ignored or boxed. Synergy in a relationship means the energy the two of you create together becomes much more powerful than either of you alone could have imagined. Tend your relationship carefully and keep putting logs on the fire.

PART V

Developing Sexual Comfort, Confidence, and Satisfaction

The first four sections of this book have hopefully given you new insight into the many factors that have contributed to your sense of being a sexual person. We have discussed the influences that have helped to shape your sexuality. We've described how your body functions sexually and changes with age. You've read about factors that can challenge sexual health, including body image, STIs, injury, illness, pain, and trauma. Because your sexuality doesn't exist in a vacuum, we've spent time describing male sexuality and presented thoughts about sexual relationships. Now what?

This final section is devoted to helping you put it all together. We want to provide you with practical steps to become more comfortable with your body, more aware of your sexuality, more confident in your ability to relate as a sexually healthy person, and more satisfied with your sexual experiences. Toward that end, we present a series of exercises that many women have found helpful in their journey of sexual growth. After describing steps for greater sexual comfort and confidence, both personally and in a relationship, we'll discuss common sexual problems, both causes and ways to overcome them. At the end of this section, we offer guidance for determining when sex therapy might be helpful and how to find a qualified therapist.

In Part V you'll find answers to these and other common questions:

- "How do I figure out what in my past is interfering with my sexual experiences today?"
- "How can I become more accepting of my body?"
- "How can I enjoy sex more?"

- "Isn't fantasizing a form of cheating?"
- "Shouldn't people who have a satisfying sexual relationship give up masturbation?"
- "How do we get the fireworks back?"
- "Who should take responsibility for initiating sex?"
- "What if one of us wants sex more often than the other?"
- "I want to feel desire for my partner—why can't I?"
- "Could my medication be causing the problem?"
- "Is there a female version of Viagra?"
- "Isn't there something wrong if I don't orgasm every time we have intercourse?"
- "Why do I orgasm on vacation but rarely at home, and what can I do about it?"
- "What is sex therapy all about, and how do I know if it can help me?"
- "How do I find a good sex therapist?"

THIRTEEN

Enhancing Your Sexual Health

Howdoes a woman become comfortable with her sexuality and satisfied with her sexual experiences? In an ideal world, starting early in childhood, an ongoing process of development would take place and culminate in healthy sexual maturity. Through childhood and adolescence, all women in this ideal world would receive sex-positive education; they would feel validated as women by their family, peers, and culture; they would be encouraged to celebrate their bodies regardless of size, appearance, or disability; they would have the opportunities, free of guilt, to explore how their bodies function sexually; they would learn to appreciate pleasure without ambivalence or guilt; they would be supported in their task of developing adaptive, healthy sexual beliefs, attitudes, and values. With healthy sexual maturity, women would then be able to interact with their sexual partners with confidence, passion, and satisfaction.

Clearly, however, we do not live in an ideal world, and for far too many women the developmental process just described becomes derailed. In Part I of this book we discussed the myriad influences that can impact and impede optimal sexual growth and development. In the real world, women are often deprived of accurate sexual education; they quickly learn that their gender puts them at risk and makes them the target of lust; they are taught that their worth is tied up with their beauty and that beauty is difficult to obtain and impossible to retain; curiosity about their bodies is discouraged; they are taught to look upon pleasure with suspicion; and they are repeatedly reminded that sex is intertwined with risk and shame. As a result, all too often women find themselves ill prepared when entering into a sexual relationship.

In this chapter, we want to help you start or resume the process of healthy sexual development that may have been interrupted during your childhood, adolescence, or young adulthood. By means of a number of experiential exercises, we hope to help you know your sexual story, better understand your body, and increase your ability to experience erotic pleasure. View these exercises as an opportunity to do something positive for yourself, something that can continue to enrich your life for years to come.

Each exercise begins with an introduction that explains the rationale for the exercise, followed by *Directions*. After you follow the directions, a *Reflection* section will help focus your attention on the key outcomes and possible sticking points of the exercise. We also suggest the *Next Steps* to be taken following the completion of the exercise.

Before moving on to the exercises, a few suggestions and cautionary notes must be made.

• If you have a physical problem, all the self-help exercises in the world won't correct that medical condition. Self-help techniques can help you increase your sexual satisfaction but cannot substitute for proper medical care. Read the suggestions offered in Chapter 15 for seeking a medical evaluation.

• Once you've made the commitment to do these exercises, try to stick with them even if you feel you're not having much success. Simply attempting the exercises is a positive step toward sexual health because, at the very least, they will leave you with a better understanding of where further growth needs to occur.

• Invest in a journal, diary, or tablet and use it to record your answers, outcomes, and reflections as you complete each exercise. You can periodically review your entries and add to them as you continue your journey to increased sexual health.

• If you find the exercises challenging, you might benefit from setting aside a regular time to work on them. Also, discuss them with your partner, making them a shared project. If any of the instructions make you feel overly uncomfortable or violate your personal or moral values, feel free to modify them to make them acceptable.

• Try to be positive and not approach these exercises as drudgery. Rather than focusing on the negative, try to view these exercises as an opportunity to do something positive for yourself, something that can continue to enrich your life for years to come.

• Finally, remember that growth is not without risk. When we examine our sexual history and experiences, we face the danger of opening a Pandora's box. As you focus on your sexuality, you may come up with insights that are hurtful or embarrassing. You may suddenly see flaws in your relationship that, until now, you have managed to avoid acknowledging. Before proceeding with these exercises, you should be prepared to take such risks. You must decide whether sexual growth is worth the awkwardness that can come from self-discovery or the tension that might arise if you and your partner become truly honest with each other. For many people, these risks are outweighed by the potential benefit of sexual growth. But you will have to decide for yourself. If you do go ahead with these exercises and suddenly feel you're in over your head, don't hesitate to seek professional help.

WAYS TO INCREASE MINDFULNESS

To start, we want to talk about a *mindset* that will be extremely valuable in helping you not only benefit from the exercises that follow but also tune in to future erotic experiences more fully.

Women are multitaskers—truly a blessing at times and, at times, a curse. Research shows that the *corpus callosum*, the anatomical structure that connects the left and right sides of the brain, is larger in women, which likely accounts for their superior ability to manage multiple tasks simultaneously. A Little League mom can prep a quick dinner, arrange a car pool over the phone, and make sure her child's dressed and ready to play—all at the same time. If the dad had to handle all of these tasks, he might end up encouraging his child to play the piano rather than baseball.

This remarkable and valuable trait, however, can become a curse in the bedroom. Many women have a difficult time giving their full attention to the eroticism of the moment rather than letting their thinking stray to PTA meetings, the ceiling needing a new coat of paint, or how their naked body looks at the present moment. Many women struggle, often with little success, when trying to immerse themselves in the passion and sensuality of the moment. To more fully enjoy a sexual encounter, they will have to learn how to check multitasking "at the door" during sex and be fully present in the moment. Unfortunately, this is easier said than done.

In recent years, the concept of "mindfulness" has gained widespread interest in the medical and psychological communities as a means of enhancing focus and minimizing cognitive and emotional distractions. It is an adaptation of Eastern meditation, especially as practiced in Buddhism. Mindfulness meditation is a way of fully engaging in the present moment without the distraction of judgments or negative emotions. Research shows that when an individual practices this focused attention for as little as 8 weeks, she actually makes changes in her brain's neural circuitry and creates healthier adaptations to her environment (Davidson et al., 2003). Therapists are now using mindfulness techniques successfully to help patients reduce stress and to treat depression, anxiety, substance abuse, and other common psychological problems. More recently, these techniques have been applied to sexual behavior with very encouraging results (Brotto et al., 2008).

What is the secret of mindfulness? In part, it is avoiding the two extreme responses to distraction—either being carried away by the distracting judgments and emotions or getting caught up in a futile battle to force the distractions out of one's mind. Instead, one practicing mindfulness meditation becomes adept at scanning her body for sensations and noting without judgment passing thoughts and emotions. Rather than creating drama out of her thoughts and emotions and getting caught up in that drama, she merely observes their presence and maintains a relaxed awareness. In reference to sexual behavior, a woman who has long struggled with a lack of sexual interest and pleasure can truly change how she experiences sex. During sexual encounters she might be bombarded with negative thoughts about previous sexual experiences, but rather than dwelling on them or trying to push them out of her mind, she merely notes their presence, as well as the presence of countless other thoughts and sensations occurring simultaneously, including the pressure on her clitoris, the feeling of fullness in her vulva, and the tingle traveling up her spine. She is aware of it all, relevant and irrelevant, but in time her awareness becomes more focused and pleasurable sensations take center stage more readily.

Over the years we have often encountered women who truly wanted to grow in their sexual comfort and therefore wanted to complete the exercises we recommended to facilitate that growth, but they found the whole experience too overwhelming. In many of these cases, mindfulness could have prevented this disappointing outcome. In the exercise that follows we will introduce you to a mindfulness meditation experience that will help you experiment with "focused attention." We're confident that by working on your mindfulness you will be in a better position to benefit from the remaining exercises in this chapter and the next.

MINDFULNESS

Directions

Begin by reading through the entire exercise.

First, plan on spending about 5 minutes doing this exercise; eventually work your way up to ten minutes. Use the timer on your cell phone or an egg timer so you will know when the time is up.

Find a quiet place, perhaps in your bedroom, where you will not be disturbed.

Get comfortable, either lying down, semireclining, or sitting up straight with your feet on the floor and hands loosely on your lap or at your side. In any of these positions, make sure you can feel your back against whatever is supporting you. Make sure your legs and arms are not crossed as this cuts off blood and causes muscles to tense.

With eyes open or closed, concentrate on your breathing. Take slow deep breaths, in through your nose, out through your mouth. As you breathe, become aware of the sound that the breath makes as it enters and leaves your body. Some women purse their lips as they exhale—they like the sound of the air escaping between their lips.

See if you can move your breathing down deeper in your body and breathe from your belly or your diaphragm. Some people get a little light-headed with this breathing. If this happens, really push all the breath out when you exhale. Light-headedness comes from not getting enough used air out of your lungs before you fill them again.

Breathe this way until you notice that you have a rhythm going.

Now take deeper breaths, breathing in as you count "one one thousand, two one thousand, three one thousand," then push the breath out, counting, "one one thousand, two one thousand, three one thousand." Repeat this rotary breathing for 20 in-and-out breaths.

After 20 breaths, you should find that your mind is focusing on your breathing. Continue in the same body posture and continue to breathe the slow, comfortable breaths.

Move your awareness to the sounds in the room. Do you hear the hard drive of a computer humming? Do you notice a faint sound outside your room? Some women notice the ticking of a clock or the sound outside a window of branches moving in the wind. Continue to notice the sounds all around you.

As you breathe and notice your breath and become aware of the sounds, you might have thoughts that distract you from your breathing and noticing. You might be thinking about what else you have to do that day. Perhaps your muscles feel a little tense and you find yourself wondering if you are going to have time to stretch before the day is over. Whatever thoughts you have, don't try to stop them. Just notice and acknowledge them. The thoughts are part of your mindful awareness. They aren't good or bad; they simply are there, along with your breathing and your awareness of your body and the support behind your back and under your feet.

Now move your awareness to all of your senses and, without judgment, notice what is going on both inside you and around you. Does something irritate you, such as sounds coming from outside your window? Try to focus again on a calm, nonjudgmental noticing of what you see, hear, smell, and feel—being aware that you sense them but that they do not necessarily have power or influence over you. You may find that there is a sensation—like the sound of birds outside or the feel of sunlight on your face—that is pleasurable. Be aware that your mind is engaging with the world around you. This too is part of your focused awareness as you steadily continue to breathe.

When you hear the timer, return to your daily activities.

Reflection

+ Were you able to get into a comfortable breathing rhythm? We breathe automatically, but being nervous or worried often makes us unconsciously hold our breath. Breath holding tenses muscles, deprives them of oxygen, and leads to light-headedness and increased anxiety.

+ What thoughts, emotions, sensations did you notice while doing the exercise?

+ Initially, did you find yourself trying to control your thinking or fighting to exclude things that felt like distractions?

+ Were you eventually able to give yourself permission just to relax and note anything and everything that crossed your sensory threshold?

+ Did you experience pleasurable sensations or comforting thoughts during this meditation exercise?

+ How did you feel at the end of the exercise? While many women report feeling calmer and more relaxed, some feel anxious or agitated. The latter reactions are often due to the newness of the experience—novelty can cause anxiety. Sometimes slowing down from 100 miles per hour to only 5 can be disquieting—constant activity can serve as a defense against having to face problems and worries. Suspend the frenetic pace, even briefly, and defenses can pop up quickly. Other women have reported feeling disappointed after completing the exercise. This is often due to unrealistic expectations. Mindfulness is not something mastered after a single exercise, but it is indeed something anyone can benefit from if practiced on an ongoing basis.

Next Steps

1. Make time to repeat this mindfulness exercise daily.

2. Check the resource section at the end of this book for more information about mindfulness. Read more about this powerful tool for increasing your physical, psychological, and sexual well-being. Consider purchasing audio recordings that can guide you through additional mindfulness meditation experiences or look for them online—some websites offer free downloads.

3. When completing each of the remaining exercises in this book, be "mindful" of mindfulness. Maintain a relaxed awareness of your breathing, thoughts, and emotional reactions as you follow the instructions. Don't fight the distractions or get carried away by them; simply acknowledge them for what they are—parts of your experiential landscape.

WAYS TO KNOW YOUR SEXUAL STORY

An important first step toward enhancing your sexual health is becoming familiar with how your past has shaped and influenced your sexual comfort and satisfaction in the present. We all have a sexual story: personal narratives about how family, culture, physical development, and experience interacted in incredibly complex ways to shape our body image, sexual beliefs and attitudes, and capacity to experience satisfying sex. Our sexual stories include how our bodies matured from newborn infants to fully developed women capable of conceiving and giving birth. Sexual experiences, positive and negative, from childhood to present, serve as critical elements of the story because they often script how we respond to sexual situations. Our sexual stories may include narratives about confusion over sexual feelings and attraction. Guilt, shame, and inhibition can be by-products of cultural influences, including both subtle and compelling messages arising from one's religious and ethnic backgrounds. Knowing your unique sexual story can help you identify and overcome barriers to sexual health and empower you to resume the sexual growth that may have been interrupted at some earlier point in your life. (If you haven't read it yet, Part I is all about how our sexual stories are written.)

Your Body's Historical Timeline

A significant part of our sexual history is the experience of our own bodies. To be oblivious of our bodies is to be insensitive to the pleasures they can produce. To be alienated from our bodies is to be deprived of a means of connecting with special people in our lives. The beginning of your body awareness will be found in memories. Whether or not you consciously recall these memories, they influence attitudes about your body, yourself, and your sexuality. By recalling and understanding these early memories, you can better understand your adult response and take action to change it.

This first exercise focuses on the history of your *body's physical changes*. The next exercise focuses on the history of your *sexual experiences*. As your body changed, so did your perceptions of your physical self. Your Body's Historical Timeline is a way of reviewing and recording your personal history. Just as researching and recording a family history can help you understand and take pride in your heritage, writing your body history can help you feel more accepting of, and grounded in, your body. This history is unique to you. It can influence not only how you feel about your body but also how you care for it now and as you grow older.

YOUR BODY'S HISTORICAL TIMELINE

Directions

You will need paper, a ruler, and a pen. Turn the paper (ideally a large sheet from a drawing pad) to a horizontal position for more space. To make a timeline, draw a long line across the center of the paper. You will need to keep expanding this line, possibly across several sheets of paper. Leave plenty of room to write along it.

At the beginning of the line, write your date of birth, the time you were born (if you know it), and whether your birth was vaginal or by Cesarean section. Now think about all the early years of your physical development and how you changed.

Note as many changes in your physical self as you can remember through the years. If you can't recall something precisely, write down your best guess about the time of the physical change.

Include physical changes that enabled you to master the new skills and abilities that became the milestones in your development. Your personal milestones will be different from everyone else's. The changes you choose to highlight may have meaning only for you, such as learning how to handle a wrench and other tools so you could fix your own bicycle or learning to swim so you could join the bigger kids at the dock.

Make sure to include sexual changes in your body, such as when you started your period or noticed breast tenderness and pubic hair. Premenstrual symptoms (PMS) and perimenopausal symptoms (if applicable) are also part of your physical self.

Try to remember when you first looked at your vulva and explored the different parts of your genitalia, including your labia, your urethra, your clitoris, and your vagina. Write down when you noticed changes in your genitals, perhaps the lengthening of your labia or the graying of your pubic hair.

Some changes aren't changes at all but simply the discovery of a quality that was always present. If you are a woman of color, for example, you may have had an early, dawning awareness that advertisements all around you were geared predominantly to Caucasian-featured people. If you were taller than your peer group, perhaps you never paid attention to your size until another girl made fun of you.

Sometimes temporary or permanent changes in the body occur because of decisions you make, such as becoming pregnant or terminating a pregnancy. The impact of these decisions can occupy a unique place in one's history. Sometimes decisions are positive and a matter of personal choice, such as beginning and maintaining an exercise program. Some decisions, such as abusing drugs or engaging in unprotected sex, are self-defeating. Some decisions can be striking in their importance, such as deciding between a mastectomy and a lumpectomy for breast cancer.

Keep noting the changes up until your present age. The list may take several days to complete. Make additions as you remember them. You may notice that there are clusters of dates that coincide with developmental milestones such as entering puberty, having a baby, or entering menopause.

Reflect on each change by asking yourself these questions:

- *"Did I understand that my body was changing?"*
- *"Did anyone give me information or talk to me to help me cope with the change?"*
- *"Was I shamed or treated negatively as a result of my body's change?"*
- *"Did I think I was the only one undergoing this change?"*
- *"Did I learn to talk to others about the body change at a later time?"*
- *"Was I kind to my body as the change occurred?"*

Reflection

✦ Reflect on your timeline by asking yourself the following questions:
  - "Have I had unrealistic expectations for my body?"
  - "Have I let social pressure or advertising negatively influence me as my body has changed?"
  - "Have I loved my body as it is?"
  - "Do I want to love my body as it is?"
  - "What will I give up by loving my body just as it is?"
  - "What will I gain by loving my body just as it is?"

✦ As you review your timeline, reflect on what the experience of moving from the body of a child to that of a woman was like.
  - Were there times of happiness as well as times of grieving?
  - Have you found positive aspects in your growth and change, or only negative?
  - Did you minimize or downplay the changes as you got older?
  - Have you given your body credit for carrying you through so much life?
  - Can you be proud of your body and your story?

Next Steps

Continue to update your body awareness timeline as you undergo more physical experiences.

If you take the time to do this exercise, you may make some interesting discoveries about your history. Earlier in your life you may have gone through important physical changes alone and without support. At those times you may have thought you weren't important or didn't matter to other people. Because of your body changes, you may have been treated negatively by others. When this happened, perhaps a part of you believed there was something wrong with you. Making a timeline allows you to look at your history more objectively and challenge unfair and hurtful beliefs about yourself. You are taking back your own history and honoring it.

Keeping your timeline current serves as a reminder that you're aware that your body changes and evolves throughout your life and that you don't have to ignore or ridicule those changes. Ultimately, you have the choice about how you feel about yourself and your body.

Sexual History Timeline

Every woman, whether or not she is sexually active with another person, is a sexual being. This next exercise focuses on experiences that helped shape your sexual identity as a woman. Over the years, as your body changed and life experiences mounted, your awareness of yourself as a sexual person continued to develop. From childhood, this awareness may have expanded from first noting that touching your vulva was pleasurable, to sexual thoughts and fantasies, to a crush on "the boy next door," to masturbating while dreaming of movie stars, to kissing and fondling your boyfriend, to sexual interaction with your partner. This expanding sexual awareness is a part of each woman's unique sexual story.

YOUR SEXUAL HISTORY TIMELINE

Directions

Turn a piece of paper to the horizontal position, ideally using paper from a large drawing tablet, and make a timeline by drawing a long line across the center of the paper. On the far left side of the line, write the date you were born. This begins your sexual history. Now note as many experiences as you can remember or were told about. As a child, early sexual awareness might have involved peeking at your baby brother's penis or rubbing your vulva. If you can't remember something exactly, just write down your "best guess" about the time. Check back with "Your Body's Historical Timeline" for reminders about physical changes that might have prompted sexual activity.

The list will take some time to complete and may become lengthy. You can work on it over a period of days or weeks. As the list develops, you may notice that clusters of dates and sexual activities center on developmental milestones. You will not have every experience on this list, nor will you have them in the order listed.

Not all sexual awareness or activity that you remember will be positive. For instance, a woman's first sexual experience with another person could have been sexual harassment or abuse. Rape or other degrading or humiliating sexual experiences may have occurred. These should be recorded on the timeline, too.

There are limitless possibilities of what could be added to this list. The following list of possible sexual activities may be useful in remembering your sexual history.

SEXUAL ACTIVITY LIST

- *Aware of the differences between female and male genitalia*
- *First time you touched your genitals*
- *First time you experienced a sexual sensation*
- *Sex play with same-age peers*
- *Discussions with parents or other adults about sex*
- *Discussions with other children about sex*

- *First time you were told about sexual intercourse and how babies were made*
- *First time you masturbated*
- *First time masturbating by slipping your finger into your vagina*
- *First time you masturbated to orgasm*

- *Sex education in school or church/temple/mosque*
- *Reading sex education materials or viewing sex education films*
- *Seeing a live birth of a baby (animal or human) in person or on TV*
- *Curiosity about sexual behavior or nudity (e.g., looking at pictures or peeking at others)*

- *Menstruation discussed with peers or adults*
- *Learning the words "masturbate" and "intercourse"*
- *Learning sex slang like "fuck" or "clit"*
- *Awareness of prepubertal changes in your body (pubic hair, breast buds, breast development)*

- *First time you fantasized about another person*
- *First daydreams that were sexual*
- *Doing something sexual that was considered "wrong" or "bad" in your upbringing*
- *First time feeling guilty about something sexual*
- *Worrying about development of secondary sexual characteristics or starting your period*

- *First time being stared at in a sexual way*
- *Being sexually molested or exploited as a child or adult*

- *First romantic feelings stirred by a book, movie, or other person*
- *Having crushes on members of same sex*
- *Realization of sexual attraction to a female*
- *Realization of sexual attraction to a male*
- *First falling in love*
- *First awareness of sexual arousal resulting in nipple hardening or "getting wet"*

- *First hand-holding and hug*
- *First kiss*
- *First French kiss*
- *First "hickey"*
- *First touching of another's body*
- *Learning about birth control*
- *First intense touching, "petting" with clothes on*
- *First intense touching, "petting" without clothes*
- *First touching of another person's genitals in sexually arousing play*

- *Seeing sexually explicit material not made for sex education*

- *Being harassed sexually*

- *Learning about the sex industry, especially about women who make their living as sex workers (strippers, prostitutes, etc.)*

- *First time masturbating by inserting an object into your vagina*
- *First use of a vibrator or other sex toy*

- *First sexual intercourse*
- *First pelvic examination*
- *First awareness of how you felt about the way your genitals looked*
- *Decision to use birth control*
- *First time spending the night with a partner*
- *First orgasm in presence of partner*

- *Recognition of self as a bisexual or lesbian woman*
- *Coming out as a bisexual or lesbian woman*

- *First oral sex given*
- *First oral sex received*
- *Masturbating partner to orgasm*
- *Masturbating to orgasm in front of partner*
- *Using sexual fantasies while masturbating*
- *Sharing sexual fantasies with a partner*
- *First anal intercourse*

- *Being drunk or high while having sex*

- *Contracting an STI*
- *First sexual difficulty*
- *First experience of low or no sexual desire or arousal*
- *First experience of not being able to orgasm*
- *Yeast infection or other vaginal problem*
- *Unable to lubricate when having sex*
- *First experience with explicit chat on the Internet*
- *Sadomasochistic (S/M) behavior in a sexual relationship*

- *Being paid for having sex*
- *Being paid for making sexually explicit photographs or videos*

- *Being beaten up while having sex*
- *Group sex or swinging*
- *Polyamory*
- *Watched by others while having sex*

- *Getting pregnant when not in a permanent partnership*
- *Having sex after decision to terminate a pregnancy—with same partner*
- *Having sex after decision to terminate a pregnancy—with different partner*

- *First sexual awareness of permanent partner*
- *Falling in love with permanent partner*
- *First sexual experience with permanent partner*
- *First intercourse with permanent partner*

- *Sex when trying to get pregnant*
- *Sex while pregnant*
- *Sex postpartum*
- *Having sex when fatigued from childrearing*

- *Sexual involvement outside your permanent partnership*
- *Your permanent partner having sex outside your relationship*
- *Falling in love outside your partnership*

- *Dating and sexual involvement after divorce*
- *Dating and sexual involvement after being widowed*
- *Continuing to masturbate after being divorced or widowed*

- *Having sex after tubal ligation, hysterectomy, or other reproductive surgery*
- *Perimenopausal symptoms depressing sexual interest*
- *Having sex after diagnosis/treatment for illness*

- *Having sex after menopause*
- *Having sex with problem of urinary incontinence*
- *Having sex after significant weight loss or weight gain*
- *Having sex with a new partner, postmenopause*
- *Masturbating to orgasm after a change in physical arousal, postmenopause*

- *Purchasing/using vibrator and lubricants in your 50s*
- *Purchasing/using sexy lingerie in your 60s*
- *Having sex or masturbating after working out (exercising) in your 70s*
- *Watching erotic movies in your 80s*

- *Asking for specific sexual activity from a partner*
- *Mutually satisfying sex in a relationship*

Reflection

✦ Perhaps you've written short phrases and dates. Maybe you've written a longer narrative. Read back over what you've written. Circle positives and negatives in your experiences. Think about the events and messages that influenced your sexual activity throughout your life.

✦ In reading through your sexual history timeline, you may recognize experiences that sadden you. You may need to take time to grieve that these occurrences happened to you.

✦ Are there other not-so-wonderful experiences in the past that you now see are important learning events in your sexual journey?

✦ Are there experiences that you can laugh about?

✦ Do you see a trend toward becoming more assertive, surer of yourself, more interested in mutual and reciprocal sexual relationships?

✦ Do you like the sexual self you're becoming? Are you continuing to value yourself sexually?

Next Steps

1. The timeline can be used in many ways; it's a journal that can be added to over time.

2. You could share your timeline with a friend who has been creating her own sexual history timeline. If you're in a relationship, you can encourage your partner to make a timeline. Consider talking about the timelines together. Have you had similar or different experiences? Can you each listen to the other's sexual experiences?

3. If you have questions about your sexual orientation, or if you want to look more closely at your orientation, go on to the next exercise, "Your Sexual Orientation." If you're comfortable in your orientation, move on to the "Influences of Color, Ethnicity, and Religion" exercise.

Your Sexual Orientation

In Chapter 1 we discussed how many women have memories of loving and being physically expressive with other women. These may be memories from childhood, adolescence, or adulthood. If you are seeking to understand more about your sexual orientation, you may find it helpful to look back over the sexual history timeline you've just made and ask yourself the questions that follow. Write out your responses in a journal or as a letter to yourself.

YOUR SEXUAL ORIENTATION

Directions

Write your responses to the following questions. You can refer to your sexual history timeline to remind you of times you felt strongly attracted to women, to men, or to both.

- *How early did you know that you felt differently from the girls around you, that you weren't attracted to the heterosexual images you saw?*
- *As an adolescent, did you date guys? Were you sexual with guys because you were trying to "prove" you had an attraction to males?*
- *Did you find that you had an attraction to boys at one time but same-sex attraction at a later time?*
- *How did you feel when you realized you did not feel an attraction?*
- *Have you fallen in love with men, women, or both?*
- *What is your history of sexual activity with others? Has it been with men, women, or both?*
- *Do you feel comfortable with your sexuality and like yourself sexually?*
- *Does your attraction to others vary depending on how you are feeling about yourself (your self-esteem)? Are there times when women just feel safer than men?*
- *What has your fantasy life been like? Is it predominantly about heterosexual, lesbian, or bisexual relationships?*
- *Do you feel mostly attracted to other women but fear the rejection of your family, friends, or coworkers?*
- *Do you feel mostly attracted to other women but fear religious condemnation or censure?*

Alfred Kinsey, the famous sex researcher, defined sexuality along a continuum from straight to gay, with 0 being entirely straight and 6 being entirely gay. This continuum, commonly known as "the Kinsey scale," allows people to think of themselves as not simply gay or straight, but instead to understand their sexuality as a blending of gradations—perhaps being a straight 2 or a gay 4. Draw a line, numbering it from 1 to 6. Draw a circle around the number(s) that reflect your feelings about yourself.

Reflection

- ✦ For many women, awareness of being attracted to other women emerges over time. Read through your responses and see how they match up with your sexual history timeline.

✦ Doing this exercise may make you think about words. It's important that you self-define—that you use words that are right for you. Some women identify as straight, others as lesbian or bisexual. Still others may say they are open, questioning, or "a woman who loves women." And others will refuse to be categorized at all.

Next Steps

1. Consider talking with others who are nonjudgmental and supportive.

2. Continue to learn about your sexual orientation.

3. Read some of the books about lesbian/bisexual identity and relationships listed in the "Suggested Resources" section and visit some of the websites listed there.

4. Many women find counseling very helpful as they explore and define their understanding of their orientation. Consider counseling as another form of support.

5. In completing this exercise, think about what you are committed to and how you lead your life. The commitments you make of your time, interests, and energy ultimately define your life; no single act, no one fantasy or relationship, defines who you are. Embrace your totality.

Color, Ethnicity, and Religion

Everyone belongs to a variety of groups based on geography, color, ethnicity, and, in many cases, religion. For example, every woman comes from some group located somewhere on the planet; African American, Asian, Indian, Scottish, Hispanic—everyone comes from somewhere. You may live in a country where your family goes back hundreds of years, or you may live in a country to which your family has recently immigrated. If you live in a country like the United States, where many races and ethnicities can be found, your family may have carefully preserved the customs of your ethnic identity, or you may come from a family of individuals who don't consider themselves ethnic at all. Even if you don't think of yourself ethnically, you may recognize that you think of yourself regionally—like "southern," "Californian," "midwesterner," or "New Yorker"—and adopt the region's values and customs. You may also identify with a religious tradition—Judaism, Christianity, Islam, or Hinduism, for instance.

We refer to the primary group you identify with, whether it's based on ethnicity, color, religion, or geographic location, as your "community." Your sexuality is influenced by your community and by the perceptions outsiders have about your community, just as it is influenced by other cultural/social influences.

In this exercise, you'll have a chance to reflect on how your community influenced your sexual development and how those influences continue to be part of you today.

INFLUENCES OF COLOR, ETHNICITY, AND RELIGION

Directions

This is a journaling exercise, so write down your thoughts as they come to you, before you have time to censor or edit. You may not think certain questions apply to you. If so, write down the question, leave a space after it, and go on to the next question. Later you may find that you have a memory that fits that unanswered question.

Now read through the questions listed below. Each question asks you to think about one aspect of how your community (based on geography, color, ethnicity, or religious affiliation) influenced your understanding and experience of sexuality. Think of an experience that reminds you of the question and write down that experience. If you're not sure of your exact age at the time, make your best guess. Because your community may have different views now than when you were growing up, we ask you to think about the influences on you as you grew up.

- *What did your community teach you about sex education?*
- *What did your religion teach about women's sexuality?*
- *Did your religion teach this through your parents at home or through your church, temple, or mosque?*
- *Did your community view sexuality more conservatively than the larger culture?*
- *Did your community have a different standard about public modesty for women than for men?*
- *Did your community let you choose whom you dated?*
- *What were the rules about dating in your community?*
- *What were the rules about clothing or showing your body in your community?*
- *Did your community place value on a woman's physical beauty?*
- *How was beauty defined?*
- *Did your community place value on a woman's size, shape, or skin color?*
- *Did your community place value on a woman's role as a family member and caregiver?*
- *What did your community teach you about women's dress and makeup?*
- *How did your community feel about women shaving their body hair? About body piercing? About tattooing?*
- *What were the rules in your community about young women flirting?*
- *What were the rules in your community about older women flirting?*
- *What were the rules about flirting with those outside your community?*
- *How did your community feel about women enjoying sexual pleasure?*
- *Was masturbation ever discussed in your community?*
- *How did your community view sexual pleasuring, including oral sex?*
- *Did your community let you choose whom you married?*
- *How did your community feel about marriage with outsiders?*
- *What were your community's views about gays and lesbians?*
- *If you are bilingual, in which language do you make love?*
- *If bilingual, in which language do you think about sexual terminology?*

- *If your community is a minority within a larger culture, how did the larger culture's standard of beauty make you feel as you were growing up?*
- *How does the larger culture make you feel now?*
- *Growing up, did the larger culture hold negative views about the sexuality of women in your community?*
- *What were the views you thought the larger culture held about women of your ethnicity or color?*
- *To what extent have your values been influenced by your community?*

On a scale of 1 to 6, with 1 being the least and 6 being the most, rate your community's influence on you now.

Reflection

✦ Looking back through your answers, do you see areas of hurt or conflict?

✦ How have you handled the injuries or conflict?

✦ Did you find support within your community during hard times?

✦ Are there women with whom you could share stories and gain support for your ethnicity and sexuality?

Next Steps

1. Your feelings about living in your skin may change over time, so periodically review these questions, perhaps thinking of other questions to ask yourself.

2. Label two columns My Community and Larger Culture. List your answers under My Community. Now speculate how someone raised in the larger culture would answer the same questions about her upbringing and write those answers under Larger Culture. Compare your answers in each column. How do you feel about any differences? How do you feel about any similarities? Do you feel that your experience has been vastly different?

3. Encourage a friend to do her own journaling about community influences. Share your notes and experiences. Even if you are of the same ethnic group, your experiences may have been very different.

4. If you are in a partnership, what beliefs about color, ethnicity, religion, and sexuality does your partner hold? Share your timeline and encourage your partner to make one too.

5. If you are in a biracial marriage, discuss with your partner how the larger culture views sexuality for biracial couples.

6. If you are a parent, what beliefs about color, ethnicity, religion, and sexuality would you like to convey to your children?

7. If you are a parent, ask your children how they experience their color, ethnicity, religion, and color.

This exercise may bring up painful memories of discrimination and misunderstanding. Perhaps this is the first time you've thought about your sexuality in this way. You may notice how different your experiences were from your parents' expectations. You may notice how much the larger culture has changed (or not changed) in relation to your color, ethnicity, or religion. By tracing the history of your body, your sexual development, and the messages from your community, you're ready to tackle the beliefs and attitudes you have about your sexuality.

Beliefs and Attitudes

Our beliefs about and attitudes toward sex are shaped over our lifetime and exert a profound influence on our sexual behavior and satisfaction. Beliefs and attitudes shaped by negative experiences or faulty education can hold you back from having a better relationship with your partner and yourself.

In this next exercise you are asked to list your attitudes and beliefs about sexuality and to think about where those beliefs came from and whether they are still meaningful to you.

BELIEFS AND ATTITUDES

Directions

Make a list of the following developmental periods:

- *Infancy*
- *Childhood*
- *Preadolescence*
- *Adolescence*
- *Late adolescence and early adulthood—18–29*
- *Adulthood—30s*
- *Early middle years—40s*
- *Middle years—50s*
- *Later middle years—60s*
- *Older adult years—70s*
- *Early old age—80s*
- *Old age—90s*

Write down any sexual beliefs or attitudes you have for each developmental period. For instance, for "Infancy" you might write: "Infants are not sexual" or "A baby's sexuality should be protected."

To help identify your beliefs and attitudes, read through your work from the other exercises ("Your Body's Historical Timeline," "Your Sexual History Timeline," "Your Sexual Orientation," and "Influences of Color, Ethnicity, and Religion"). Think about the beliefs and attitudes you learned or developed as a result of these experiences.

Next to each belief or attitude, write down where you think it came from—who or what influenced this belief or attitude?

As you look at your list, do you see attitudes and beliefs that you'd like to revise, perhaps based on your life experience, reading this book, or talking with others?

Reflection

✦ Reading through the list can be a periodic activity that recharges your awareness. You may want to ask a friend what she was taught and what she believes now about sex. If you're in a relationship, you can ask your partner about his or her attitudes and beliefs. If you're in contact with your siblings, ask them how their attitudes and beliefs were shaped by your family's environment. Try to be nonjudgmental in sharing and listening to yourself and others.

Next Steps

1. Because attitudes and beliefs may change over time, periodically review your list and note any changes, even small ones.

2. If you're in a partnership, try to come up with a shared list of attitudes and beliefs.

3. If you're a parent, ask yourself what beliefs you would like to convey to your children about female sexuality and sexual interaction. Think about initiating conversations with your children on this topic.

4. If you're a parent, use your own sexual journey as an opportunity to provide sex education and values clarification for your children. Ask your children to articulate their views about sex. Discuss different sexual scenarios and how their beliefs about sex would apply. Share your own thoughts and beliefs in relation to the scenarios. Remember that this is a discussion in progress, not a one-time-only opportunity. When talking with anyone about his or her attitudes and beliefs, you are treading near the very core of that individual's personality and identity. You'll need to move gently, avoid preaching, and revisit the discussions regularly.

WAYS TO UNDERSTAND YOUR BODY

As we stated in Part II, our bodies are central to our sexuality. They make possible the experience of pleasure and the yearned-for connection to our lovers. Being familiar with our bodies not only helps de-mystify sex but also makes it easier to relax and feel confident in sexual situations.

Following are three exercises to help you become more familiar and comfortable with your body.

Body Language

How you experience yourself as a person begins with the words you use to describe your body. Though everyone has a general language of body terms, we've discovered that some women have never developed an intimate, private language for their bodies, and many women never learned the proper terms for the sexual parts of their bodies. Some haven't taken time to think about what parts of their bodies are sexually responsive. When you think about and name the sexual parts of your body, you are acknowledging the importance of your sexuality. The following exercise is designed to help you develop your own body language.

BODY LANGUAGE

Directions

Find a comfortable place to sit or stretch out. Have a pad of paper and a pen ready. Beginning with your toes, think of each part of your body, perhaps even touching that part, and then write down the name you use for that part of your body. Don't type this assignment—your own handwriting is important.

Look at your list, studying each word carefully. Did you leave any words out? What words did you use for your genitals? What do you call other sexual parts of your body?

Circle any word that is a put-down or a negative word. Remember that words can be negative for some people, but not for others. For example, boobs or pussy may seem negative for one woman but very natural and positive for another woman.

Cross out negative words and substitute more positive ones. Referring back to Chapter 3 may help you come up with alternative words.

Take the words for the sexual parts of your body and rewrite them, putting the word my in front of each. Look at your list again. Do you like these words? If there are still words that you don't like, cross them out and write in the words that you want to start using for your body. There is no objective standard of right or wrong, only the words that are right or wrong for you.

Trace your finger across each word in the completed list. These are the words that you use to describe your body. This is your personal body language.

Reflection

+ Are the words on your list ones you would want a lover to use?

+ When you're mad at yourself, do you use negative or positive words for your body? For example, do you use "cunt" or "asshole" as a way to put yourself down?

+ Make an effort to use your positive body language all the time.

Next Steps

1. Review your list several times over the next few weeks. Make a conscious effort to use your body language when you talk to yourself about your body. Use these words with your lover as well.

2. A further idea might be to ask a friend what words she uses in her body language.

3. Continue to think about and use your body language to gain increased comfort with your sexual self.

Hands-On Exploration

The exercises you've completed thus far have asked you to look inward, remember, and reflect on the meaning of life experiences, beliefs and attitudes, and sexual language. The next two exercises move from the realm of thoughts, ideas, and words to the world of flesh and blood. We ask you to get close and personal as you examine your body.

First we're going to have you focus on your genitals. Many women have been conditioned to have negative or even phobic reactions to their genitals—which, not surprisingly, often results in sexual avoidance and dissatisfaction. Knowledge of, and familiarity with, your genitalia can help desensitize these reactions.

EXPLORING YOUR BODY

Directions

Undress from the waist down and make yourself comfortable on your bed or sofa. Prop pillows behind your back. Spread your legs apart, and with a small mirror, study your vulva. Have this book alongside you, opened to the diagrams in Chapter 3.

Identify your clitoris, labia majora, labia minora, perineum, and anus.

After propping the mirror to free your hands, spread the labia apart and look for the urethra and examine the introitus (vaginal opening). Take your time, paying attention to the texture of the skin and whether the opening of your vagina is moist or dry.

Slide back the prepuce (clitoral hood) and examine the exposed clitoris.

Moisten a finger with saliva or a water-soluble lubricant and insert your finger in your vagina. Explore the interior of your vagina. Notice its ridges and wetness. If you have the physical flexibility to do so, press the upper wall of your vagina, about 2 inches inside, toward your pubic bone. Try rubbing back and forth. You may feel some pressure to urinate, and you may feel pleasant sensations. If you continue the stimulation, you may experience sexual arousal. The level of arousal will be different for different women and will depend somewhat on how much experience you have had with stimulating your G spot. The goal is to be aware of the different areas of arousal of your body, not to achieve a specific level of stimulation.

With your finger inserted in your vagina, contract your pelvic muscles. Note the pressure of the muscular contractions around your finger.

Experiment with the sensation of contracting and relaxing the pelvic muscles.

Reflection

+ For many women, this exercise may be the first time they have closely examined their genitals or perhaps the first time they have touched their genitals directly without using a towel, washcloth, or tissue. This can be a big step, and initially it may feel uncomfortable.

+ If you find yourself becoming anxious, stop for a few moments, close your eyes, do some deep breathing, and remind yourself that your exploration and touching are really no different from examining your nose or ear. Remember, this is your body.

+ If you find this exercise overwhelming at first, break it down into steps that seem more manageable. For example, the first time, simply study your vulva in the mirror until you feel more comfortable. Perhaps the next time you repeat the exercise, add touch, but touch only your pubic hair and surface skin. Later, when you feel ready, you can explore the opening of your vagina. By slowly phasing in all the steps as you repeat the exercise over time, you will probably reduce your uncomfortable feelings.

Next Steps

1. Continue strengthening your sense of ease with your body. Each time you bathe or take a shower, rather than rushing through the process of washing your genitals, take a moment to pull back your clitoral hood and spread open your labia, study your exposed genitals, touch and stroke them lovingly as you rinse, and review your body language.

2. Continue to the next exercise, which focuses on your pelvic floor muscles.

In addition to your genitalia, your pelvic floor muscles are a very important source of sexual pleasure and arousal. Contracting and relaxing the pelvic muscles can actually promote lubrication and increase arousal. The sensations of sexual activity can be heightened by consciously pulsing these muscles.

Gaining voluntary control over the pelvic floor muscles can have additional benefits to increasing sexual satisfaction. As women age and lose estrogen, the elasticity of the muscles can be affected. Strengthening these muscles not only counteracts this loss of elasticity but also can help with involuntary urine loss that some women experience.

PELVIC FLOOR MUSCLES EXERCISE

Directions

Identify the pelvic floor muscles and how you control them. As a first step, when you are urinating, start and stop the flow of urine. When you have accomplished this, you have begun to isolate control of the pelvic floor muscles.

Find a comfortable place and time where you can lie back and use a hand mirror to see your vulva. Contract and relax your pelvic floor muscles. You may be able to see the perineum (the area between your vaginal opening and your anus) move in and out as you contract and relax these muscles. Your buttocks may squeeze together, but the goal is to notice the sensation of contracting the muscles around the vulva rather than the butt muscles, stomach, or thigh muscles. Depending on your body size and flexibility, you may not be able to see much, but you should be able to feel whether your muscles are contracting appropriately. Place your hand gently against your vulva and contract your muscles. You'll feel them move.

When you are doing this exercise, note which parts of your pelvic region are contracting. Don't just tighten the muscles. Alternately push out, as if you were trying to expel a tampon. Notice the differences in the sensation of contracting and relaxing the muscle.

Moisten a finger with saliva or a water-soluble lubricant and try inserting it in your vagina. With your finger inserted, contract your pelvic muscles. Note the pressure of the muscular contractions around your finger.

Experiment with the sensation of contracting and relaxing the pelvic muscles. Exercising the pelvic muscles can be sexually arousing. Focus on your arousal. Try contracting the muscles in brief, short pulses and in longer, more concentrated contractions. See which is the most satisfying and arousing to you. This exercise may remind you of the description of Kegel exercises in Chapter 8.

Try lying on your back while tensing and relaxing your pelvic muscles several times. Then proceed to rock your pelvis up and down, as if mimicking intercourse in the missionary position. Try 10 "rocks" followed by 10 pelvic muscle exercises.

Reflection

+ Did your pelvic floor muscles feel strong or weak?

+ Do you feel much control over these muscles? Many women have weak control of these muscles and have never attempted to increase voluntary control of them. At first it may seem like these muscles have a mind of their own, but don't become discouraged.

+ Did this focus on your pelvic muscles make you feel aroused? Like any exercise program, don't expect that you will gain dramatic control or feel the sexually arousing aspects of pelvic muscle exercises immediately.

Next Steps

Practice the tightening and relaxing exercises frequently during the day. You can do pelvic floor muscle exercises anywhere without anyone being aware of what you are doing.

WAYS TO MAKE PEACE WITH YOUR BODY

In Part III of this book, we examined some of the challenges that can alienate a woman from her body—low body esteem, illness, disability, genital pain, STIs, and trauma. This alienation often prevents a woman from experiencing sexual pleasure and satisfaction. As a result, making peace with their bodies is a crucial step for most women when striving for sexual health. The following exercises add to the ideas in Part III for making peace with your body, regardless of the cause of alienation, by presenting strategies for increasing body acceptance and expanding your capacity to experience pleasure.

Liking What You See

To enjoy sexual feelings, it's important to be firmly rooted in your body—not a perfect body but *your* body. All too often women become alienated from their bodies because they don't conform to Madison Avenue's definition of beauty. If they don't dwell on their bodies, they decide, they won't feel ashamed or disgusted. Other women are alienated from their bodies because of their upbringing. They learned at an early age that nakedness was bad and sensual pleasure was shameful. This exercise is designed to help you make peace with your body. The more often you look at your body, the less foreign it will be to you. What at first you considered to be flaws or imperfections should become, to you, aspects of your uniqueness. By becoming more accepting of your body, you'll feel less self-conscious during lovemaking; you'll be less distracted and more capable of focusing on erotic cues.

LIKING WHAT YOU SEE

Directions

Find time alone when you have privacy and no concerns about being interrupted. First take a leisurely bath or shower to unwind and relax. Afterward, stand before a full-length mirror and study your naked body. Talk out loud to yourself, describing what you see, what you like, and what makes you feel awkward.

Highlight and let yourself feel good about features that please you—perhaps the shape of your calf, the curves of your breast, the profile of your face, the muscle tone of your arms, the softness of your thighs, or the texture of your nipples.

Note your negative reactions and recognize that these reactions are probably based on society's obsession with the perfect body. Refer to the cognitive work section ("The Solution, Not the Problem, May Be in Your Head") in Chapter 15 for guidance on challenging and revising any negative thoughts you have.

Reflection

+ If you find it difficult looking at yourself nude, perhaps try the exercise in your underwear or fully clothed. Start by restricting your focus to just one part of your body. Repeat the exercise over a number of days, carrying on a healthy dialogue with yourself. Identify the thoughts that make nakedness threatening and process them by using the suggestions provided in the section "Challenging Our Thinking: Moving from Punitive to Positive Awareness" in Chapter 6.

+ It can be difficult to downplay the constant hype about perfect bodies. It's important to confront Madison Avenue's beauty bias and not allow it to rob you of the pleasure you can feel in your body.

Next Steps

1. Work on analyzing and revising negative and inaccurate thinking.

2. Move on to the next exercise.

Sensory Journey

When sex becomes a source of conflict, fear, or discomfort, you may learn to distance yourself from all physical feelings, not just sexual sensations. But even if you're not alienated from your body, you may have similar difficulties with being out of touch with physical sensations. Do you take pride in being able to do two or three things at once, like entertaining your toddler with funny faces as you talk on the phone and empty the dishwasher? That's great in terms of efficiency, but it also means you've probably become an expert at ignoring your sensory cues in favor of outside demands and responsibilities. While making funny faces and managing the phone and dishwasher, you may have ignored the fact that your feet hurt, that you are bone-tired, and that you want to lie down. You tune *out* what your body is saying and tune *in* to what the outside world is demanding of you.

The goal of this exercise is to reverse the process of blindly responding to outside demands by ignoring physical sensations. Instead, you will be encouraged to respond to what your senses tell you.

SENSORY JOURNEY

Directions

This exercise focuses on your five senses, beginning with sight, then sound, smell, taste, and touch. You may want to read through it first so that you can plan this exercise in advance. You will need to gather different objects, and you'll need a place where you can relax undisturbed. You should allow at least an hour for this exercise.

In advance, collect the following items: mirror, radio or music player with favorite music, and a clock that ticks. Put together some favorite scented items like incense, scented candles, perfume, a favorite bar of soap, a small pine or cedar branch, an orange, and cinnamon or some other spice. Gather a few favorite tastes like fruit or chocolate.

To begin, undress slowly and take a leisurely bath or shower, noticing the feel of the water on your skin. Press your face against the cool side of the tub or shower, contrasting the soft warmth of the water with the hard coolness of the tile. Slide your hands gently all over your body, consciously focusing on the water wrapping around you.

When you decide to end your shower or bath, move out of the tub slowly, noticing the feel of the air against your damp skin. Dry off carefully, focusing on the rough texture of the towel against your skin and the tingling feeling where rough and smooth meet.

SIGHT

Now you're ready to begin the sensory exploration. While still naked, stand in front of a mirror and stretch both hands over your head and reach for the ceiling, first with one arm, then with the other. Notice the comforting stretch of your muscles and watch in the mirror as your body moves with your arms.

Let your arms come down to your sides and study your head and face. See your hair wet from the shower or bath. Look into your eyes and smile, really smile, at yourself. Think about how happy you were when there was a snow day and school was canceled, or when you found your favorite childhood doll in a box in the attic, and smile like you did then. Let your eyes look at all of you and, for once, just let your body be. This exercise is not about shape; it's about sense.

Slowly turn around in front of the mirror, letting your eyes roam over all of you. Find the hollow where your shoulder blades meet. Look at other special places on your body. Find places you can affirm and, for once, don't criticize any part of you. This exercise is about your ability to see and enjoy the sense of sight.

SOUND

Move over to a soft place where you can sit or lie down. Concentrate on listening to the sounds around you. Are they familiar sounds? Listen to the sounds of a clock ticking, of noises coming from outside the room, of the stillness in the room. Listen to the sound of your body moving on the fabric where you are lying. Listen to the sound of your feet as you move them against each other.

Listen to the sound of your fingers as you brush them against your skin. Listen to the sound of your own breathing. Try breathing in slow, even breaths.

Put on a recording of your favorite music or nature sounds. Listen to the blends of sounds and how the music is soft at times, then louder, sometimes gentle, and sometimes urgent and compelling.

Check out the sound of your own voice. Start by saying your name out loud. Say a few other things like the names of your favorite foods, your best friends, or places you want to visit.

Now focus on finding the range and variations of your voice. Hum a brief passage of the music you just heard. Next, softly hum a steady note with your lips closed. Now open your mouth and see how the sound changes.

Make soft "la-la" sounds with your mouth open. Change the sound as your tongue taps the roof of your mouth. Change the pace of how fast you sing "la-la-la" and let a little more sound out.

Sing "Doe, a deer . . . " Each musical note in the song has a different vowel sound. Skip the words and concentrate on the sounds. For example "doe" becomes "ooohh," "ray" becomes "aaaehh," "me" becomes "eeeee," and "fa" "aaaaah." Think of how the sounds are similar to lovemaking sounds. Practice whispering the sounds as well as saying them out loud.

Now try saying sexual words out loud. Maybe these are words from your body language list, or things you'd like to try with your lover. Saying the words out loud when you're alone is good rehearsal for asking for what you want when you're having sex with your partner. If you feel self-conscious about saying the sex words out loud, practice whispering them.

SMELL

Remember those items you collected in the smell category before beginning this exercise? Now's the time to focus on them. Notice the different scents and concentrate on your responses to each one. Let your mind wander freely. What do the scents remind you of? Where were you when you last smelled that scent?

Now take your fingers and slowly slide them over your vulva and into your vagina. Let your fingers come into contact with your vaginal secretions.

Now bring your fingers to your nose and inhale. This is your body's natural human scent. What does this smell like to you?

TASTE

Repeat the last exercise using the foods you've selected. Roll these foods around in your mouth. Concentrate on their unique flavor and the way you respond to them. Let your mind wander to other times you've enjoyed tasting these particular flavors.

If you're comfortable with this, insert your finger into your vagina and then slide your finger into your mouth. What do you taste like? Some women say this is a chalky taste. Others think it's slightly salty. You get to be the expert on yourself.

TOUCH

Take time to touch yourself slowly and carefully, starting with your toes and ending by sliding your fingers through your scalp. Concentrate on your response to this touch. Where do you like to touch yourself? Are there places that are ticklish or uncomfortable? Are there places that you're comfortable touching but don't want a partner to touch?

End the touch exercise by gently touching and massaging your face. Stroke your eyes, your forehead, your cheeks, and finally your mouth.

Reflection

✦ As you moved through each section of the exercise, what were your reactions? Was it hard to move from the more "passive" part of the exercise involving sight to the more active parts, like making sounds and singing? What thoughts crossed your mind as you did this exercise? Was any part of the exercise distasteful?

✦ Were your thoughts strongly negative (e.g., *I hate doing this*, or *This is disgusting*, or *I just can't do this*)? If so, where do you think the response came from?

✦ If you want to work on the negative thoughts or feelings, you can try substituting more positive thoughts, like, *Even though this feels a little funny at first, I can do this*, or *I can try it a few times and if I don't like it, I'll try making up some sensory experiences that are more comfortable for me.*

Next Steps

1. If you liked increasing your sensory awareness, make up some of your own exercises using your five senses.

2. Make a point every day to take time to tune in rather than tune out the subtle signals registering in your senses. Enjoy seeing, smelling, tasting, feeling, and hearing things that you have normally missed in the past.

WAYS TO INCREASE EROTICISM

Thus far the exercises have guided you in becoming more aware of your sexual history, more knowledgeable about your body and comfortable with it, and more sensitized to physical sensations. All of these objectives are important prerequisites for sexual health and satisfaction. Now we want you to focus on ways to heighten your eroticism—your ability to experience sexual thoughts, desire, and sensations.

Get Attitude

Probably the most important ingredient for heightened eroticism is not technique but attitude. With the right attitude—the sense that you are comfortable with your body, interested in eroticism, and ready to pleasure and be pleasured—you create a sexual aura around yourself. You bring to lovemaking a sensuality and energy that can excite and fulfill both you and your partner. Interestingly, women with this type of attitude are often found to be attractive and desirable, regardless of body type or the presence or absence of physical features society associates with beauty. On the other hand, classic beauties who lack this attitude are often found to be neither sexually desirable nor sexually fulfilled.

Admittedly, "getting attitude" can be easier said than done. It would be nice if all we had to do to escape self-defeating attitudes about sexuality was to tell ourselves, *Don't think that way!* Unfortunately, it's not that easy. As we discussed earlier, changing sexual attitudes takes self-examination, ongoing awareness, and hard work. The good news is that it can be done, and the fact that you're reading this book shows that you've begun the process. Chapter 6 on body image is one good place to start, and making a commitment to work on your sexuality by doing the exercises in this chapter is a good way to continue.

Fantasy

Sexual fantasies can play an important role in heightening eroticism. They are perfectly normal and, indeed, a part of the sexual experience of people everywhere. It is important to note that some people find the idea of sexual fantasies awkward; during sex they rely solely on the physical and emotional sensations of the moment. Still others may be intrigued by the idea but feel too conflicted about sexual fantasies to experiment with using them. Perhaps they were raised with the belief that sexual thoughts—which are fantasies—were sinful and to be avoided. This type of upbringing can create confusion, conflict, and even shame about having sexual fantasies. For vast numbers of people, however, fantasies freely accompany sexual arousal without reservation or guilt.

What goes through your head during lovemaking will impact how pleasurable and satisfying the experience will be. Research has shown that the most common cause of loss of physical arousal in healthy people is the loss of erotic focus. *Erotic focus* means being fully mindful of the sexy, arousing thoughts and sensations during lovemaking. Assuming you're in good physical health, if during lovemaking you focus on the pleasant tingling radiating from your vulva, the feel of your partner's skin, or mental images that are sexual, nature will take its course. If, on the other hand, during the midst of your partner's passionate foreplay you're trying to remember whose turn it is to pick up the kids from soccer practice, you can say good-bye to arousal. Remember, women are often conditioned to be much more attentive than men to the little distractions that can pop up during sexual situations. Sexy thinking and imagery can help a woman maintain the erotic focus that is critical for sexual arousal.

Why does sexual fantasy "work"? Remember that your mind has an extremely powerful influence over your body. When you see a movie where the hero is dangling over a cliff, your heart races, your breathing speeds up, and your body tenses. You know it's make-believe, but for a few moments you suspend your critical judgment and allow this two-dimensional picture to become your reality. Your body reacts accordingly. The same thing happens with sexual fantasy. This is why sexual fantasy is one of the most powerful (and free) aphrodisiacs available to us.

Fantasies Unlimited

Because people are unique, there will be a great deal of variability in what each person finds arousing in a sexual fantasy. Fantasy is an adaptive resource that can serve as a rehearsal for how you want to change something in your life, or it can be a fleeting, fictitious time-out from reality. Some people enjoy having the same sexual fantasy every time they make love. They say it is a sure way to arousal. Some have a smorgasbord of fantasies. Some draw upon passionate scenes from a book or movie, some recall past experiences with their partner, and others create imaginary scenes involving strangers or people they know only in passing.

Imagining sex with someone other than one's partner is a concern for some people. It's important to remember that fantasies are not necessarily wishes. As a matter of fact, research has shown that people often fantasize about things they would never act on in real life, even if the opportunity presented itself. Heterosexual women and men may, on occasion, fantasize about a homosexual encounter. In real life they may have no interest in making love to someone of the same sex, but within the safety and anonymity of fantasy the unthinkable can lead to novel excitement. Women and men may fantasize rape (sexual force is a common fantasy theme), but this does not mean they would want to sexually exploit or be exploited in real life. Within the safety of make-believe, however, sex without consent may be an exciting image for some people.

Fantasy Detractors

When you fantasize, you're taking advantage of the novelty that imagination can create to heighten your sexual excitement. Fantasy allows you to flirt with outrageous and totally out-of-character sexual behavior without any risk of harm, whether alone in masturbation or with your partner. "But doesn't this distract from the intimacy of the moment?" some people ask. We think not. During the act of making love, you are choosing to share your body with your partner. Using a mental image to heighten your arousal is no different from stroking your own genitals during lovemaking.

Intensifying your own excitement doesn't detract from the basic significance of the fact that you are freely choosing to share with your partner one of the most personal and intimate ways of experiencing pleasure.

As we have discussed earlier, sex makes us vulnerable. Egos can be fragile. We wouldn't suggest that after the next act of lovemaking, as you lie with your partner in a brief postorgasmic glow, you say, "That was great! Between you and Brad Pitt, that was one incredible experience!" Your sexual fantasies belong to you. Fantasies are not wishes or intentions. Some couples enjoy sharing fantasies; others wisely agree to respect boundaries in each other's private world. You can certainly discuss with your partner how you want to handle talking about sexual fantasies.

Like any resource, you can use fantasy in an adaptive or maladaptive way. When it comes to sexual fantasy, we think there's a big difference between lusting after every warm body that walks by and making use of thoughts and visual imagery to enhance a moment of shared pleasure with a sexual partner.

Some professionals have questioned whether encouraging people to use fantasies will leave them dissatisfied with the real thing. It's similar to the fear that if a woman uses a vibrator, she might end up preferring it to the real thing. We don't believe either possibility is a realistic concern, with one important caveat. If a couple has good communication, works hard at developing a relationship characterized by mutual respect and sensitivity for each other, and approaches sex in a loving way without hidden agendas, neither fantasies nor vibrators will ever compare to the real thing.

FANTASY

Directions

Explore your capacity for fantasy. Try the following:

- *If you ever had an exciting sexual experience in the past, recall it in vivid detail. Write about it in your journal. Embellish the details to make it even more dramatic, romantic, and arousing.*
- *Read examples of other women's sexual fantasies. (There are many excellent books and magazines featuring women's sexual fantasies and erotica. See the "Suggested Resources" section at the end of the book.)*
- *Take a shot at writing your own sexual fantasy. Remember, just because you fantasize about someone or something doesn't necessarily mean that you would ever act out the fantasy in real life.*

Reflection

✦ If you read samples of female erotica, you may find that many of the fantasies have little effect on you. That's fine. Fantasies are highly personal and can be incredibly diverse. Even if you find only one or two intriguing or exciting examples of fantasy when reading these books, your time will have been well spent. The object is to expand your horizons, to come up with imagery that can excite and arouse rather than depress and discourage you.

Next Steps

1. Make time to let your mind wander to sensual thoughts.

2. If you watch a movie or read a book that has a scenario you find sensual and exciting, replay it in your mind, casting yourself as a main character.

Masturbation

Masturbation is an ideal learning environment for increasing eroticism; it provides a safe, private, relaxed opportunity for you to explore your body and how it responds to stimulation. Most men benefit from this learning opportunity during adolescence. Many women don't have this advantage. From an early age they're taught that good girls don't touch themselves "down there." Because early in life many women are told that menstruation is "the curse," their genitals become guilty by association.

Masturbation is one of those sexual practices that has long carried a social taboo. People often blush when the topic is raised, yet as many as 95% of all men and 71% of all women have masturbated to orgasm at some point in their life (Gerressu et al., 2008). And the practice of masturbation isn't restricted to adolescents who have hormones bursting out of their ears. Research has suggested that more than a third of women between the ages of 60 and 69 and almost one in five women over the age of 70 continue to masturbate on occasion (AARP, 2010). We're therefore talking about a very common practice, despite a history of social and religious condemnation.

Even though masturbation is so common, many people are troubled if they learn that their partner is doing it. Perhaps priding themselves on being open-minded, they concede that masturbation is okay for adolescents, single adults, and even married adults when separated from their spouse. But, they argue, masturbation shouldn't be necessary if you're in a satisfying sexual relationship. *If my wife's happy with our sex life*, a man might reason, *why would she want to masturbate? Why settle for a substitute*, a woman might argue, *when he can have the real thing?*

Yet despite these common misgivings, in a large survey of a representative national sample, 85% of the men and 45% of the women living with a sexual partner had masturbated during the preceding year (Laumann et al., 1994). For many men and women in a relationship, masturbation is not a rejection or an avoidance of the partner, but an enjoyable erotic practice that can produce a very powerful orgasm. If you think about it, masturbation represents the perfect touch—you know exactly where to touch, how to touch, and how much to touch. The amount of pressure and the speed of the stroking are continually adjusted to match your growing level of excitement until you climax. Emotionally, masturbation may not compete with the joy of making love to your partner, but that doesn't mean that masturbation can't be enjoyed in its own right.

It's unfortunate that masturbation has such a bad name. We believe that self-pleasuring is a positive thing in our lives and should be enjoyed and valued. Consider the fact that we feel no shame when taking delight in any of our senses. We relish the aroma of fresh bread baking in the oven, the melody of a musical score, the feel of silk against our skin, the subtle aftertaste of a fine wine, the eye-pleasing hues of a sunset. How fortunate we are as human beings to experience these simple pleasures in life. And, we would argue, isn't it also wonderful that we can touch certain parts of our body and produce immense pleasure? Why should this pleasure be considered as different from any other pleasure we derive from our bodies?

MASTURBATION

Directions

Before attempting this exercise, read and reread the following set of instructions to minimize any distractions such as wondering, What am I supposed to do next? Once you understand the steps, go ahead and enjoy.

Find a time when you're home alone and won't be interrupted. Consider turning the ringer off on your phone. If you want, start with a leisurely bath or shower. Set a comfortable, sensuous mood with lighting and music. For this exercise you can either be nude or wear underwear or lingerie that makes you feel sensual. Lie down and make yourself comfortable. The following steps are suggestions—feel free to improvise:

- *Lightly touch your face with your fingertips. Lightly stroke your cheeks and draw your fingers across your forehead. Rub your temples; massage your scalp. Slow down, take your time. Notice the texture and the temperature of your skin. Pay attention to your breathing. Take long deep breaths and tell yourself to relax; try to make your entire body go limp each time you exhale.*
- *Now move your hands up and down your arms, across your shoulders, and behind your neck. Note your muscle tone, especially any sign of tension or tightness. Vary your touch by rubbing, lightly stroking, and kneading your muscles. Continue to slow your breathing; take long, deep breaths and tell yourself to relax.*
- *Move your hands to your breasts; cup them, stroke them, play with them. Lightly roll your nipples between your fingertips. Gently pinch them, pull on them, stroke them.*
- *Continue down, massaging your abdomen, hips, and thighs. Slow down; vary your touch; keep your breathing slow and even. If you want, you can sit forward and massage your calves and your feet. Whatever you do, don't rush.*
- *When you're ready, move back up your body to your pelvis. Place both hands over your vulva and apply gentle pressure. Barely move your hands in small, slow circles as you again tell yourself to relax.*

- *Position your hand so you touch your clitoris, rubbing it gently between your thumb and fingertips. Now stroke the shaft of your clitoris, the part that is below the surface of your vulva; lightly stroke the entire length of your clitoris with slow up-and-down movements. Experiment with speed and the amount of pressure.*
- *While stroking your clitoris, with your other hand explore your labia, rubbing and stroking gently. Touch your introitus. Experiment with pressing your thighs together as you stroke your vulva to apply more pressure. Try gently rocking your hips up and down as you stroke. Using a lubricant may make it easier to glide your fingers along your clitoris, over your vulva, and into your vagina.*
- *If you have the flexibility to reach two inches or so inside of your vagina, stroke along the front wall. It may take some minutes of direct stimulation and firm pressure in this area before the stimulating effects are evident. Experiment with speed and amount of pressure.*

From here you're on your own. Self-stimulation is a highly personalized experience in self-loving. Experiment by searching for movements and touching that create the most pleasurable sensations. Give yourself permission to abandon yourself to your sensations. Indulge yourself in fantasy to help heighten your focus and arousal. For a few moments forget about your scrutinizing self— there will be time later for that.

Stop when you feel satisfied. Don't wait for an orgasm. If one comes, fine. If you don't orgasm but find the stimulation pleasurable, that's equally fine.

Reflection

+ Were you able to relax enough to allow yourself to experience the sensations? If not, look for possible reasons and distracting thoughts. Write them down and speculate on any steps you might take to overcome these challenges. As before, make use of your cognitive restructuring skills.

+ Don't expect a specific outcome on your first attempt. For some of you, the exercise may seem quite radical and may take a number of times before you become sufficiently relaxed to enjoy the experience.

+ As you repeat the exercise, don't be restricted by our instructions. The steps are not meant to be a cookbook recipe for sexual arousal. Experiment, follow your instincts, do what feels good.

+ If this exercise seemed overwhelming, break it down into more manageable parts. Perhaps start fully clothed, wearing loose-fitting, comfortable garments. The first few times you do the exercise, restrict your focus to nongenital stimulation.

+ If masturbation is an unacceptable behavior for you, consider making use of this exercise by restricting it to nongenital touching to learn more about deriving pleasure from your entire body. Contrary to popular opinion, the clitoris and vagina are not your only sex organs. Your mind and your skin, whether on your face or the soles of your feet, function as vital sex organs, capable of producing intense sexual arousal.

✦ Even if religious or personal reasons prohibit you from performing this exercise, don't worry. These steps can be incorporated later in an exercise with your partner. That way, you will still have an opportunity to explore ways of arousal without using masturbation.

Next Steps

1. Negative thinking is self-defeating. Follow through by cognitively restructuring negative thinking (see "The Solution, Not the Problem, Might Be in Your Head" in Chapter 15).

2. Repeat this exercise, modifying and customizing the steps until you become comfortable and find the experience pleasurable (not necessarily orgasmic, but pleasurable).

3. Go on to the next section for thoughts about how to further let yourself go so you can more fully enjoy sexual sensations.

Letting Go

Many women find it difficult to let go and experience sexual arousal with abandon. Whether making love with their partner or self-pleasuring, they find themselves holding back, if ever so slightly. Sexual arousal and orgasm can be powerful experiences involving involuntary sounds and movements. Some women fear losing control during sex and appearing foolish. Play-acting can help you to loosen up and desensitize you so the prospect of being really turned on or experiencing a dramatic orgasm won't seem so threatening.

AN ACADEMY AWARD PERFORMANCE[1]

Directions

When the house is empty, lie back and relax. To help create a sensual mood, you may want to read erotic literature or fantasize about a sexy scene. You may want to listen to music. Some women prefer quiet music; others prefer high-energy, get-the-body dancing music.

Role-play the most dramatic, violent orgasm imaginable. Pull out all the stops. Start by moving your hips, rocking them up and down or side to side. Press your thighs together and tense your muscles in your feet, legs, and arms. Try quickening the pace of your breathing. Begin making sounds—moaning sounds, groaning sounds, sounds of unendurable pleasure. Try to let go and roll and thrash about; claw the sheets or pillow with your fingernails; moan, groan, and yell in fake ecstasy.

---

[1] This exercise has been adapted from the work of Julia Heiman and Joseph LoPiccolo (1988) in their book *Becoming Orgasmic: A Sexual and Personal Growth Program for Women.*

Reflection

+ Most women who do this exercise at some point start laughing at themselves, feeling ridiculous as they go through such dramatics. Laughing at yourself is great; sex needs to be more playful. More important, succeeding in this exercise, despite feeling mildly embarrassed and self-conscious, serves as good practice for loosening up internal control over your behavior.

+ If propriety and a sense of decorum prevented you from doing this exercise, even though you were alone and no one could observe you, you have highlighted a possible barrier to experiencing orgasm. You may choose to do further work to loosen up, to allow yourself to feel freely and express your pleasure and joy without fears about appearance or criticism. Take some time to analyze your hesitation. Try to identify self-defeating thinking and read "The Solution, Not the Problem, May Be in Your Head" in Chapter 15.

Next Steps

1. Keep working on cognitive restructuring until you feel more comfortable role-playing a dramatic orgasm.

2. After feeling more comfortable letting go, move on to the next exercise, which incorporates a vibrator for intensifying sexual arousal.

Vibrator, Anyone?

Many women find that vibrators can increase sexual arousal, during both masturbation and partnered sex. Although some women will resort to using vibrators due to difficulties experiencing orgasm or medical conditions that have led to decreased genital sensitivity, most women use vibrators for increased pleasure, novelty, and enjoyment. In a study conducted at Indiana University, more than half of the women surveyed had used a vibrator in the past, and regular vibrator users tended to be more proactive about their gynecological health and reported more positive sexual function than non-vibrator-users (Herbenick et al., 2009).

Sometimes a partner can feel threatened by the woman's use of a vibrator and worry that somehow he or she is failing or that the woman is losing interest in him or her in favor of a mechanical lover. In such instances, dialogue and reassurance are important. The partner needs to be reassured that the use of the vibrator is not an indictment of him or her as a lover. It should be pointed out that plastic and batteries can never compete with flesh-on-flesh contact and emotional intimacy.

GOOD VIBRATIONS

Directions

Purchase a vibrator. You can purchase an all-purpose vibrator (the kind that straps on the back of your hand) at major retail stores, or you can mail-order a wide variety of vibrators specifically designed for genital stimulation (see the "Suggested Resources"). A vibrator should be kept clean with soap and water. Consider a vibrator as private and personal as a toothbrush. Never transfer stimulation from the anus to the vagina or vulva without thoroughly cleaning the vibrator first.

Before attempting stimulation with a vibrator, take time to relax. Use the masturbation techniques from the previous exercise to become aroused.

Experiment with applying the vibrator to different parts of your body. The guiding principle is: if it feels good, do it more before moving on. The type of genital stimulation you get will depend on the type of vibrator you use. All vibrators allow direct and indirect stimulation of the clitoris. Use varying degrees of intensity until you identify what works best for you. Some vibrators not only allow you to stimulate your external genitalia but are designed for vaginal penetration; you can also stimulate the inner walls of the vagina. Using a vibrator in this way makes it easier to reach the G spot and experiment with sustained, applied pressure. As with any sexually pleasuring activity, there may be times when this stimulation is effective for you and times when you may prefer another type of stimulation.

Reflection

✦ Were you comfortable or awkward using the vibrator? Why?

✦ Do you have any concerns about using a vibrator? Some women fear developing a dependency on a vibrator to the point that it becomes the only way they can respond sexually. No scientific foundation supports this concern; you will not become addicted to your vibrator!

✦ How did the sensations resulting from the use of the vibrator compare to sensations when masturbating without a vibrator? How did the sensations compare to when your partner stimulates you?

✦ If you are in a relationship, how does your partner feel about your experimenting with a vibrator?

Next Steps

1. Continue to experiment with the vibrator, varying the speed, pressure, and location.

2. If you are in a relationship, discuss your experience with the vibrator and listen to your partner's reaction. Discuss how the vibrator might be incorporated into your lovemaking.

3. Talk to trusted girlfriends about their experiences with vibrators.

WAYS TO KEEP IT GOING

If you have completed all of the exercises in a thoughtful, conscientious manner, congratulations. Reading this book and doing the work in this chapter represents strong motivation and a significant commitment to sexual growth. Chances are good that your efforts have already begun to pay off in terms of increased sexual knowledge, improved body esteem, greater sexual comfort, and an expanding capacity to experience and appreciate physical pleasure. But please don't stop here.

An important part of enhancing your sexual health is actively seeking out, rather than shying away from, opportunities to be sensual. The more intentional, or thoughtful, you are about your sexual expression, the more satisfaction you will experience from it. Many women fear that if they plan their sexuality they'll lose spontaneity. Just the opposite is true: with planning, more opportunities become available for spontaneous things to happen. Planning time for your sexuality doesn't mean you are overvaluing sex, and being intentional about sexuality is not just for women with partners. Learning to take time for your sexuality is important to all women.

INVESTING TIME IN YOUR SEXUAL SELF

Directions

Think realistically about how often you'd like to feel sexual pleasure in a day, in a week, in a month. Decide how often you'd like that sexual pleasure to come through fantasy, how often through sensual touch or masturbation, and, if you have a partner, how often you'd like to include your partner. Can you find sexual pleasure in sensual thoughts and feelings, or must orgasm be present to qualify as sexual pleasure? Each woman is different.

Once you've decided how often to have a sexual experience, you can figure out where you can schedule time for it during the course of a day or week. Most women's lives are busy, and it will take prioritizing and determination to increase your time to be sexual. Keep in mind that you can vary the time you spend on a sexual activity. Not every sexual interlude needs to be two hours! If necessary, make a list of these times as a reminder of your priorities.

Reflection

✦ After a week of planning and prioritizing sex, evaluate your response. Did you like knowing when you were going to have time to concentrate on sex? Did you feel disappointed that the element of unplanned spontaneity was missing? Or did you enjoy the pleasure of anticipation as well as the pleasure of the event? Did you find yourself feeling that it was okay to plan some things, like sex with your partner, but not okay to plan other things, like sexual fantasies or masturbating?

✦ Pay attention to your thoughts and reactions. Were you critical or judgmental about yourself? If you were, it may be helpful to read Chapter 15 on analyzing, challenging, and modifying self-defeating thinking.

Next Steps

1. Continue to find time each week to explore and enjoy your sexuality.

   - If you're enjoying this sexual growth, here are some additional ideas to try over time:
   - Read other books about sex.
   - Try using a vibrator while masturbating.
   - Develop favorite sexual fantasies. If you're passive in the fantasy, try being active. If you're always the active one, try reversing the roles.
   - Rent an erotic movie.
   - Read a romance novel.
   - Write yourself a letter expressing appreciation of your sexuality.

FOURTEEN

Strengthening Your Sexual Relationship

"Some nights, I want passion and excitement—I want fireworks. I settle for Jimmy Fallon."

Most couples want a satisfying, perhaps even a vibrant and exciting sex life. They may be willing to settle for periods of abstinence, delays in frequency, and even a few boring interludes, but overall they want sex to be an enjoyable, fulfilling part of their relationship. Unfortunately, however, many of us feel that our sexual relationship has become routine, or a source of conflict, or a low priority, or a constant reminder that we're somehow sexually inadequate.

What does it take to create a more satisfying sexual relationship? What creates passion is *involvement*. To experience loving sex, it's important for both partners to commit themselves fully to talking honestly and openly about sexuality, being respectful of each other's sexual needs and vulnerabilities, and making sexual intimacy a priority in their relationship.

In this chapter we build on Chapter 12, making a series of suggestions and proposing exercises to help you and your partner enrich your sexual relationship. This is a chapter you will want to read with your partner, discuss together, and plan for together. We encourage you to keep open minds and approach this chapter like you would a trip or vacation. Enjoy not only the actual trip but also the anticipation as you plan it and the memories that remain long after the trip is over. Take time to plan the exercises. Be curious about them, talk about them, even laugh about them. When doing the exercises, involve yourselves fully. Tune in to each other and tune out extraneous distractions. Most important, try to let go of or set aside long-standing disappointments and resentments. Enjoy the fact that you are doing something sensual together. Afterward, share your reactions to the exercises and take pleasure in the memories.

If there's tension in your relationship, we would advise moving slowly, being clear with each other about what you want out of each exercise, and keeping expectations reasonable. Finally, remember to keep trying. Patience, respect, and mutual commitment can create important change in a relationship.

CREATING THE RIGHT MINDSET

Before we make specific suggestions about how to enliven your sex life, we want to take just a moment to focus on the importance of having the right mindset when it comes to a sexual relationship. We offer three simple suggestions: lighten up, get real, and get over it. Please don't skim over this section in a rush to get to the exercises, but read it carefully and talk it over with each other.

Lighten Up

Now hear this: Sex is not serious business!

It's amazing how our society has made sex—this simple, beautiful gift in life—so terribly complicated. Sex can certainly be profound—it can be a powerful means of communication; it can be a sign of commitment; it can even generate life. But it doesn't have to be serious. Sex can occur during serious moments, such as when partners seek comfort from each other during times of personal or family crisis. But, for the most part, sex can be joyful, playful, and perhaps on occasion even slapstick.

Hopefully, there is always a place for humor in a healthy sexual relationship. When we can laugh at ourselves, enjoying our own quirks and foibles in the bedroom, we reduce the destructive impact of self-criticism, performance anxiety, and resentment. A couple might mentally catalog their own sexual bloopers and, as the years pass, recount them with delight. They can revel in retelling the time that the husband woke up his in-laws by falling off the bed during lovemaking; the time that the 5-year-old thought Mommy was praying because she kept saying, "Oh God"; the time that the 6-year-old took Daddy's "balloons" to school for a classroom party; and the time that, in the midst of beautiful lovemaking, complete with body oil, lit candles, and soft music, one partner unexpectedly made the wind rather than the earth move. Sex can be a source of great humor and joy—it doesn't have to be serious business!

Get Real

There's a host of sexual gurus out there today who proclaim on talk shows and in books that they can tell you how to have stupendous sex. Even if you have a good, loving sexual relationship, if you listen to these "sexperts" long enough, you'll start to wonder whether you're missing out on something. The truth is, sex can be wonderful, but not every time. Sex can be beautiful, but it will never become the center of the universe. Sex brings us moments of pleasure, but it doesn't ensure happiness. This may sound strange coming from a trio writing a book about sex, but we feel that it's important for people to have realistic expectations. On some occasions, everything—mood, energy level, events earlier in the day, the ambience—will line up perfectly, and as a result, lovemaking *clicks*. And on those occasions every nerve ending explodes upon touch and the resulting orgasm rivals those described in the sexiest paperbacks. Those experiences, if and when they occur, should be enjoyed and cherished. But these magic moments are the exception, not the rule.

Sex between lovers varies dramatically from one occasion to the next. Sometimes you'll climax; sometimes you won't. When you do orgasm, one time it might feel like a tidal wave crashing over you, and the next like a quiet ripple washing gently across your body. On one occasion you'll feel incredibly connected with your partner, and perhaps on the next you'll feel that he or she merely came along for the ride.

Disappointed that there are no secrets to nonstop, earth-shattering sex? Or perhaps relieved? Well, it's reality. If we approach sexuality with realistic expectations, we spare ourselves the pressure of trying to perform like Olympic athletes. Instead, with each sexual encounter we can try to approach our partner with an attitude that says: *Well, here we are. The next few moments may be great, or they may be just okay, but because we're sharing them together, they'll feel good. Let's speak to each other with our bodies rather than with our words. And whether we climax or not, whether the earth moves or not, we'll try to hear each other's message—I love you.*

Get Over It

Sex can be a two-edged sword in a relationship. It can serve as a profound act of love between two people, but it can also serve as the flash point for conflict. Sex is a common trigger for conflict because of our increased vulnerability when dealing with sexual issues. Our partners can disagree with us about the weather, the economy, politics, or religion, and unless the disagreement is particularly vicious and personal, it's unlikely that we'll feel deeply wounded. We may become irritated and conclude that our partner can be a real jerk at times, but these areas of dispute seldom touch close to home. But when our partners challenge our sexual beliefs, criticize our performance, or make light of our desirability, look out—they're venturing into a minefield. Because we live in a culture that equates appearance and sexuality with personal worth, any ridicule of our bodies or criticism of our lovemaking strikes at the very core of our self-esteem.

Conflict over sexual issues can be highly toxic to a relationship. Far too often in our work we see couples wanting to strengthen their relationship and increase their sexual satisfaction, but they just can't let go of long-standing resentment and disappointment. Positive steps can be made toward addressing sexual problems, and then suddenly one or the other partner will utter something like "You never really liked sex" or "You never follow through" or "My needs have never been important to you" or "You're never satisfied," and all efforts to improve the sexual relationship come to a screeching halt.

If you and your partner are serious about improving your sexual relationship, both of you will need to find a way to address your *relationship* concerns. Chapter 12 offers information about typical relationship challenges and effective ways to approach those challenges. If there is an unresolved sexual issue in the relationship, you will need to understand the issue, talk about it with open minds and mutual respect, avoid games and power plays, and work toward a win-win solution. Only then will you be in a position to focus on strengthening your sexual relationship with trust, affection, and goodwill.

STARTING WITH THE BASICS

With the right mindset, you are ready to work on strengthening your sexual relationship. We always suggest starting with the two basic ingredients for a satisfying sexual relationship—communication and touch.

Discuss, Discuss

Many couples have been together for years or decades, yet in all that time have never openly discussed sex with each other. Talking about sexuality can make people feel vulnerable as no other topic can. When sharing what turns them on and what turns them off, they might feel they're exposing too much about their identity, quirks, hang-ups, and insecurities, that they're standing psychologically naked in the presence of their partner. "So why get naked?" you might ask. Because getting emotionally naked is like getting physically naked—it may not be absolutely essential, but it can make sex much more rewarding and enjoyable. More important, it helps to prevent misunderstanding and fosters greater intimacy in the relationship.

It is important for couples to communicate about sexual issues such as their wishes, fears, and insecurities. We're aware that this type of dialogue is challenging, but discussing sex openly with your partner is a critical ingredient for a satisfying sexual relationship.

WHAT'S IN A NAME?

Many of us have been raised to believe that nice people don't talk about sex, certainly not in a way that might sound "vulgar." The following exercise is designed to help desensitize sexual language. You and your partner will be encouraged to say aloud every sexual slang word or phrase you can think of. The purpose is to "break the ice" so that you two can begin to build a framework for healthy sexual communication.

Directions

Schedule time alone together when both of you are feeling relaxed and unrushed. Start with the word penis *and brainstorm for slang terms. Go back and forth, taking turns voicing slang expressions. When you run out of ideas, repeat the exercise with each of the following words:* vulva, vagina, breasts, masturbation, intercourse, *and* oral sex.

When you finish going through all of those terms, take turns answering the following questions:

- *How did I feel about doing this exercise?*
- *Were there any slang expressions I didn't like or found offensive? Which ones?*
- *Which words do I feel most comfortable using when talking about sex and body parts?*

Reflection

✦ When doing this exercise, did you feel embarrassed or ashamed? If so, can you trace these reactions back to earlier experiences in your life? Share your reflections with your partner.

✦ Some people may find this exercise exciting. The excitement can come from the novelty of using language that may have been forbidden during childhood. There is often a natural attraction to outrageous and risqué behavior. Also, feeling liberated from a long-standing sexual prohibition can be exciting.

Next Steps

Be sure to respect each other's sensitivities about language. If you or your partner finds certain terms demeaning or offensive, it's important to respect these responses in future discussions.

So the ice is broken: you can use the anatomical words, including the slang versions. But can you express the feelings—the wants, the fears, and the excitement—that sex brings out in you? For many couples, that's a big challenge. Just starting this type of conversation can seem daunting. *How do I bring the subject up? What if I shock him? Will she think I'm obsessed with sex?* This next exercise has been designed to help the two of you start talking about sex. By answering the questions listed in the exercise and sharing your answers with one another, you will begin to explore issues important in all sexual relationships. Our hope is that you'll continue throughout your lives to talk openly and honestly about your sexual relationship.

CAN WE TALK?

Directions

Make two copies of the following open-ended questions:

- *The thing I most admire about you is:*
- *My most exciting sexual moment with you was:*
- *The part of my body I feel most self-conscious about is:*
- *The sexiest part of your body is:*
- *The thing about sex that I am most uncomfortable with is:*
- *The most exciting place for us to make love would be:*
- *My favorite part of lovemaking with you is:*
- *You make me feel special when:*
- *Things that make lovemaking exciting for me are:*
- *The sexiest thing about you is:*
- *The thing you do sexually that turns me on the most is:*
- *If you weren't a part of my life, I'd feel:*

Make a date with your partner for a quiet, romantic dinner at home or at a restaurant where there'll be enough privacy to do some serious talking. Before the dinner date, write down your answers to the questions above and bring them to the dinner.

On your date, after both of you have had a chance to relax, pull out your answers. Read the first question aloud and then your answer. Allow your partner to respond; be prepared to elaborate. Then ask your partner to read his or her answer. Before moving to the second question, be sure both of you have had ample opportunity to talk about the answers.

For the remaining questions, alternate who reads his or her answer first.

Reflection

✦ Honest communication is critical for a successful relationship, yet it can be difficult and scary. The communication sparked by these questions should be nonthreatening—the questions were designed to elicit flattering feedback, not criticism. You and your partner will also have to talk about the rough spots in the relationship, but for right now, enjoy hearing and giving positive feedback.

✦ If you and your partner find it difficult to do this exercise and you're having sexual difficulties, you may have an answer to why. If as a couple you can't discuss issues raised by these simple questions, you probably don't have much communication or mutual expression of affection as part of your lovemaking. Working on the relationship will probably be productive, as is the case if this exercise leads to criticism rather than compliments. You may want to review Chapter 12 on relationships.

✦ Reflect on the following questions and share your responses with one another:

- How difficult was this exercise?
- As the two of you went back and forth sharing your answers, did the exercise become easier?
- Were you surprised by anything your partner said?
- What can both of you do to ensure that more talks like this happen in the future?
- Based on what you heard from your partner, are there any action steps you want to take to help make sex more exciting and satisfying for both of you?

Next Steps

1. If problems become obvious, consider steps to help improve and strengthen your relationship (e.g., counseling, marital enrichment weekend, communication course, etc.).

2. Keep talking, honestly but lovingly.

Touch

Far too many couples have lost their ability to fully enjoy lovemaking. Rather than making sex an exciting experience that awakens and stimulates all of their senses, couples often fall into a predictable routine. To make matters worse, the routine often deprives women of the emotional and physical stimulation that is most effective in leading to their sexual excitement and satisfaction. The following exercise is designed to help you and your partner return to the basics. Rather than focusing on genital arousal, the two of you are encouraged to rediscover the joy that can come from flesh touching flesh, using all of your senses as you enjoy quiet, intimate time together.

LET'S KEEP IN TOUCH

Directions

Find quiet, private time together and go through the following steps:

- *Set a comfortable mood with music, soft lighting, scented candles, and perhaps wine, or special mineral water, or sensuous fruit. Make sure the room temperature is at a comfortable setting.*
- *Undress each other, taking your time and focusing on your senses.*
- *Have your partner lie face down. Begin a slow, sensuous body massage. If you want to, experiment with body oil. Pay attention to all of your senses. Take in the scent of the burning candles*

(if you're using them to create a mood) or the essence of your partner's cologne. Feel the texture of your partner's skin. Hear the music; listen to your partner's sighs and moans. Look at your partner's face, hair, and body and appreciate the curves, lines, angles, and shapes that make him or her unique.

- *After slowly moving from head to toe, have your partner roll over. Repeat the massage, starting with the facial muscles and working your way down to the feet. For now, skip the genital area.*
- *When finished providing a massage, switch roles and allow your partner to massage you, back and front. Give yourself permission to relax and to indulge in pleasure. This is not the time to worry about whether your partner is enjoying him- or herself—these are a few moments for you to be selfish.*
- *When your partner is finished, take a few more moments and hold each other. Enjoy the silence together or talk about your reactions to the experience you just shared.*

Reflection

✛ Reflect on the following questions, and if you are willing, share your reflections with your partner.

- Did you feel self-conscious while doing this exercise? If so, what may have caused your feelings of awkwardness or discomfort?
- Were you concerned about your appearance?
- Were you afraid that your partner was not enjoying the exercise?
- Did you feel like you were doing something wrong?

Next Steps

On a different occasion, repeat the steps, adding genital stimulation. Experiment with ways of stimulating each other without relying on intercourse. Try using your hand, tongue, thigh, breasts, a feather, or a vibrator.

STIMULATING THE MIND, NOT JUST THE BODY

Lying on her side, Laura hugged her pillow. As she drifted off into that twilight state between consciousness and sleep, she was startled by a body pressing up against her. Clearly Larry was aroused—his firm penis poking her buttocks left no doubt about that. Not an unpleasant way to end the day, she thought.

"Are you trying to tell me something?" she asked playfully.

Larry answered by reaching under her nightshirt and cupping her breast. As he gently pinched her nipple, Laura felt a warm rush radiating from her pelvis. Very definitely a nice way to end the day, she decided.

Despite her fatigue a few moments ago, she rolled on her back and began kissing and stroking Barry's body.

Larry shifted so his penis could penetrate her; she was amazingly moist, given the brevity of the foreplay. Within seconds of him entering her, Laura picked up the tempo of his thrusting and began moving in concert with his body. She was immersed in pleasurable sensations until she suddenly heard the telltale moan forming deep in Larry's diaphragm.

No, not yet, she thought.

Larry began to shudder, then his body went limp and lay heavy on top of her. Laura couldn't move; breathing became an effort. Fortunately, within seconds of his climax, Larry rolled off her.

"Thanks, Hon," he whispered.

"You're welcome," Laura answered, trying to mask her disappointment.

"That was really nice," he sighed before drifting off into blissful sleep.

Yeah, I guess it was, Laura thought without conviction. *But am I wrong to want more than nice?* she wondered. *Sex has become so ordinary, so predictable. We never try anything new or different. God, when we first made love years ago, it was always an adventure. When he touched me, every nerve ending exploded. There were times when we'd be in public and just looking at each other would drive us crazy—we wanted to rip off our clothes and do it right there. But after 15 years and doing it at least a thousand times together, I'm probably being silly wishing for more. I guess we're lucky that we're still doing it at all.*

Today, unlike 50 years ago, the media bombards us with suggestions that sex should be breathtaking and exciting. Against this standard we look at our actual experience, and especially if we have been with the same person for many years, odds are the sex just doesn't match up in comparison.

"What do you expect?" many people will argue. Like Laura, people often assume that once the novelty of a new relationship wears off, sex between the same two partners is destined to become routine and boring.

But is this necessarily so? Is a new partner a prerequisite for sparks to fly in a sexual relationship? Do partners in long-term relationships inevitably lose the ability to have great sex together? We don't think so. As one colleague confided, "Each time my partner and I can get away for a weekend—without pagers, telephones, car pools, and deadlines—we rediscover that there's actually nothing wrong with our sex life." Many couples have made the same discovery. If your routine sexual encounters lack excitement, it doesn't necessarily mean that you and your partner have lost the potential or capacity for exciting, satisfying sex with each other.

So why does sex become boring in a relationship? The answer is that exciting sex is the result of more than just physical stimulation—it requires stimulation of both the body and the mind. That's why sexual encounters with a new partner can be so exciting. It's not the novelty itself but the intellectual and emotional stimulation that the novelty creates. With a new partner, there is the excitement of discovery and the satisfaction and validation that come from feeling desired. With a new partner, there is intrigue and the possibility of previously unknown pleasures. There is also a sense of intimacy created when two people allow each other to move beyond private boundaries, such as seeing each other naked for the first time.

For many couples, sex over time ends up on autopilot. To their credit, they find time for sex in their busy schedules, but they rely too much on stroking the vital spots for arousal. Sex becomes an exercise in stimulating the body with little attention given to stimulating the mind. That's the problem with many "how-to" sex manuals; they teach three ways to stroke the clitoris and six variations of oral sex, but they often overlook the importance of bringing one's mind and emotions into the sexual experience.

Before going into specific suggestions for bringing more excitement into your sexual relationship, we want to make two points. First, while we are saying that a long-term sexual relationship does not have to be boring, it doesn't mean that every sexual encounter has to have nail-digging intensity. Sexual encounters, like orgasm, vary from the dramatic explosion to the quiet shiver. Not every sexual encounter has to be dramatic or explosive for a sexual relationship to be exciting and satisfying.

Second, it's important to be able to trust the relationship enough to take chances, to try new behavior, to stretch oneself in pursuit of growth. You may feel self-conscious the first time you suggest making love in the shower or the back seat of the minivan, but it can be worth the initial uneasiness if the resulting novelty sparks a moment of excitement and passion. Remember to voice your wants and needs and suggest variations. Take a risk and try something new.

Now let's look at ways to stimulate the mind and create sexual excitement.

Foreplay

This is probably not the type of foreplay you're thinking of—we're not talking about the hugging, kissing, and stroking that precedes intercourse. Instead we're talking about what occurs before the clothes come off—the intellectual and emotional stroking that can precede lovemaking.

One colleague described foreplay as "offering to take the garbage out after dinner." Foreplay is two lovers taking the time to talk, and listen, about each other's day. It's laughing over some silly occurrence. It's doing a favor, offering praise, saying thank you. Foreplay is breaking out of the daily routine long enough to share a quality moment together; foreplay is any moment that heightens the couple's sense of connectedness. When this type of sharing and caring occurs, the mind and emotions are stimulated, and any physical contact that follows is all the more likely to be exciting and fulfilling.

That's why so many couples find sex more enjoyable when they run off on a lovers' weekend. Yes, part of the reason is that they're escaping the stress of their daily routine, but an even bigger part is that they have the time to reconnect with each other and rediscover the qualities that first brought them together. Both find themselves saying, "Oh, yeah, *this* is why we fell in love."

Unfortunately, there can never be enough run-away weekends in our lifetime. Foreplay allows us to create at least run-away moments, which serve as a great prelude to loving sex.

Positions for Penetration

Experimenting with positions for penetrative sex is a valuable way of stimulating both the mind and the body. Being on top, underneath, or beside your partner; facing or away—each of these options affords variations in what you see, where you can touch and be touched, and how your body is stimulated. Although these positions may be associated with intercourse, they can be adapted to other forms of penetration between partners as well—with fingers, dildos, and vibrators.

Missionary Variations

The most familiar position for making love is the "missionary position," in which the woman lies on her back with her partner positioned over her—the epitome of conventional sex. Its very name reflects Western restrictions in regard to sex: it was the only position that missionaries would condone for their unenlightened converts. (Today one might question who the unenlightened ones were.)

There are variations of the missionary position that can be quite pleasurable. In the normal missionary position, the woman typically spreads her legs wishbone style. Placing pillows under her hips and buttocks can be a nice variation, allowing deeper penetration and additional stimulation to the front wall of her vagina. The woman can also bring her legs up and wrap them around her partner. This movement repositions the pelvis, creating both a variation in stimulation and the sense of being physically entwined with each other. Finally, for those yoga-esque women who are sufficiently limber, bringing their knees up to their chest and looping their ankles over the partner's shoulders can permit deep penetration and intense vaginal stimulation. If the man kneels when his partner is in this position, the G spot can receive exquisite stimulation.

A nice feature of the missionary position is that it allows partners to make eye contact during lovemaking. If you haven't tried it before, the next time you're about to orgasm, look directly into your lover's eyes. There can be an intense feeling of shared union when eyes are locked at the moment of climax.

Female Superior

The female superior position, in which the woman and man switch positions so that the woman is on top, allows the woman to take a more active role during intercourse. She can position her body to maximize stimulation and control the tempo of thrusting so that it matches her growing arousal. With the woman riding atop her partner, the man's hands are free to caress her breasts, face, arms, and buttocks. An equally arousing advantage is the visual stimulation this position provides. Not only can the lovers admire each other's naked bodies, they can also make eye contact.

The female superior position can also take on subtle but enjoyable variations. The woman can either kneel over her partner or, with her feet flat on the surface, crouch over him. Kneeling is more common and comfortable, but crouching and rocking up and down can be great exercise and provide a subtle variation in vaginal stimulation. The woman also has the option of facing her partner or having her back to him. In the latter position, the woman's hands are free to stimulate both her clitoris and her partner's scrotum. Finally, with all the options above, the woman can further modify the position by remaining upright, leaning forward, or arching backward. Each option varies the stimulation, makes different body parts available for caressing, and provides different visual perspectives of your bodies.

We've had a number of our cancer and heart transplant patients, both men and women, report that a variation of the female superior is particularly helpful. The man lies in a semireclining position with pillows propping up his back. The woman then kneels astride and upright. The couples report that this position maximizes accessibility for penetration while minimizing pain and discomfort.

Rear Entry

With the rear-entry position, the man approaches the woman from behind (not to be confused with anal sex). In this position, the woman is on her hands and knees or lying with her head and shoulders on the bed and her buttocks in the air. The position allows deep penetration and intense vaginal stimulation. Also, if her shoulders and head are resting on the bed, the woman has a free hand and can reach back and stimulate both her clitoris and her partner's scrotum. This position minimizes any visual stimulation for the woman, but she may enjoy her partner caressing her buttocks. This position is particularly valuable when the woman has back problems or other physical difficulties that would make it painful to have her partner lying on top of her.

Spoon

The spoon position is an option when both partners are tired and looking for a nice, leisurely paced coupling. In this position, both are lying on their sides with the woman's back to her partner. If they were upright, it would look like the woman was sitting on the man's lap. Lying on their sides demands minimal energy. The couple can gently rock in a mutual rhythm that's pleasurable for both. The man has at least one free hand to caress his partner. The woman can reach down between her legs and stimulate her clitoris, her partner's scrotum, or both. Women often find this position emotionally appealing because it creates the sense of being held or cuddled during lovemaking.

The spoon position may require some practice, flexibility, and good humor. One difficulty is that the man's penis can slip out easily, and alignment must be done by touch—neither the man nor the woman is in a position to view the genitals. Heavier couples may have to improvise if they find it difficult for their bodies to fit together like spoons. As a variation, they can position their upper torsos into a V shape, with their penis/vagina connection being the base of the V.

The four positions described above are hardly an exhaustive list. Feel free to experiment. Depending on your physical flexibility, turn and twist, rise up and lower as you search for new variations that might lead to a different angle of penetration, a different view of your partner, or a better vantage point for caressing both your and his genitals. Enjoy the variety!

New Ways to Make Love

"It was a nice evening," Josef said as he removed his tie.

"And it's not over yet," Carla answered with a coy smile.

Josef looked surprised. "With that medication I'm on, I don't know if I can do the job." He tried to sound matter-of-fact, but his awkwardness was apparent.

"Oh, I don't want to screw," Carla said. "I've got other ideas."

Seductively, she pulled him toward the bed and removed his shirt. Josef's reluctance melted away as Carla's tongue traveled from his lips to his nipples. Finally she looked up. "Undress me, handsome," she said playfully.

Lying naked together, Carla took Josef's hand to her mouth and then guided his moistened fingers to her vulva. Satisfied that he would follow her cue, she shifted her attention to his penis. They explored each other's mouths with their tongues and pressed against each other in every conceivable way.

Josef slid his hands along her vulva, fingering her labia and clitoris. With his other hand he touched her breast, circling it with his fingertips. When his teeth pressed firmly but gently against her swollen nipple, Carla felt a warm wave of pleasure wash over her.

She reached down and took his scrotum and penis in her hands. His penis was swollen, but lacked hardness. As she continued to stroke and caress him with her hands, she reveled in his moans of pleasure. *We made love*, she thought, *such beautiful love.*

Another way to stimulate the mind as well as the body is by experimenting with new ways to make love. We're not referring merely to different positions for intercourse but to a broader definition of lovemaking, one that's not synonymous with intercourse. Contrary to popular thinking, lovemaking without intercourse is not second-rate, incomplete, or flawed. Once a couple understands and accepts this premise, a whole range of options opens up for them. They are no longer shackled by a rigid formula involving mandatory groping, penetration, thrusting, orgasm, and sleep. They become more open and eager to experiment. Even couples with sexual problems such as erectile difficulty or pain with penetration can still have hot sex when they follow this broader notion of lovemaking.

Ready to experiment with making love without intercourse? Try the following exercise.

NOW THAT'S WHAT I CALL MAKING LOVE!

Directions

Working on your own, start with each of you taking some time to write down answers to the following questions:

- *What joint activities would be a great prelude to making love? (e.g., out on a date, watching a sunset, attending a concert, sitting in a hot tub)*
- *What locations, types of lighting, music, props, etc. would create a sexy background for us to make love?*
- *Without intercourse, how and where would I like my partner to touch me, play with me, tease me, pleasure me?*
- *Without intercourse, how and where would I like to touch, play with, tease, and pleasure my partner?*

Make time to sit down together and share your answers to these questions. See if your partner suggested things you didn't have on your list, or vice versa. Let your partner know if anything on his or her list falls outside your comfort zone.

Agree to find a private time when you can make love without intercourse, using the results of your discussion for planning the prelude and ambience. When that time comes, go ahead and make love, in Carla's words earlier, such beautiful love. Remember, no intercourse; instead use with abandon any combination of suggested caresses and techniques that came up during your earlier discussion.

Afterward, share with each other your reactions to the lovemaking experience.

Reflection

+ Are you and your partner getting better at discussing your sexual relationship?

+ Was the lovemaking experience comfortable or awkward? Boring or hot?

+ Did you miss intercourse?

+ What could have made the experience more exciting?

+ Did you learn anything new about your sexual relationship? Things that you and your partner need to work on further?

Next Steps

1. If the experience did not go as well as you hoped for, talk over ways that might make lovemaking without intercourse more comfortable and sexually satisfying.

2. Keep thinking of new ways to surprise, excite, and pleasure each other.

DEVELOPING A SENSE OF ADVENTURE

There are a number of erotic practices that some people find to be enjoyable enhancements to their lovemaking repertoire, but others find disagreeable. We've made frequent reference to the sexual negativity that exists in our society. There's a widespread tendency to label any form of sexual variation as abnormal or perverted. The long-standing assumption going back more than a thousand years in Western culture is that sex, and all pleasures of the flesh for that matter, is essentially immoral. Early philosophers and theologians were faced with a dilemma, however. Even though they were inclined to condemn sex as the number-one evil of the flesh, the future of humanity would be short-lived without it. Their solution was to condone sexual intercourse for procreation. Sexual activity not directed to that end (masturbation, oral sex, anal sex, protected sex, homosexuality) was considered evil. Times change. Or do they?

More than a thousand years later remnants of this thinking continue to subtly, and sometimes not so subtly, influence our beliefs and attitudes about sex. For many, anything that hints at being sexually unconventional leads to feelings of awkwardness and shame. People are often quick to use labels like *perverted* and *sick* for anything that falls outside their comfort zone. As a counterpoint, we would like to suggest that *any consensual sexual practice among adult participants that does no harm and provides mutual pleasure is fine.*

As we discuss how to expand one's sexual horizon in the next few sections, we remain respectful of people's individual preferences and moral beliefs. We do not advocate engaging in sexual activity that you find distasteful or morally objectionable.

What we do advocate is openness and a nonjudgmental attitude. It's one thing to say, "I'm not comfortable with masturbation because I believe it's morally wrong"; it's a whole different ballgame to say, "Masturbation is disgusting, and anyone who does it is sick!"

Let's look at common sexual practices that may add variety to a sexual relationship.

Oral Sex

Oral sex refers to stimulating your partner's genitals with your lips, mouth, and tongue. *Cunnilingus* is the Latin word for when a woman's genitals are stimulated orally; *fellatio* is the Latin word for oral stimulation of a man's genitals. Oral sex can lead to orgasm, or it may be used to heighten arousal before switching to intercourse or some other variation of lovemaking. It's a common sexual practice; studies report that as many as 90% of all couples have engaged in oral sex as a part of their love-making experience (National Center for Health Statistics, 2004).

Some people fear that oral sex is unhealthy. They assume that the genitals are somehow less clean than the rest of the body. Because sexual matters are often labeled "dirty" (as in dirty pictures, dirty movies, the dirty deed), the genitals end up taking the same rap. Another common objection is "I'm not going to put my mouth there—that's where he [she] pees." Assuming that neither partner has an STI and that both practice good hygiene, oral sex should not present a health concern. The genitals should be as clean as any other part of the body, and unless there's an infection, urine is sterile. Still, some people find that they are more comfortable with oral sex if their partner showers prior to lovemaking.

Women often have many questions about oral sex before deciding whether or not to try it. Here are answers to some of the more common questions about fellatio and cunnilingus:

- *Will fellatio make me gag?* If the penis hits the back of the throat, it can trigger a gag reflex. The woman can prevent gagging by positioning her hand on the shaft of the penis, which gives her control over how much of the penis enters her mouth.

- *How much semen is ejaculated?* On average, a man's ejaculation will produce about a teaspoon of semen. The amount varies depending on genetics, age, and the recent frequency of sex. A man ejaculates less semen as he grows older. If he ejaculates more than once over the course of a few hours, the amount of semen will decrease with each successive ejaculation.

- *What does semen smell and taste like?* The smell of semen makes many people think of ammonia. Taste varies from man to man and can be affected by diet, but in general, it will be salty and mildly acetic. One woman compared its consistency with a light white sauce she makes by mixing flour, milk, and butter.

- *Does ejaculate have calories?* Semen contains about 5 calories per teaspoon, hardly a diet buster.

- *Can the force of ejaculation make me gag?* Although the force of ejaculation is not enough to make a woman gag, if she's not prepared, the sudden squirt of semen can startle her. Some women enjoy orally stimulating their partner's penis but dislike swallowing semen or being caught off guard by the ejaculation. If this is the case for you, share your preference openly and tactfully, and ask your partner to signal you when he's about to climax. You can then stroke his penis with your hand until he ejaculates, or take the ejaculate in the front of your mouth and spit it out.

- *If I want to perform cunnilingus, where do I put my mouth and what do I do with my tongue?* Try positioning your mouth and lips over a portion of the vulva, like the clitoris or introitus (opening) of the vagina, rather than trying to cover everything. Move your tongue around, stroking along the shaft of the clitoris, around the tip of the clitoris, across the vestibule (the area between the inner lips), and in and out of the introitus. Alternate the speed with which you move your tongue and the pressure you apply on the vulva. And don't rely solely on your tongue to stimulate your partner—you can use your lips to caress and lightly suck swelling tissue, and even your teeth to gently tease and excite.

Many women and men highly value oral sex as part of their lovemaking. Some women report that their most intensive sexual arousal occurs when their partner's tongue strokes their clitoris and probes the opening of their vagina. Most men not only enjoy the physical sensation of their penis being orally stimulated but also find great psychological satisfaction from the act. They have been conditioned to interpret oral sex as evidence that they are attractive and that they excite their partner. They figure, *when my partner is doing this for me, I must really turn her on.*

In straight and lesbian relationships, many women can understand their partner's interest in oral sex, but may wonder why the partner seems so intent on performing cunnilingus on her. *As long as I'm satisfied,* they reason, *what difference does it make whether or not oral sex is performed on me?* What these women fail to take into account is that it feels good for some people to perform oral sex. Because oral sex can produce intense arousal, it can make the partner feel valued as a lover.

This does not mean that a woman must perform oral sex to prove that she's attracted to, or in love with, her partner. Nor should she feel pressured to receive cunnilingus simply to soothe her partner's ego. There are numerous other ways for partners to pleasure each other. In healthy sexuality, choices such as whether or not to practice oral sex are made through open communication and by partners' honesty with each other and with themselves.

Oral sex, when performed out of desire for mutual pleasuring, can introduce an exciting variation in lovemaking. If it's been a while since you considered oral sex—giving or receiving—we encourage you to revisit this with your partner.

Anal Sex

Anal sex involves any stimulation of the anus. This particular form of eroticism not only carries the cultural bias against sex but also collides with our cultural fetish for cleanliness. Nevertheless, anal eroticism is a popular form of sexual stimulation in mainstream America; 30–40% of American women have experimented with anal intercourse (National Center for Health Statistics, 2004), and about 10–12% of American women regularly engage in it (Reinisch, 1991).

What's the attraction to anal sex? One factor is physical pleasure. For men, stimulation of the prostate gland, which is next to the rectum about 2 inches past the anus, is highly arousing and can quickly trigger orgasm. Inserting a finger in the anus and rubbing or applying gentle pressure on the front wall of the rectum can stimulate the prostate gland. In both women and men, the anus has abundant nerve endings that make it an exquisitely sensitive area of the body for sexual stimulation.

In addition to the physical pleasure, anal sex can create psychological stimulation. First of all, there is the novelty of making love differently. Perhaps even a greater factor than novelty, however, is the stimulation that comes from doing the forbidden. Forbidden fruit has always held a strange lure for people, and because anal sex has long been considered in polite circles to be dirty and unthinkable, it easily qualifies in the minds of many as forbidden. Another source of psychological stimulation is the sense many people have that the more unconventional the sexual act is, the more exclusive the relationship. The man might reason, *Not only am I the only person she will have intercourse with, but I'm so special to her, she's even willing to allow me to penetrate her in the most private of places.* The woman might think, *There's no part of my body I'm unwilling to share with him.* For both of them, this sense of exclusivity might be highly erotic and satisfying.

Unlike oral sex, anal sex does present some health issues that should be considered. Bacteria reside in the anal area as well is in the rectum. Unprotected sex exposes the man's penis to these bacteria, which can enter the body either through breaks in the skin of the penis or through his urethra. This danger can be minimized but not eliminated by thoroughly washing the anus prior to lovemaking. Using a condom during anal sex is the best way to avoid the risk of infection. Because of the bacteria, the penis should never be moved directly from the anus to the vagina. Following anal activity, the penis should be washed thoroughly and a new condom applied before vaginal contact. Otherwise, the woman will very likely develop a vaginal infection.

Unlike the vagina, the anus does not secrete natural lubrication. With a lack of lubrication, small tears in the rectum can easily occur with penetration, making the person more susceptible if exposed to an STI. When attempting any form of anal penetration, precautions must be taken to prevent tissue damage. The use of saliva or, even better, a good water-soluble lubricant, can make anal penetration far more comfortable and less harmful to the rectal lining. And, most important, penetration needs to be slow and unforced.

So much has been said about AIDS being transmitted through anal sex that AIDS and anal sex have become synonymous in the minds of many. Anal sex itself does not cause AIDS—HIV can be transmitted only if one of the partners is already infected with the virus. Because anal sex has been shown to be the easiest way for an infected partner to spread the virus, however, this sexual behavior should be reserved for long-term monogamous relationships, or at least for relationships where safer-sex practices are followed (see Chapter 9).

Anilingus and digital penetration are two additional variations of anal eroticism. Anilingus is the stimulation of the partner's anus with the tongue. Proper hygiene, which includes a thorough washing of the anus and the surrounding area, is essential to minimize the risk of infection during this activity. The use of a dental dam is an even more effective way of preventing infection. When both individuals are comfortable, anilingus can be a highly personal, intense form of pleasuring. A more commonly accepted form of anal stimulation is digital penetration—the insertion of a finger in the partner's rectum. Both women and men report that during sexual arousal, touching the anus or having a finger inserted can greatly intensify arousal and often trigger orgasm.

Although many men are fascinated with anal sex, some are quite threatened by penetration of the woman's finger. Many men in our society are phobic about anything resembling homosexuality. Because anal eroticism has been associated with male homosexuality, some men are afraid to acknowledge that they find pleasure in anal stimulation. It's important to note that anal stimulation is pleasurable regardless of gender or sexual orientation. Enjoying stimulation of his anus implies nothing about a man's sexual orientation.

Sexually Explicit Media

It is not an uncommon Friday night ritual in many homes for moms and dads to watch the latest Disney release with the kids, then send them off to bed and come back to watch their own X-rated movie together.

Before we wade into the controversy involving pornography, a clarification of terms might be helpful. First of all, when we talk about material being sexually explicit, we're talking about the graphic depiction of sexual activity. When considering sexually explicit videos, some people will use the terms *soft porn* and *hard porn* to distinguish just how graphic the sex is. With hard porn, nothing is left to the imagination—the viewer sees the erect penis and swelling clitoris. Soft porn, on the other hand, involves frontal nudity and depicts couples having sex, but actual genital contact is not shown.

There are critics who insist that all sexually explicit material is obscene and should be banned from the marketplace. Legally, however, material is considered obscene only when it intends to arouse the reader or viewer by depicting actions that most people find offensive and shameful. In other words, obscene material attempts to sexually excite by glamorizing behaviors most of us would find to be unacceptable and disgusting. Examples of obscenity would include children being sexually abused, graphic rape scenes, and sex with animals.

Erotica is the artistic depiction of love and sex. Erotica can be quite explicit, but unlike obscenity, the intent is not to use lewd material to arouse its audience. It attempts to inspire its audience by capturing in word or image the sensual quality of our existence. Although some might argue that X-rated DVDs or adult content on premium television channels are erotica, anyone who has viewed much of this material would have to agree that we're definitely not talking about art.

Pornography is a drawing, song, book, or movie that attempts to sexually excite its audience through the graphic depiction of "socially acceptable" sexual activity. Under the law, there is a wide range of behavior that is considered "socially acceptable" but may not be acceptable to a particular individual or couple. What one person finds acceptable may not be acceptable to another. Some people find pornography to have erotic power while others do not. For some, pornography is disgusting and unacceptable; for others, it is the graphic depiction of actions in which they have engaged or about which they have fantasized.

The issue of pornography is certainly complex. From the papers to the pulpits, from courtrooms to coffeehouses, it is hotly debated. In this book we have no intention of offering the final word on this controversy. We believe that there are sexually explicit videos that couples can view as an enjoyable source of variety for their sexual relationship. We also believe that there are sexually explicit videos that are degrading and negative to both women and men.

Does erotica or pornography have any merit? For some couples, viewing sexually explicit material is exciting. Other couples feel it objectifies sex and dilutes the intimacy between them. It's entirely personal. If you do decide to watch a DVD and find it offensive, turn it off.

Sexually explicit material is not for everyone, and your values, attitudes, and beliefs should be respected. If you're curious, consider experimenting with sexually explicit material. If you're not interested in hard core, find a sexy, R-rated movie. Have a movie night with your partner. Enjoy the raw eroticism depicted on the screen. Enjoy the fantasies and desire the movie might conjure up within both of you.

Erotic Power Play

Bondage and discipline, sadomasochism, and fetishistic activities aren't just for the guys. Many women enjoy dominance/submission play in the bedroom. This may vary from talking dirty to acting out fantasies. If you're interested in trying and want to keep it fun, we suggest that you learn about the basics. There are several books describing erotic power play in the "Suggested Resources" at the end of the book.

Erotic power play can be aggressive or gentle; the line between pain and intense sensation is different for everyone. Many couples engage in occasional "light bondage" by gently tying hands or feet. They find the novelty exciting and feel it increases their erotic focus. Because household items like scarves or neckties can cut off circulation, we suggest investing in Velcro ties made for the occasion and sold through the companies listed under *sex toys* in the "Suggested Resources" list. Remember to establish a word for *stop* and another for *lighten up*. Most people don't mean stop when they say it during the heat of erotic power play. Find a different word that is guaranteed to slow down the action if needed.

People who are involved in "heavier" sadomasochism usually find an S/M group or club and meet regularly. If you decide to get involved, remember that you need to set up careful boundaries with others and avoid being exploited by anyone. It's important that you have the freedom to choose the type of activities and the pace that works for you.

Most people use the rule "safe, sane, and consensual" when engaging in erotic power play. If your partner is pressuring you and you're not interested in this kind of thing, tell your partner no. Sex has to be consensual, especially sex that flirts with aggression.

Toys and Other Props

Vibrators, dildos, sexy lingerie, body oils, and a host of other sexually oriented items are now part of a multimillion-dollar industry. Many couples find that such toys and props bring a touch of novelty to their lovemaking. We've already made the point that lovemaking can be playful and that making use of fantasy and creativity can heighten pleasure for lovers of all ages.

The only point we wish to add when considering toys and props is the importance of not being taken in by the myth that "natural is best." Somehow many people have gotten the idea that an orgasm should come only from a penis or vagina, or if they're very progressive, perhaps also from a finger and a tongue. *Heaven forbid*, they reason, *that an orgasm ever be triggered by something inanimate or mechanical. And if love is not enough to stimulate passion*, they conclude, *the relationship must be in trouble.*

Why? If your partner stimulates you to climax with an electric vibrator, is his desire to pleasure you any less than if he had used his finger, his tongue, or his penis? Is the mood set by your partner wearing sexy briefs or your wearing flimsy lingerie any less legitimate or meaningful than the mood set by candles and music? If you suggest a sensuous massage with body oil, are you implying that your partner is a lousy lover and you need more to be satisfied? If you want to wear 6-inch heels into the bedroom to excite your partner, are you turning yourself into an object? We think not. Sex provides the opportunity for two people to play, to harmlessly indulge their own and each other's fantasies. When toys and props are used playfully by a couple, they can provide novelty, excitement, and fun.

Mutual Masturbation

Mutual masturbation involves partners masturbating in each other's presence. Initially this practice can seem awkward and embarrassing. Most of us are accustomed to viewing masturbation as highly personal and private. When we were younger, the act was done quickly and quietly to avoid detection. The thought of being caught by anyone—parent, sibling, or playmate—was horrifying. Yet despite these initial inhibitions, many couples find mutual masturbation exciting and informative. They report feeling a unique intimacy that results from watching each other engage in what has traditionally been such a highly personal act. By watching each other self-pleasure, couples can learn how to more effectively stimulate their partners during lovemaking.

Now It's Time to Experiment

One valuable way to avoid letting your sexual relationship drift into autopilot is to add variety and excitement to your lovemaking. By making use of your imagination, creativity, and sense of adventure, you and your partner can introduce playful, sensual, mutually enjoyable variations into your sex life. The following exercise provides a safe format for you and your partner to look at a range of novel sexual experiences without having to feel particularly threatened. If you identify only one new mutually acceptable behavior as a result of the exercise, wonderful. Try it, enjoy it, and learn from it. Over time, keep revisiting this exercise. Things you would never consider doing right now may become more acceptable in the future as both your sexual comfort and your sexual relationship continue to grow.

A final note about experimentation. It's important that both people want to try the new behavior. If one person is turned off by the idea but agrees to try it to accommodate the partner, trouble is inevitable. Remember, the goal of experimentation is to keep excitement and passion alive, not to create resentment and discomfort.

LET'S EXPERIMENT

Directions

Take two sheets of paper and make three columns on each sheet. Above the first column, write "**New Activity**," *above the middle column, write* "**Let's Try It**," *and above the third column, write* "**Pass**."

- *Underneath the first column list the following:*
- *Shower together*
- *Perform fellatio*
- *Perform cunnilingus*
- *Masturbate in front of each other*

- *Have anal sex*
- *Try new positions for intercourse*
- *Play strip poker*
- *Have phone sex with each other (explicit talk about sex over the telephone)*
- *Role-play a fantasy*
- *Watch an erotic movie*
- *Watch an erotic dance performance*
- *Use sex toys*

Both of you take a copy of the list and check off which of the activities you're willing to try (second column) and which you want to skip (third column).

Compare your lists and see which activities both of you want to try. Neither of you has to explain or defend his or her choices.

Pick an activity you're both willing to try and start planning when and how to do it.

Reflection

✦ Did you feel that you had to defend any of your choices? It is important that each partner's personal tastes and comfort level be respected. If you're feeling pressured or criticized by your partner, try discussing these feelings with him or her—and be sure to monitor your own responses to your partner for any stray criticalness or pressure.

Next Steps

1. Periodically revisit this exercise. Options you decline now may become more acceptable in the future. Perhaps the two of you will think of additional possibilities to put on the list.

2. Continue to be open to experimentation and novelty, but never allow yourself to be pressured into trying something that exceeds your comfort level or violates your values—and never allow yourself to pressure your partner.

ADDRESSING TWO COMMON PROBLEMS

Let's look at two of the most common sexual conflicts that arise in sexual relationships.

Who Initiates

A common source of conflict in a relationship is the issue of who initiates sexual contact. Surveys show that most people believe that ideally both partners should initiate sex with equal frequency. Surveys also show, however, that in the vast majority of relationships, this equality doesn't occur—usually one person initiates sex much more frequently than the other.

Even when the noninitiating partner readily accepts the invitation to make love and participates enthusiastically, his or her failure to initiate can create tension in the relationship. The offended party (the usual initiator) is often tempted to read significance into his or her mate's failure to reciprocate. He or she may reason that if two people are attracted to each other and enjoy being sexual, both should be equally inclined to initiate sex; because the partner doesn't initiate, deep down he or she must not really enjoy their lovemaking.

Although the preceding reasoning appears to be logical, when it comes to sex, the rules of logic don't necessarily apply. Yes, normally when people want something, they take steps to get it. But because sex is such a loaded issue in our society, many people find it awkward to initiate lovemaking, even when they desire it and thoroughly enjoy it. Many women and men who have been raised with the belief that sex is dirty, for example, may shy away from suggesting erotic behavior. They may enjoy lovemaking, but the burden of feeling awkward or ashamed of wanting it too much inhibits them. If a woman or man feels sexually insecure, initiating sex can be intimidating. The ever-present possibility of being turned down or ridiculed makes the overture too scary. In both cases the noninitiator may gladly accept when his or her partner takes the initiative.

Surveys show that men are initiators more often than women. We suspect that this trend (and it is only a trend, because in many relationships women are the primary initiators) may be due to upbringing and different arousal patterns. Many women were raised hearing the message that good girls don't ask for sex or that sex should be reserved for special moments of intense emotional intimacy. On the other hand, cultural myths give men permission to initiate sex without shame or remorse. Unlike women, they have not been conditioned to associate sex with special moments of emotional intimacy but instead have been taught that "real men" will try to have sex whenever possible.

In addition to upbringing, differences between women and men in their patterns of sexual arousal may account for men being more inclined than women to initiate sex. First of all, in an erotic situation a man may become more quickly aware of his arousal than a woman. A man's major physical sign of arousal, the erection, is more apparent than the more subtle signs for a woman, such as genital swelling, warmth in the pelvic area, and vaginal lubrication. The more readily a person becomes aware of arousal, the more readily he or she will tend to act on that arousal.

Another difference may come from what causes a man to become sexually aroused, in contrast with what arouses his partner. It appears that, in general, men are more responsive than women to visual cues. A man watching his partner undress is more likely than a woman to feel arousal. Some professionals believe this is due to differences in culture and upbringing. They point out that women's bodies are more often glamorized, and exploited, in our culture. Peepshows, "girlie" magazines, topless bars, and stag films are ever-present messages to young boys and men that seeing a woman's naked body is something to be desired. It is a highly valued experience, even something to brag about. Other professionals have suggested that the different ways many women and men respond to visual cues may be due to minor differences in the structure of their brains. They suspect that cues from a man's visual cortex (the part of the brain that mediates vision) may be connected more directly to the sex center of the brain. Whether it's due to nurture or nature, men are often trained or conditioned to respond to visual cues more quickly than women.

Regardless of the reasons, it's dangerous to overinterpret the meaning of a partner shying away from initiating sex. It isn't proof positive that the partner doesn't enjoy sex. Instead, it's usually a reflection that the partner's arousal pattern is different from the initiator's. The partner is just more comfortable being the pursued than being the pursuer. As long as a couple can enjoy physical intimacy, our response to the initiator who complains that his or her partner doesn't initiate is "So what?"

Frequency

Two people can have perfectly normal sex drives yet differ dramatically on how frequently they want sex. There is no ideal or correct frequency that applies for all people. Among normal, healthy, well-adjusted adults, there can be a wide range in sexual desire, with some people desiring sex every day and others desiring sex weekly or less often. The desire for sex can also vary dramatically over time in response to factors such as stage of life, quality of the relationship, level of fatigue, and the presence or absence of stress or illness. As we discussed earlier in the book, however, it is not due to inherent gender differences. Because of this variability in sexual desire, it's inevitable that most couples will, at times, face a discrepancy in their preferences for sexual frequency.

The reasons that frequency of sex can become a major issue for couples are varied and complex. At the most basic level, people tend to get upset if they're deprived of something they want. If another person repeatedly tells us, "No, you can't have it," chances are we'll become resentful over time.

For some people, being denied sex goes beyond the simple disappointment of being deprived a moment of pleasure. For many people, sex has a lot of symbolic significance. Some people, for example, equate having sex with being desirable. As a result, if they're told "No sex!" they hear "You're not desirable." Other people may believe that the true sign of love and a strong relationship is the presence of a torrid sex life. It's not surprising if, after being turned down by their partner enough times, these folks begin to question the merits of their relationship.

At a deeper level, a couple's struggle over the frequency of sex may really be a reflection of a struggle over more basic issues.

Diane and Mariana are a couple who have been feuding for months. Rarely home, Diane has been immersed in a project at work. Mariana complains that Diane is so wrapped up in work that little or no interest is shown to her. Diane dismisses these complaints and accuses Mariana of being hypercritical. Against this backdrop, each time Diane turns away from sex, the anger Mariana ends up feeling does not simply come from "not getting any" but from feelings of being ignored, minimized, and unimportant.

Tal has strong emotional needs and looks to Alison as a substitute mother—he wants her to constantly hold his hand as he encounters life. Alison, however, feels as if a noose is tightening around her neck. She loves Tal, but his dependency is suffocating her. For survival, she pulls back at times to create distance. Saying no to his frequent requests for sex permits her to keep that distance; otherwise, lovemaking would become one more way for Tal to cling to her emotionally.

What steps can a couple take if one partner consistently wants sex more often than the other? Because the causes can be varied and complex, the solution is usually not a simple one. Having sex with your partner out of a sense of obligation is not the answer—resentment will surely be the long-term result. Likewise, shaming the partner with the less-intense sex drive, or the one with the more-intense sex drive, trying to make him or her feel guilty, will inevitably create tension in the relationship.

The challenge of addressing this discrepancy in desire is often part of the larger challenge in any relationship: two people trying to meet their individual needs while respecting the needs, values, and sensitivity of the partner.

Saying "No" Nicely

Dressed only in his boxers, Riad leaned over the sink and vigorously brushed his teeth. *I think I'm ready for tomorrow*, he thought. *The slides are done and the handouts are in my briefcase; the boss should be impressed by my presentation.*

Hands came from nowhere and began to play with the thick, black hair on his chest. Startled, he looked up and, in the mirror, saw Rana peering over his shoulder with an impish grin.

"What's a girl gotta do to get laid around here?" she asked playfully.

Riad rinsed out his mouth and turned around. Taking her hands, he said gently, "Normally that would sound great, but tonight's a bad night."

"Seems like there's been a lot of bad nights lately," Rana said, the smile now replaced by a look of disappointment.

"I know," he sighed. "I guess I've been in a slump lately. But I do love you."

"I was starting to wonder," she said, her smile returning.

"Don't ever question that," Riad said, squeezing her hands for emphasis. "I'm not up for sex tonight, but it would be nice to hold you."

Riad didn't want to have sex. While making clear his own preference, he acknowledged the validity of Rana's request. Instead of becoming defensive or resorting to sarcasm, he reaffirmed his love and desire for his wife. He attempted to come up with an alternative—holding each other—that would at least partially meet her needs as well as his own. This vignette shows how any disagreement, whether it involves sex, money, in-laws, or parenting, can be handled better when the communication is marked by honesty, sensitivity, and mutual respect.

The preceding vignette models what we call "saying 'No' nicely." We believe if you reread this little story periodically and attempt to model Riad's way of saying no, you'll find that a great deal of misunderstanding and hurt feelings will be avoided. When our partner says "No thank you, but let's hold each other," or "I'm not up for tonight, but how about if we plan some special time this Saturday?" we're much less likely to feel shot down or rejected.

Passive Lovemaking

"Good night, darlin'," Patrick said as he kissed Kathleen on the forehead. Reaching for the lamp, he turned the lights off and settled back to fall asleep.

"Tired?" Kathleen asked in the darkness.

"Yeah, it's been a hell of a day."

"Too tired to make love?" she asked.

After a moment of awkward silence, Patrick answered, "The way I feel tonight, it would be more like work than fun."

"Do you mind helping me?" she asked.

"Not at all," Patrick answered, rolling over toward Kathleen.

Laying her head on his shoulder, Kathleen cuddled against her partner. Through the thin cotton of her nightgown, Kathleen lightly traced the lines of her labia.

With his free hand, Patrick stroked her cheek. Kissing the top of her head, he whispered, "I love you, darlin'. Enjoy."

By now, she could easily feel the fullness of her vulva as she became more aroused. When she felt moisture coming through the material, shivers of excitement began racing from her vulva and up her spine.

Reaching inside her nightgown, Kathleen spread open her labia and slid her fingers along the shaft of her clitoris with short, rapid strokes. Still aware of Patrick holding her next to him, she slowly, rhythmically rocked against her lover's body.

Her breathing quickened as excitement continued to build. Her pelvis felt full and her vulva was wonderfully sensitive and swollen. She could sense that her orgasm was coming. She changed her pace of self-caressing, her strokes now longer and more deliberate. Finally, as the sensations and excitement built, she felt the spasms of her orgasm.

She lay against Patrick, completely content. Patrick hugged her and kissed her hair, then rolled over on his side. Within moments, he was asleep.

Kathleen lay silently, feeling spent but invigorated, relaxed but wide awake. *How wonderfully different tonight turned out*, she thought, *compared to what would have happened just a few years earlier.*

Kathleen's sex drive had always been stronger than Patrick's. This discrepancy often resulted in tense moments, especially when she wanted to make love and he didn't.

Fortunately, things were different now. A few years ago, Kathleen asked Patrick if he would like to watch her masturbate. Even though she was comfortable with self-pleasuring, it had always been something she had done in private. She was fearful Patrick might be shocked by her question, but to her pleasant surprise, he agreed. Dim lights and soft music helped her overcome her initial embarrassment. After coming to orgasm, she was pleased to find Patrick aroused rather than disgusted.

In later discussions, Kathleen asked Patrick how he would feel if she masturbated on those nights when she was turned on and he wasn't in the mood. She explained that having him present would make it feel much more special than if she went off by herself in another room.

Fortunately, he was open to the idea. After the first few times, he told her that he was enjoying being part of her self-pleasuring. He appreciated no longer feeling pressured or guilty. And best of all, on those occasions when he was a passive partner, he felt a loving connection to her. Since that time, Patrick and Kathleen have continued to enjoy intercourse once or twice a week, but to the satisfaction of both of them, they now make love almost daily.

This vignette demonstrates a strategy many couples have found to be a creative response to a desire discrepancy in a relationship. If your partner invites you to make love and you are not in the mood, passive lovemaking provides you an alternative to always saying "No" (albeit nicely). Instead, you can say something like, "No, but I can help you."

As you read in the vignette, Kathleen masturbated. Usually masturbation is considered a solitary act, but in this case Patrick was very much a part of the self-pleasuring, even if his role was relatively passive. For Kathleen, the arousal and pleasure came not only from her physically stimulating herself, but from the emotional connection with Patrick. He held her, gently caressed her, whispered love and encouragement. Both Kathleen's desire to make love and Patrick's fatigue were respected. And as passive as Patrick was during this lovemaking scenario, chances are high that he felt connected to Kathleen, pleased that he could selflessly contribute to her pleasure without overexerting or stressing himself.

PASSIVE LOVEMAKING

Directions

Over the next couple of weeks, try passive lovemaking two times. Alternate being the passive participant.

When you are the passive participant, determine how you want to support your partner. Try laying your head on your partner's shoulder or holding your partner. Gently touch your partner's face, play with his or her nipple, stroke your partner's hair, caress her breast or rub his chest, lightly scratch his scrotum. Say nothing or gently whisper reminders that you love your partner and encourage him or her to enjoy.

For the person who is self-pleasuring, allow yourself to indulge in the pleasurable sensations of masturbating while being encouraged and supported by your partner.

Afterward, discuss your reactions to the experience, either as the passive participant or as the participant who self-pleasured.

Reflection

+ What were your reactions when you were the passive participant? Did you feel burdened? Did you enjoy seeing your partner's pleasure? Was the experience physically taxing?

+ What were your reactions when you were the participant who self-pleasured? Did you feel self-conscious masturbating? Did you wonder whether your partner felt bored or imposed upon?

Next Steps

Try using passive lovemaking as an alternative when you don't feel up for a big romantic interlude but want to be close and responsive to your partner's sexual needs.

PRIORITIZING PHYSICAL INTIMACY

As we bring this chapter to a close, we want to suggest one last exercise that will hopefully become a regular routine in your relationship. Incorporate this exercise into your relationship and your chances for keeping passion and intimacy alive for the duration increase.

NAKED EMBRACE

Directions

For the next 2 weeks, make a commitment to go to bed together each night. If one of you is a night owl, you only have to remain in bed for 10 minutes before going back to your nighttime activities.

Undress and, lying down in your bed, hold each other face to face, spooning, or side by side, joined at the hip.

You can talk about the day or say nothing at all.

Focus on the flesh-on-flesh contact. Remind yourself that this simple act is nevertheless a highly intimate act that you would never think of sharing with any other person.

After no more than 10 minutes, feel free to put on your night clothes (or leave them off), turn off the light, and go to sleep unless you want to get back up while your partner sleeps.

Sex is not the objective of this exercise. If on any given evening you both choose to make love at bedtime, spend time holding each other afterward before falling asleep or getting back up. If your partner is not interested in sex that evening, be respectful of his or her wishes.

If lying naked creates too much sexual tension, alter the exercise so that you embrace while dressed in your street or night clothes. In that case, we'll change the name of the exercise to "Wish-We-Could-Be-Naked Embrace."

Reflection

+ How comfortable was this intimate time each evening?

+ Did being naked each night create tension because it prompted sexual expectations? If so, were the wishes of the person not desiring sex respected? Were you able to talk this issue through?

+ Over the course of 2 weeks, did you feel a closer connection?

Next Steps

1. Make an ongoing effort to regularly make use of a naked embrace at night to maintain physical intimacy as an ongoing priority in the relationship.

2. Don't become complacent. Keep working on your sexual relationship. Periodically reread Chapter 12 on relationships and review the information and exercises in this chapter.

If you and your partner have worked your way through this chapter, taking the time to carefully read the instructional material and making the effort to complete each exercise, you have truly taken a journey together. The journey is far from over; hopefully it will be a lifelong journey of ever-deepening love and physical intimacy. One of the biggest challenges your sexual relationship will face as time goes by is complacency. Life will happen, responsibilities will tax your energy and compete for your attention, and your sexual connection can easily be sidelined. We encourage you to resist that complacency and continue to prioritize the role of physical intimacy in your lives.

FIFTEEN

Overcoming Sexual Difficulties

Throughout this book, we have discussed factors that influence our sexuality, including childhood events, cultural messages, relationship issues, previous sexual experiences, life stressors, and physical health. When these influences don't encumber us—when our bodies are working normally and our minds can focus on eroticism without distraction—nature is free to take its course and we should be able to respond normally to sexual cues. On the other hand, when there is a medical problem, or when psychological issues distract us from the eroticism of the moment, our bodies often fail to function normally in a sexual situation.

There are many ways the body can fail to function sexually; that is, there are many different types of sexual dysfunction. You may have lost interest in sex or hate sex. Perhaps you can't lubricate or find you can't stay focused on your sexual feelings. Maybe you're unable to orgasm at all, or only in very specific situations, like when you're alone or drinking. You may have pain before, during, or after sex. Or you may have nongenital pain, such as cramps, headaches, or back pain, that occurs during or after sex.

> "I thought my low sexual desire was due to working and having a baby, but I asked my doctor, and she found out that I have a thyroid problem and needed medicine."

> "I was sure my sexual pain was some awful disease, but my gynecologist did a careful exam, and there was nothing wrong with me physically. She did a good job of explaining how my body can have a real physical problem, like muscle spasms and pain, but not have a medical cause for that problem. She was the first person to tell me about sex therapy."

"I was never able to get aroused even though I wanted to want sex. Every time I talked to a physician about my problem, I felt like he or she was telling me that it was 'all in my head.' I was so ashamed."

Do you believe you have a sexual problem? Some people would say that if your sexual behavior, or lack of it, causes you no distress, you have no sexual problem. This "no harm, no foul" line of thinking makes a lot of sense in many cases, but there is a potential flaw in its logic (Sugrue & Whipple, 2001). Sometimes a person may avoid sex due to physical discomfort, fear, lack of confidence, or past trauma. For years this person may convince herself that she doesn't need sex or that it's not important to her. As a result of long-standing denial, she may not experience distress, but clearly emotional or physical barriers have prevented her from experiencing sexual pleasure and satisfaction. One could argue that this is a problem, regardless of the absence of distress.

On the other hand, you may believe you have a sexual problem when in reality your sexual response is a variation of normal. Only because you are misinformed or your expectations are unrealistic do you experience distress, in all likelihood avoidable distress. In such cases, accurate information and reassurance often go a long way toward resolving the distress, thereby freeing you to enjoy your sexual experiences.

Again, do you think you have a sexual problem? For starters, go ahead and ask yourself the following three questions:

- Are you interested in sexual activity, do you desire it, and do you have sexual thoughts or fantasies?
- Do you find sexual activity pleasurable?
- When all the circumstances are right (e.g., absence of distractions, feeling sensual and aroused, adequate physical stimulation), are you satisfied with your ability to experience orgasm?

Could you answer "yes" to all three questions? According to a large national survey, more than 40% of adult women between the ages of 18 and 59 could not (Laumann et al., 1999). Before we take a closer look at each of these questions and what it means if you answered "yes" or "no," we're going to provide some foundation for dealing with sexual problems in general. We will talk about how to assess your sexual problem, how to get a medical evaluation, the importance of finding accurate information, and the value of including your partner in efforts to overcome a sexual problem. We will also introduce a valuable technique to combat the distracting and negative thoughts present in almost all sexual problems. After providing you with this foundation, we'll return to these three questions and the three most common sexual difficulties women encounter.

PRELIMINARY CONSIDERATIONS

Check It Out: Doing a Self-Assessment

Some women know right away that something has gone wrong sexually, but for others the awareness dawns gradually. We think you should do a self-assessment of your sexual functioning as soon as you become concerned that something might be wrong. You'll notice that the self-assessment gives you valuable information that will help you make decisions on how to address the problem and whether or not to get help.

> "When I discovered I couldn't even do the self-assessment, I realized I had another problem besides sexual pain. I'm going to see a counselor because I'm scared to even think about sex."

> "It wasn't until I wrote down my answers to a self-assessment that I realized I had low sexual desire only at home. I felt great about sex when we were away."

Take a look at the list of questions that follows. If you're comfortable expressing yourself in writing, you may want to write your answers on a piece of paper or in a journal. You'll be amazed by the insight you gain when you go through the effort of trying to capture thoughts, feelings, and experiences in written words. Recording your thoughts will also give you something to refer to when you see your healthcare provider.

- *What is the problem?* Give a full description of what happens or doesn't happen for you in sexual situations.

- *Is the problem physically painful, or does it cause bleeding, chronic itching/sore-ness, or infection?* If your sexual problem has immediate medical implications like the ones suggested in the question, make an appointment with a healthcare provider as soon as possible.

- *When does the problem occur?* All the time? Only in certain situations? These questions are designed to help you determine what might be triggering the problem, such as stress, fatigue, disagreements, interest in someone other than your partner, shame about being sexual, or resentment over being pressured to have sex.

- *When did it first happen?* Has the problem been lifelong? If not, what was going on in your life when the problem first appeared? These questions may also help you understand what is causing your sexual problem. For instance, if you lost your sexual interest around the same time you were going through a marital crisis, perhaps the low desire is related to a lack of trust in the relationship.

- *If the problem is lifelong, can you write down why you want to address the problem now?* Is it because you want to correct the problem, or is someone else pressuring you to change? We have found that change is very difficult when we're doing it not for ourselves but to please someone else.

- *What thoughts go through your head when you're being sexual?* This is a great question because it helps you gain insight into your current feelings about sex. For instance, if you discover that your thoughts during sex involve self-criticism for being overweight or unattractive, then you have a good idea about what is preventing your erotic focus during sexual activity. More important, you also have an idea about where to direct your attention when trying to resolve your sexual problem. Strategies for overcoming negative thinking are presented later in this chapter.

- *How comfortable are you with sex?* If you're not comfortable, where is the discomfort coming from? Are there things in your past that might make sex a problem? Look back through Part I, "Knowing Your Sexual Story," and be sure to complete the timeline exercises in Chapter 13 to pinpoint a time when you were comfortable with sex. For instance, some women say they felt good about sex until they had kids. From that point on, they felt self-conscious and more like a "mommy" than a sex partner.

- *Do you avoid relationships that have the potential to become sexual?* Here again is a place to examine your reactions to Part I. By reflecting on your sexual story, you may come up with insights into why a sexual relationship might be threatening. Upon reflection, you may discover that past abuse prompts you to avoid sexual relationships. In that event, reading Chapter 10 may be helpful.

- *Do you have certain beliefs and attitudes about sex that might not be helpful?* Think about what sexual messages you have been exposed to, both now and in the past. Pay particular attention to the stereotypes for your age and stage in life. Do you believe that there is something wrong with you if you're 21 and not oozing raw sexuality all the time? Are you expecting yourself to be over the hill sexually just because you're over 40? Part I, "Knowing Your Sexual Story," and Chapter 6 can help you identify many of the common myths and stereotypes that follow us throughout our lives.

- *Do you have accurate information about sex in general and about your problem in particular?* If you are like most women, you've been given few specifics about how your body functions sexually. This would be a good time to review Part II, "Understanding Your Body," which provides a wealth of practical and useful information.

- *What impact does this problem have on your partner and your relationship?* Review the suggestions in Part IV, "Creating a Better Sexual Relationship," to gain general information about couples and sex. Although you might think the problem is just yours, we have found that a sexual difficulty always affects both the partner and the relationship, making it a shared problem. The exercises in Chapter 14 can help enrich a sexual relationship.

• *How are things going in your relationship, both sexually and nonsexually?* This is an elaboration of the preceding question and encourages you to think about your overall relationship. Couples have challenging times together. Is this one of those times for you right now? How much are you enjoying each other? Do you spend quality time together? Do you have a sense of goodwill toward each other? When you argue, are you both trying hard to resolve the problems? Have you considered specific strategies to help your relationship, like reading self-help books or going to couples counseling?

• *How are things going in your life in general?* Are there current major or chronic stressors in your life? Do you escape from problems by drinking or taking drugs, reasoning that you "deserve" a drink or must have a drink to have a good time? Do you chronically yell at people you love and then have to apologize later? Are you continually worried about money or upset about your work? Have there been serious problems with your children? If you answer yes to any of these questions, we recommend that you contact a counselor and discuss these stressors in your life. A counselor will be able to do an in-depth evaluation with you and can recommend strategies to help you cope.

• *How's your health?* Are there any health problems that could be contributing to your sexual problem? Are you worried about your health? When was your last physical? Do you feel healthy? Are you getting exercise, sleeping well, and following a healthy diet? Your lifestyle is fundamental to taking care of yourself. It may be time to contact your healthcare provider and share your concerns about your health or lifestyle.

"Tell Me It's Not in My Head"

As sex therapists we encourage every woman we see to stay current in her healthcare. We encourage our patients to have yearly physical exams and to see their healthcare provider more frequently if they experience medical difficulty. Good healthcare is essential for good sexual health. Failure to detect and treat medical conditions such as thyroid problems, diabetes, or high blood pressure can affect your sexual functioning. A healthcare provider should always be consulted when there is a sexual dysfunction, both to determine whether or not there is a medical cause and also to make sure the dysfunction is not signaling the presence of a potentially serious health problem.

If you don't have a healthcare provider, you will need to choose one. Many women have a primary care physician or nurse practitioner. These are professionals trained in the comprehensive care of the patient. Some women also have a gynecologist, a physician who cares for the woman's reproductive system and hormonal balance. Many women ask their friends for advice about how to find a good healthcare provider. If you don't know whom to ask, call a local hospital for names of healthcare providers in your community.

In choosing your healthcare provider, you'll need to find out whether you can use your health insurance or will have to pay out of pocket. Ask what the normal fees and lab test expenses will be for a general physical or gynecological workup and how long you'll have to wait for an appointment.

When making the appointment, the receptionist will probably ask why you want to see the healthcare provider. If you are not comfortable providing details over the phone, you can simply answer, "I have some sexual concerns that I would like to discuss with the doctor." You may be asked if you want a full physical examination or just a gynecological (pelvic) exam. If you've recently had a complete physical, you can opt for the pelvic exam only. Ask the receptionist if the healthcare provider will have time on the day of the exam to discuss your questions or if you should schedule a separate appointment.

When you go for your appointment, have your questions written down. Mention to the medical assistant who puts you in the exam room that you have several important questions for the healthcare provider and would like to ask them while you're still dressed in street clothes. Remaining dressed until you've discussed your questions helps you feel more comfortable while discussing your sexual concerns. Doing so lets the healthcare provider know, right from the start, that you have concerns you wish to discuss, and it prevents you and the healthcare provider from having to dash through the questions because they had been left to the final moments of the appointment.

Begin your discussion with the healthcare provider by saying, "I have some questions about my health—in particular, my sexual health." Some women find it helpful to use the following outline in succinctly presenting their problem:

- Description of the problem
- Onset of the problem (when and under what circumstances the problem started)
- Your understanding, if you have one, of the problem
- What, if anything, you've done to try to correct the problem
- What your expectation is

Using this outline, some women may write a script for what they want to say when they meet with the healthcare provider. Here's an example:

"Doctor, I wanted a chance to talk to you at the beginning of the appointment. I have a problem that seems to happen only during sex. I get pain in my abdomen [description]. It started about three months ago [onset] and happens every time I have sex. I don't know why it happens [understanding], but I have tried relaxing more and using different positions [past experiences in trying to help yourself]. I want to have sex without pain [expectation]."

If your healthcare provider is not helpful, you have to decide whether you want to find another provider or want to try to work things out. If you decide to try to work it out, you may find it helpful to take your partner or a close woman friend with you to the next appointment. Your friend or partner can be an objective observer and give you valuable feedback following the session. His or her presence in the room will demonstrate to the healthcare provider your seriousness about getting help for your problem. Some women have found it helpful to make statements like the following to an unhelpful healthcare provider:

> "I realize that you're quite busy today. Why don't I make an appointment for a different time? I really need your expertise."

> "When you say 'There's nothing wrong,' can you tell me what possible medical problems you've already considered?"

If you continue to be dissatisfied with the healthcare provider, ask to speak to another provider in the group or ask for a referral elsewhere.

Experiencing a sexual problem can be distressing and confusing. If you go for a medical evaluation, you may be like many women who hope that a straightforward and easy-to-treat medical condition will be found. If you're told that everything is medically normal, you may feel that the implication is that the problem is all in your head. Nothing could be further from the truth. Regardless of whether or not a medical diagnosis is made, your sexual difficulty is real, not imagined. As we've pointed out throughout this book, powerful social influences from the earliest days of our lives impact our sexual knowledge, attitudes, and self-esteem. It's this impact, not the problem, that ends up in our head, and as we discuss later in this chapter, so is the solution.

Information/Education

Accurate sexual information is critical for overcoming sexual difficulties. After our many years of clinical work, we continue to be impressed by how often sexual problems develop as a result of misinformation or a lack of information. Most adults today, even young adults, received sexual education that was far from stellar. Discussions at home were likely to be rare and painfully awkward or infuriatingly condescending. Little practical information was provided in the classroom. In church, temple, or mosque we were told what not to do rather than how to do it successfully. For most of us, our primary sex educator was a girlfriend who claimed to be experienced, an older sister, or a nameless, faceless writer of an advice column for a teen magazine. As a result many, perhaps most, of us were deprived of basic information necessary for healthy sexual growth and adjustment. If we don't know what a normal sexual response is, what sexual wishes and behaviors are common in the general population, or how we can make lovemaking more satisfying, we are susceptible to developing sexual problems.

The problem, of course, is finding good sources of information. Frank discussions with family and friends can sometimes be helpful, but there is always the danger of people merely sharing their own misinformation. Articles in popular magazines may help, but they vary in quality. Some magazine articles are superb, but others end up being mostly hype with little substance. Beware of syndicated radio and television programs that focus on sex. Some provide a true public service, but far too many place entertainment and ratings ahead of solid education. Websites and self-help books like the one you're reading right now are important sources of adult sexual education, but be sure the websites are reliable and that book authors have solid credentials in the area of human sexuality. Things to look for in so-called sexperts are advanced degrees in relevant fields like medicine, nursing, psychology, social work, or counseling; professional certification as sex educators or therapists; and/or affiliation with a reputable university. Adult education classes or sexuality courses at a local community college are additional sources of valuable information. For still more ideas, consult the resources at the end of this book. The important message here is to seek accurate information. What you don't know can hurt you.

The Solution, Not the Problem, May Be in Your Head

Do any of the following statements sound familiar?

- "No one could ever love me with this body."
- "The only way I can keep a partner is by being good in the bedroom."
- "Sex is dirty."
- "Women shouldn't enjoy sex too much."
- "I'm just not a sexual person."
- "I could never learn to be sexual."
- "I have to keep control at all times."
- "Sex is for the young and beautiful."
- "No one is sexy after menopause."
- "Everybody has better sex than I do."
- "If he's ready, I should be.

Can you imagine the effect these beliefs might have on a woman's sex life? There's an old saying in mental health circles: "How you think, so shall you feel." This adage applies not only to conditions like depression but also to sexual dysfunctions. Negative thoughts and misinformation can, in the short term, distract us during sexual activity and, in the long term, cause chronic problems with desire, arousal, and orgasm. Fortunately, we have found that by helping people challenge these negative thoughts and replace them with more positive, reality-based ones, called "positive cognitions," we can often help them overcome their problems.

Negative thoughts that affect sexuality can range from self-criticism to unrealistic expectations to outright misinformation about sex. Sometimes the problematic thinking during sex may not be negative but distracting. For example, thinking about work or unpaid bills during lovemaking can have a disastrous effect. Remember, for normal sexual functioning the mind must be free to focus on the eroticism of the moment. If the mind is preoccupied with mundane or critical thoughts, is it any wonder that the person has difficulty experiencing a hunger for sex, arousal during sex, or the contentment that comes with orgasm? That's why cognitive work is so important for overcoming sexual dysfunctions: your mind has to be free of distraction to enjoy erotic sensations.

In the next few pages, we describe three steps for overcoming distracting and negative thoughts. If your self-assessment uncovered distracting or negative thinking, you may want to try these steps to change or revise the thoughts.

Step 1. Identifying Distracting and Negative Thoughts

You need to identify what goes through your head when you encounter sexual cues. What messages are you hearing in the background when you see yourself naked, when your partner touches you, or when you feel a warm tingling in your genitals? Although there is a multitude of possible distractions, here are five of the most common varieties.

- *Distractions of daily life.* Some distracting thoughts are the result of the challenges of daily living. Parenting concerns, deadline pressures, the long-term illness of a parent, the threat of job loss, and financial worries are examples of daily life issues that can preoccupy you, follow you into the bedroom, and distract you from responding sexually.

- *Performance pressure.* You might feel pressure to please your partner. If you think your partner views your orgasm as a measure of his or her success as a lover, you may feel a strong obligation. Natural body responses can be disrupted when you feel pressure to perform. The harder you try to do something, the more difficult it can be to accomplish.

- *Self-esteem issues.* As we discussed earlier, sexuality has a powerful ability to bring our insecurities to the surface. Sex tends to highlight issues about competence and desirability that can trigger distracting thoughts and worries. Sexual behavior puts your body at center stage; if you're not happy with your body, sex can be intimidating.

- *Sex-negative thoughts and beliefs.* For most of us, sex-negative messages were plentiful during our upbringing. Even though sex is glamorized in the media and exploited in advertising, the messages that sex is shameful, that sex is dangerous, and that sex is impure can remain ever-present in our psyche. The media can also portray sex as suitable for a certain few—the beautiful people. Ignoring these messages, especially in the midst of sexual activity, can be very difficult.

- *Reliving past trauma.* Have you ever heard a song from the past and immediately been flooded with images, sounds, and even smells from that era? The song served as a memory link; it was a common denominator between the present moment and some moment in the past when you were listening to that song. Just like hearing an old song, sex can serve as a potent memory link.

Consider a woman who was sexually traumatized in the past. Years later, in a wonderful relationship, she becomes confused by her negative reactions to sex. When she makes love, she tenses up. Images from the past assault her. *Why is this haunting me?* she wonders. *My partner is kind and gentle, nothing like the man who abused me. I shouldn't feel this way. What's wrong with me?*

What this woman doesn't realize is that sex, like an old song, has become a bridge linking her past with the present. Unfortunately, as long as the resulting thoughts and recollections remain in the forefront of her mind, a natural sexual response will be very difficult to achieve.

Step 2. Sidestepping Distracting Thoughts

Once you've identified distracting thoughts that pop up during sex, the next step is to take a close look at them to judge their accuracy and validity. Some distracting thoughts may accurately reflect current life issues. *I can't forget to pick up the kids*, *There's a rumor about layoffs at work*, and *Right now I'm furious with my partner* are examples of thoughts that may accurately reflect reality. When that's the case, your task is either to change the reality or improve your ability to cope with it. Having a backup plan for the kids, researching new job opportunities, and heavy-duty communication and problem solving with your partner are examples of trying to minimize the impact of distracting worries.

When you have little control over stressful issues, your task is to come up with strategies for checking troublesome thoughts at the door before entering the bedroom. Unfortunately, putting such thoughts aside is easier said than done. If you realize that you're putting pressure on yourself to perform during sex, it won't be enough to simply decide *I won't think that way!* Most people don't have that kind of control over their thinking.

Picture a beautiful sun-swept beach with white-capped waves crashing against the shore. Make the image as vivid as possible. Got the picture in your mind? Now get rid of it—don't think about or imagine the beach.

What happened? If you're like most people, an image or thought is not easily willed away. More likely, the more you tell yourself not to think about the beach, the more resilient the image becomes. So how do you get the image of the beach out of your mind? Thought substitution. Odds are that as you read on, by the time you finish the next paragraph or two, you'll no longer be consciously aware of the beach. The beach image will be gone, not because you told yourself to stop thinking about it but because other thoughts will have replaced it.

Freeing yourself of distracting thoughts is a paradoxical process. Rather than directly trying to rid yourself of the thoughts, you are more likely to be successful if you go about this indirectly. In the example of being plagued by performance worries, rather than thinking, *I won't think about trying to perform well*, you'd be better off thinking, *I'm going to focus on the great sensations in my body*.

Step 3. Challenging Unhealthy Thinking

Some distracting thoughts may be accurate reflections of reality. But self-defeating thoughts, when placed under the light of scrutiny, always prove to be unfounded, unfair, and irrational. *I look hideous, Sex is disgusting*, and *I'll never be able to enjoy sex* are examples of thoughts usually based on emotion rather than reason. Because they pop up so easily and naturally, we rarely challenge them. We often conclude, *Because I've felt this way for so long, it must be true*. When you're burdened by inaccurate and unhealthy thoughts, it's not enough to sidestep them. It is important to challenge these thoughts with healthier and more accurate alternatives.

You are hardly an impartial judge in this area. Still, how can you determine whether your thoughts are accurate reflections of reality or self-defeating distortions? One simple approach is to write the thoughts down on paper and next to them list facts supporting each thought. If you're still not convinced that the thought is irrational, play devil's advocate and, for each thought, write down an alternative, "rational" thought.

As an example, say you are tense and ill-at-ease during lovemaking. Upon reflection, you realize that whenever you're undressed in front of your partner you think, *I look disgusting*. Is that accurate? Highly unlikely. But at first glance you may insist it's true. Going through the exercise described above, you might write, as "proof" of the accuracy of your beliefs:

- I'm 35 pounds overweight.
- My breasts are sagging.
- I have stretch marks.

Your reasoning has been contaminated by many of the cultural influences discussed earlier in this book. After writing down supporting arguments for your belief, you may feel even more strongly that your self-criticism is accurate. But is it?

The next step is to challenge this distorted logic. If you make an honest attempt to play devil's advocate, you can come up with statements like the following:

- A model's figure is not essential to being worthwhile.
- Sensuality goes far beyond body type.
- There are parts of my body that bring me great pleasure, parts that, if I choose to share, should make my partner feel privileged.
- There are parts of me as a person that, if I choose to share, should make my partner feel even more privileged.

Left unchallenged, self-defeating thoughts like *I look disgusting* can have a devastating impact on both you and your sex life. Upon examination, however, the bedrock of negative and irrational convictions can begin to crumble. This may take time to change, especially if you've practiced unhealthy thinking for years. But we have seen many women learn to steadily dismantle their negative thoughts and replace them with more positive ones.

If you need additional guidance for doing this kind of cognitive work, check out *The Feeling Good Handbook* by David Burns (1999), an excellent resource to help you identify and change unhealthy thinking.

Bringing Your Partner "Up to Speed"

It has been our experience that people can best address a sexual problem when they feel they have their partner's support. Even when only one person in a relationship has a sexual problem, both people are involved. Without realizing it, the partner may be reinforcing the problem or making it worse. Certainly the partner will be affected by the symptoms of the problem. He or she will often feel disappointed, resentful, inadequate, or insecure. An attitude of "It's your problem, so you fix it" doesn't help anyone. It's important for you and your partner to approach a sexual difficulty as a shared problem needing a shared effort to resolve it.

When your partner participates in the healing process, you both become a source of support and encouragement for each other. If you decide to attempt the behavioral exercises throughout this book, knowing that your partner understands what you are doing and why can be a positive support. By making the healing process a joint project, both of you are less likely to feel that either one of you is somehow defective or solely responsible for the sexual problems in the relationship. Your partner's participation also makes it possible for both of you to openly discuss ways to make sexual encounters more relaxed and arousing.

There are a number of ways your partner can be an active participant in resolving a sexual dysfunction. First, by discussing sex in general and the sexual problem in particular, both you and your partner can become sensitized to each other's sexual issues, needs, and concerns. Second, by reading this book, your partner can become better educated about female sexuality. People need to know more not only about their own sexuality but also about their partner's sexuality. Third, some of the behavioral exercises in this book are designed for couples (see Chapter 14). By doing these exercises together, both of you may find it easier and less awkward when you make the transition into an active sex life. Finally, you can work together in strengthening the nonsexual dimensions of your relationship. It's not uncommon for a relationship to take some hits when a couple is facing a sexual problem. Taking time to work on better communication, to ensure that there is quality time together, and to resolve areas of disagreement, are valuable ways to help the relationship grow and to counteract the strain created by the sexual problem.

If your partner is unaware of or uninterested in your sexual concerns, here are some suggested ways to bring him or her "up to speed":

- At a nonstressful and nonsexual time, tell your partner you'd like to discuss your sexual relationship.
- Begin by describing the problem as you see it. Avoid blaming ("It's all your fault") or generalizing ("You've never been a good kisser").
- Ask your partner to repeat what you have just said. This allows for early corrections of any misunderstandings.
- Explain what you've learned from your self-assessment and medical evaluation.
- Ask your partner for feedback as you discuss your concern and answer his or her questions.
- Explain this book and the self-help exercises.
- Suggest that your partner might want to read this book to find out more about women's sexuality (this applies to lesbian couples as well).
- Explain that there are some exercises that will require your partner's cooperation and participation.
- Ask your partner directly for respect and emotional support in this process.
- Tell your partner what steps you plan to take to address the problem and when and how you would like to involve him or her.
- End the discussion by assuring your partner that you will talk about this concern again and set a date for the next discussion, if that feels comfortable.

Now back to the three questions we asked you to answer at the beginning of the chapter. Your answers to these three questions will help you identify whether your interest in sex, your ability to experience pleasure, or your capacity for orgasm is problematic. If so, you'll find valuable information about possible causes for these common problems and, more important, specific steps you can take to resolve them.

SEXUAL INTEREST

Question 1: Are You Interested in Sexual Activity, Do You Desire It, and Do You Have Sexual Thoughts or Fantasies?

For the past 40 years the answer to this question often determined whether or not you were considered to have low sexual desire. The majority of adults will answer "yes" to this question, but many men and women will not. As we discussed in Chapter 4, since the 1970s we had been operating under the assumption that sexual response was a linear chain of events starting with desire, followed by arousal, and culminating in an orgasm—the triphasic model of sexual response. If a person did not think or fantasize about sex, hunger for it on occasion, or ever feel horny, we concluded that there must be a problem. The assumption had been that unless there were catastrophic life circumstances overriding basic biology, everyone should be naturally responsive to sexual cues and, under the right circumstances, biologically receptive to acting on them.

Today our thinking has changed. We no longer assume that sexual desire necessarily precedes sexual activity. We understand that sexual desire is a *receptivity* to sexual activity and a responsiveness to sexual stimulation. For some people, this receptivity and responsiveness is evident much of the time. They think about sex often, have an active fantasy life, easily become distracted in the presence of a sexually attractive person, and feel frustrated and agitated when they are sexually inactive for an extended period of time. For other people, this receptivity and responsiveness is not always apparent, or may become apparent only under very specific circumstances.

When we have men and women coming into our office complaining that they lack sexual desire, the real moment of truth occurs when we ask the next question.

Question 2: Do You Find Sexual Activity Pleasurable?

When those complaining of low sexual desire answer "yes" to this second question, we can assume that they do indeed have sexual desire. The fact that they can derive pleasure from sexual activity suggests both a receptivity to sexual activity and a capacity to respond to sexual stimulation. As we said earlier, sexual desire does not always precede sexual activity but, instead, may become evident only during actual sexual stimulation.

Consider Marie and Stacey. Both women are in their mid-forties, married, and have sought therapy for low sexual desire. We ask each woman, "If your partner invites you to make love and you agree, what happens?" Marie says that if she accepts the invitation, it's usually a conscious decision to appease her partner. Once they get going, however, she becomes aroused, finds the experience pleasurable, and afterward feels emotionally closer to her partner. Stacey, however, unlike Marie, derives nothing from the experience and marks time until the act is over, comforted only by the thought that she is now off the hook for at least another month.

Based on our earlier discussion, we would conclude that Marie does indeed have sexual desire, even though it does not take form in the version glorified by Hollywood. She doesn't necessarily pine for her partner's touch or feel moist when gazing into his or her eyes. Desire for Marie does not typically precede sexual activity, but it clearly kicks in once the caressing and stimulation begin.

As for Stacey, the jury is still out as to whether she has low sexual desire. She clearly lacks sexual desire in response to her relationship, but that lack of desire may not be across the board. Low sexual desire can be situational—confined to specific circumstances—or global, a lack of receptivity and responsiveness regardless of the circumstances.

We don't understand why some people experience strong sexual desire prior to sexual activity while some people do not. Or why some people may at one point in their life experience strong sexual desire as a prelude to sexual activity and at another point experience desire only when they are in the midst of sexual arousal. Our sexuality is complex, and many biological and psychological factors influence and shape how we experience and respond to sexual cues.

Going back to Marie for a moment, she might feel reassured to learn she is not abnormal—that is, that her sexual desire is merely a variation of how people experience their drive to be sexual. Nevertheless, she may still wonder whether there is anything she could do to experience and enjoy her sexuality in broader and more fulfilling ways. The answer is yes.

We often encourage people like Marie to make a conscious decision to be more aware of their sexuality on a daily basis. It's easy for people to become so caught up in their day-to-day world that they miss the joy that can come from the subtle sensual cues surrounding them. They unintentionally tune out the pleasure that can come from sight, sound, touch, taste, and smell. They fail to savor the pleasant memory of recent lovemaking. They deprive themselves of the excitement of planning and anticipating erotic encounters with their partner. The exercises in Chapters 13 and 14 can be very helpful in awakening and enhancing sensual awareness.

We also find it helpful when people realize that sexual desire can take shape in more than one way. Sexual desire can be a biological experience—a powerful drive that propels us into sexual behavior. But sexual desire can also be an intellectual experience—a conscious, willful decision to initiate or accept an invitation to make love. We may not always feel a compelling, visceral drive to be sexual, but we can make a conscious decision to initiate a physical connection with our partner, confident that once the touching and caressing begins, a pleasurable emotional and biological response will occur. In this latter case, we initiate or agree to sex not because we feel obligated, but because we *intellectually* desire it.

What about people who answered "no" to the second question above—that they do not find sexual activity pleasurable? When we look at the first two questions together, we come up with two groups of people who answer "no" to the second question—people who report no sexual interest and no sexual pleasure and people who report interest but don't find it pleasurable. Let's look more closely at both of these groups.

NO INTEREST AND NO PLEASURE

"Everyone makes such a big deal about sex, but in all honesty, it does nothing for me."

When a person reports having no interest in sex and finding no pleasure during sexual activity, we can safely say he or she has low or no sexual desire. Low sexual desire is one of the most common reasons women seek help for sexual concerns. In an American survey of adults between the ages of 18 and 59, researchers found that 33% of women reported that they lacked sexual interest (Laumann et al., 1994). In a 29-nation study of 13,882 women between the ages of 40 and 80, the incidence of low sexual interest ranged from 26 to 43%, depending on the geographic region (Laumann et al., 2005).

In the Symptom Lie the Clues

Low sexual desire comes in different varieties. For example, it can be a lifelong problem or a recent one. It can also be a global problem (you have no interest in sex regardless of the partner, circumstances, or timing) or a situational one (it occurs only in certain situations).

"I have zero interest in having sex with my partner. I feel guilty because I masturbate frequently and I notice I get turned on by looking at other guys at the gym where I work out. I can't seem to feel any desire for my partner! I know we have our ups and downs, but honestly, I'm not trying to sabotage our relationship!"

By determining whether or not your low sexual desire is lifelong, and whether it is global or situational, you gain valuable clues about its cause and possible solution. If the problem is lifelong, sex-negative influences dating back to your childhood may be contributing to your low sexual desire. If, on the other hand, the problem appeared after you started taking medication for depression, there is a good chance that your low desire is a medication side effect. If your problem is situational, you can probably learn a great deal by carefully analyzing the circumstances associated with the symptom. You can also be fairly confident that if there is a medical problem it is not the sole or major cause for the low sexual desire. If it were, your desire would probably always be low, not just under special circumstances. When low sexual desire is global, we often find general, pervasive difficulties like depression, chronic fatigue, disillusionment, sexual conflict, or a medical problem.

A Word about Asexuality

> "I've never been interested in sex and can certainly live without it. I think I'm one of those people born without a sex drive."

We've heard countless patients make statements similar to the one above, suggesting that they might be asexual. With appropriate treatment, however, most of these patients proved capable of being receptive and responsive to sexual cues and experiencing pleasure during sexual activity. It's easy to confuse low sexual desire and arousal with asexuality. *Asexual* in its broadest definition describes a person who has never felt a sexual attraction to another person. In its strictest definition, "asexual" excludes any interest in sex, including masturbation.

If you have long struggled with low sexual desire, you may be tempted to give up and declare yourself asexual—that is, born without a sex drive, with sex having no place in your life. In reality, asexuality is rare, maybe 1% of the population (Bogaert, 2004); it's observed far less often throughout the world than cases of low sexual desire, which occurs in at least a quarter to a third of all women (Laumann et al., 2005). The odds, therefore, are much greater that medical or psychological factors account for your long-standing lack of sexual interest and arousal than that asexuality does. Given that a lack of sexual interest often can be treated successfully, close examination is warranted before writing off your sexuality as nonexistent. The information and suggestions that follow may prove to be very helpful for understanding your lack of interest and pleasure.

"Is Something Physically Wrong with Me?"

Certain medical conditions and drugs can directly affect sexual desire by altering hormone levels or disrupting the normal function of the limbic system, sometimes referred to as the sex center of the brain. Table 15.1 provides a list of conditions and medications that are known to have a direct impact on sexual response.

Having one of the illnesses or taking one of the medications listed in this table doesn't mean you'll necessarily have low sexual desire. And to make matters more complicated, not appearing on the list doesn't mean a medical condition or drug can't affect sexual desire. The stress and fatigue that often accompany illness can dampen or shut down the sexual drive, even if the illness does not directly affect hormonal

TABLE 15.1. Medical Conditions and Drugs That May Affect Sexual Desire, Arousal, and Orgasm

Medical conditions	Possible impact on		
	Sexual desire	Arousal	Orgasm
• Addison's disease	✓		
• Adrenal disease		✓	✓
• Alcoholic neuropathy		✓	✓
• Amyotrophic lateral sclerosis (ALS)		✓	✓
• Chronic renal failure	✓		
• Cushing's syndrome	✓		
• Depression	✓		
• Diabetes		✓	✓
• Epilepsy		✓	✓
• Estrogen-producing tumors	✓		
• Head trauma	✓		
• Hepatitis	✓	✓	✓
• Herniated lumbar disk		✓	✓
• Hypertension (high blood pressure)		✓	✓
• Hypothyroidism	✓		
• Kidney disease		✓	✓
• Lactation (breast feeding)		✓	
• Menopause	✓	✓	
• Multiple sclerosis		✓	✓
• Oophorectomy	✓	✓	
• Parkinson's disease	✓		
• Pituitary diseases	✓	✓	✓
• Postradiation treatment of the vagina		✓	
• Radical pelvic surgery		✓	✓
• Severe malnutrition		✓	✓
• Spinal cord injury			✓
• Stroke	✓	✓	✓
• Temporal-lobe epilepsy	✓		
• Thyroid deficiency		✓	✓
• Vaginitis		✓	
• Vascular disease		✓	
• Vitamin deficiency		✓	✓

Drugs	Possible impact on		
	Sexual desire	Arousal	Orgasm
Blood pressure and heart medication			
• Aldactone (spironolactone)	✓	✓	✓
• Aldomet (alpha-methyldopa)	✓		✓
• Catapres (clonidine)	✓	✓	✓
• Corgard (nadolol)	✓		✓
• Digoxin (lanoxin)	✓		

(cont.)

TABLE 15.1. *(cont.)*

Drugs	Possible impact on		
	Sexual desire	Arousal	Orgasm
Blood pressure and heart medication *(cont.)*			
• Hygroton (chlorthalidone)	✓		
• Inderal (propranolol)	✓	✓	✓
• Ismelin (guanethidine)	✓		✓
• Minipress (prazosin)	✓		
• Oretic (thiazide)	✓	✓	
• Serpasil (reserpine)	✓		✓
Cancer medication			
• Nolvadex (tamoxifen)	✓	✓	
Minor tranquilizers/sleep medications			
• Ativan (lorazepam)	✓	✓	✓
• Halcion (triazolam)	✓	✓	
• Klonopin (clonazepam)	✓		✓
• Librium (chlordiazepoxide hydrochloride)	✓		
• Tranxene (clorazepate)	✓		
• Valium (diazepam)	✓		✓
• Xanax (alprazolam)	✓	✓	✓
Major tranquilizers/antipsychotics			
• Clozaril (clozapine)	✓		
• Compazine (prochlorperazine)	✓		✓
• Geodon (ziprasidone)			✓
• Haldol (haloperidol)	✓		✓
• Mellaril (thioridazine)	✓		
• Navane (thiothixene)	✓		
• Prolixin (fluphenazine)	✓	✓	✓
• Risperdal (risperidone)	✓	✓	✓
• Seroquel (quetiapine)	✓		
• Thorazine (chlorpromazine)	✓	✓	✓
• Zyprexa (olanzapine)	✓		
Mood medications (antidepressants and medication for bipolar disorders)			
• Anafranil (clomipramine)	✓	✓	✓
• Asendin (amoxapine)	✓	✓	
• Aventil, Pamelor (nortriptyline)	✓		✓
• Celexa (citalopram)	✓	✓	✓
• Cymbalta (duloxetine)	✓		✓
• Effexor (venlafaxine)	✓		✓
• Elavil (amitriptyline)	✓	✓	✓

(cont.)

TABLE 15.1. *(cont.)*

Drugs	Possible impact on		
	Sexual desire	Arousal	Orgasm
Mood medications (antidepressants and medication for bipolar disorders) *(cont.)*			
• Eskalith (lithium)	✓		
• Lexapro (escitalopram)	✓		✓
• Luvox (fluvoxamine)	✓		✓
• Nardil (phenelzine)		✓	✓
• Paxil, Pexeva (paroxetine)	✓	✓	✓
• Prozac, Sarafem (fluoxetine)	✓	✓	✓
• Tofranil (imipramine)	✓	✓	✓
• Zoloft (sertraline)	✓	✓	✓
Sedatives/anticonvulsants			
• Depakote (divalproex)	✓		✓
• Dilantin (phenytoin)	✓		
• Luminal (phenobarbital)	✓	✓	✓
• Neurontin (gabapentin)			✓
• Topamax (topiramate)			✓
Ulcer medication			
• Tagamet (cimetidine)	✓		
• Zantac (ranitidine)	✓		
Birth control			
• Depo Provera	✓	✓	
• Lo/Ovral	✓	✓	
• Cyclen, Tri-cyclen, Ortho-Cyclen	✓	✓	
Over-the-counter medications			
• Antihistamines		✓	
• Decongestants		✓	
• NSAIDs (ibuprofen, indomethacin)		✓	
Recreational drugs/abused substances			
• Alcohol (chronic use)	✓		✓
• Amphetamines			✓
• Cocaine	✓		✓
• Marijuana		✓	
• Methadone (dolophine)	✓		✓
• Narcotics	✓	✓	✓

or limbic functioning. (We discuss illness and disability in detail in Chapter 7.) Some medications are highly idiosyncratic—that is, they can affect certain people in unique ways, unlike their effect on most other people. If you're experiencing low sexual desire and have a medical problem or are taking medication, regardless of whether or not the medication or illness is listed in the table, discuss your symptoms with your healthcare provider. Be sure to review the suggestions at the beginning of this chapter for how to talk with your healthcare provider about sexual concerns.

Counteracting Drug Effects

If you're taking a medication that is affecting your sexual desire, your healthcare provider may have a number of options for correcting the problem. In some cases, changing the dosage of the medication can lessen the side effects without compromising the medication's effectiveness. Substituting medications is another possibility. For example, while some antidepressants may decrease sexual desire (Prozac, Zoloft, Paxil), other antidepressants tend to leave sexual response intact (Wellbutrin, Serzone, Desyrel, and Remeron). Another possible way to counteract a medication's side effects is by adding an antidote. For example, preliminary research findings suggest that the addition of Wellbutrin or BuSpar may eliminate or minimize sexual side effects caused by popular SSRI antidepressants like Prozac, Zoloft, or Paxil. Drug "holidays" are another strategy that can be helpful, but only under the supervision of your healthcare provider. For some drugs that are neither very long- nor very short-acting, patients can, for example, discontinue taking them after their Thursday or Friday morning dosage and resume taking them Sunday morning, allowing them to be sexual Saturday evening with minimized medication interference.

Drugs for Desire: What's Out There?

For thousands of years people have sought out aphrodisiacs, ranging from oysters and ground beetle shells to vitamin E and ginseng. Despite all the hype and dramatic claims made by herbalists and health food stores, we still lack scientific evidence that any vitamin, herb, food substance, or drug is the perfect aphrodisiac. Researchers are finding some substances, however, that show promise in certain cases.

Testosterone

Even though testosterone is often referred to as the "male hormone," it is present in both men and women and plays an important role in generating sexual desire for both genders. Testosterone has been shown to boost sex drive in women, but questions remain about its long-term effectiveness and safety. Canada, Australia, England, and a number of other countries have formally approved the use of testosterone for women who are naturally or surgically menopausal. At the time of this writing, no testosterone treatments for women with low desire are approved by the U.S. Food and Drug Administration (FDA)—although a testosterone gel (LibiGel) is undergoing clinical trials that appear promising. Nevertheless, many postmenopausal women in the United States have been treated with testosterone "off-label," that is, testosterone is prescribed for them in a manner other than the ones for which it has been approved. Women who experience a drop in sexual desire with menopause often find it helpful to include a small dose of androgen (a naturally occurring testosterone in women) in their hormone therapy (HT). Testosterone can be administered as a pill, a patch, a subcutaneous pellet, an injection, or a cream/gel that is applied topically to the vulva, wrists, or thighs. Because the administration of testosterone during pregnancy can cause serious birth defects, physicians are reluctant to prescribe testosterone for women of childbearing age. Testosterone treatment is not advisable for women with a history of breast or ovarian cancer, cardiovascular problems, or liver disease. Chapter 5 provides additional information about menopause, hormones, HT, and sexual desire.

Wellbutrin

Unlike many antidepressants that cause low sexual desire as a side effect, Wellbutrin has been proven to be effective in treating depression without sexual side effects. Recent studies suggest that nondepressed women with low sexual desire may also benefit from this medication. It appears that Wellbutrin differs from many other antidepressants because, rather than focusing on increasing available serotonin levels, a neurotransmitter that can decrease sexual desire, it focuses on dopamine and norepinephrine, neurotransmitters that support sexual desire. The FDA has not approved the use of Wellbutrin for low sexual desire and further research is necessary, but the preliminary findings are encouraging.

Bremelanotide

Lab animals are routinely used to test the safety of new drugs before they are made available to the public. Bremelanotide, also referred to as PT-141, looked promising as a tanning agent until all those little lab rats kept mounting each other nonstop. Further research showed men getting vastly improved erections and women experiencing increased vaginal arousal and sexual desire. It appears that bremelanotide ignores hormones and, unlike Viagra, has nothing to do with the vascular system but goes to work directly in the sex center of the brain. To get this peptide to the brain quickly and efficiently, the medication was initially designed as a nasal spray. The research and development project came to a crashing halt, however, when some of the subjects experienced dangerous spikes in blood pressure. Clinical trials have resumed, now with the medication being administered through injection just beneath the surface of the skin. Observers are optimistic that this tanning agent will one day bring sunshine into the lives of many, including women experiencing low desire and arousal.

Herbal and Other Remedies

Some women report being helped by herbal remedies like ginkgo biloba, ginseng, DHEA, *dong quai*, or L-arginine. Researchers are reporting promising results from their initial investigation of DHEA, a hormone that is transformed into testosterone and estradiol. Currently DHEA is considered an herbal supplement and is sold at health food stores. Two other over-the-counter (OTC) products also boast scientific evidence supporting their effectiveness. *Argin Max for Women* is an oral supplement that includes L-arginine, ginseng, ginkgo biloba, damiana leaf, and a number of other vitamins and minerals. L-arginine in particular has been studied extensively and has been shown to be a precursor of nitric oxide, a chemical that signals blood vessels to relax and that allows increased blood flow. *Zestra* is a topical oil that is applied directly to the vulva. It is a proprietary blend of botanical oils and extracts that appears to increase blood flow to the genitals and enhance genital sensitivity. Research has shown that women using either of these two products often report increased sexual interest, pleasure, and satisfaction.

It's important to realize that, with the exception of the few products mentioned above, to date there is little or no scientifically controlled research on the multitude of sexual enhancement products on the market and no real understanding of their safety or effectiveness over long-term use. If you're considering any OTC product, be cautious and educated in your decision making and be sure to discuss your decision with your healthcare provider.

You may find that the most effective medical intervention for low sexual desire is optimizing your health. Many women report that they experience increased sexual desire when they get enough rest, eat a healthy diet, and exercise regularly.

If It's Not Physical, Then What?

> "I totally lost interest in sex and went to see a doctor. Guess what? Nothing wrong physically, and no medication that will take the rap. That left me with my relationship and myself. Because I didn't think I had the time or even the interest to fix it, I put my low desire back on the shelf and ignored it for a long time."

If, after a medical evaluation, it appears that your problem is due to psychological rather than physical factors, don't panic. Many women face this problem at some point in their lives, and most find ways to increase their sexual desire. In this section we present examples of psychological causes for low sexual desire, ranging from deeply hidden issues that have been around for a long time to issues of a more recent vintage that are fairly apparent and easy to identify. We encourage you to think about these examples and consider whether any might apply to you. With this insight, you'll be in a better position to make good use of the suggestions found throughout this book.

Self-Protection

Sometimes the mind unconsciously decides that, for reasons of safety and self-preservation, sex must be avoided at all costs. For example, if you were sexually molested in the past, avoiding sex in the present may serve as a way to avoid a repeat of the past trauma. Because these efforts at self-protection are often unconscious, it may be very difficult to figure out what's going on. It may be helpful to pay close attention to thoughts that go through your head when you encounter sexual situations. They can provide clues to why you're avoiding sex. But there is a good chance you may never know whether or not your lack of sexual interest has an unconscious or hidden origin.

The good news is that we can often overcome an unconscious barrier, even if we don't know what that barrier is. In many cases doing exercises like the ones in Chapters 13 and 14 can help make sex feel more comfortable and less threatening, which in turn lessens the unconscious mind's need to self-protect. If you find that doing the exercises makes you feel uncomfortable and anxious, however, consider seeking professional help to explore your low sexual desire more closely and finding ways to overcome it.

A Stranger to Pleasure

Some people are raised in such a way that they have a very difficult time experiencing pleasure. We see this most often in people who come from emotionally constricted backgrounds. If you were taught from early childhood to ignore sensory pleasure, you may not be accustomed to enjoying the beauty of a sunset, taking time to appreciate beautiful music, or reveling in the fragrance of a fine wine. In short, you've been programmed to live life in as conservative, modest, unassuming a manner as possible. You've been taught that if you expect little, you'll seldom be disappointed.

This way of approaching life can influence your sexuality. You can become so successful at ignoring the simple pleasures of the body that you end up minimizing the pleasure of sex.

If you're a stranger to pleasure, begin with the sensory journey exercise in Chapter 13. Try a facial, pedicure, manicure, or massage as a way of experiencing pleasure in your body. Complete the other exercises in Chapter 13, always reminding yourself to stay in your senses.

If, despite your best efforts, you can't seem to awaken pleasure in your body, consider consulting a sex therapist, who can help you uncover other conflicts that may be getting in the way of pleasure (see Chapter 16).

Competing Priorities

Sometimes you can get so caught up with all the challenges and responsibilities in your life that you let sex drop to the bottom of your priorities. For instance, you may be juggling your career and parenting obligations and feel so overwhelmed that you put all thoughts of sex on the back burner. If you have a sexual stirring, you dismiss it, telling yourself, "Some other time—I'm too busy right now." After doing this time and time again, you may become insensitive to any sexual stirrings. It isn't that you make a conscious decision to become nonsexual; instead, your loss of sexual interest happens by default.

Fortunately, recognizing competing priorities is the gateway to overcoming low sexual desire. Start by listing what your priorities are and looking carefully at how you spend your time. Do you have time for sex? If not, how can you make time? Rather than trying to radically change your lifestyle all at once, try starting slowly. Begin by inserting small segments of "pleasure time" into your schedule throughout the day—2 extra minutes of touching your body in the shower, 2 minutes of deep breathing and massaging your temples at midday, 3 minutes of sitting quietly in your car and relaxing tensed muscles before driving home from work. These snippets of time will help you refocus on your body. Once you can accommodate these time-outs in your schedule on a regular basis, you'll be ready to carve out the 20- to 30-minute segments necessary to do the exercises in this book.

Fatigue

This is another outcome of a busy and complex lifestyle. It's difficult to think about sex when you feel sleep-deprived or sapped of all your energy. Sex is a basic instinct, but it waits in the background until other bodily needs, including rest, are met. If you have low sexual desire but find that you're interested in sex when you're on a restful vacation, your low sexual desire is probably due to fatigue.

There are a number of things you can try to overcome this difficulty. Start by setting realistic expectations. For instance, plan sex for the weekends, when you have more time to rest. Start exercising. Sometimes exercise actually reduces fatigue. Even a brisk walk for 10 minutes can infuse you with new energy. Try walking before you do the self-help exercises in Chapter 13 and see if that helps your energy level.

If your fatigue is linked to having young children, you'll have to tailor your downtime to the needs of your situation. Make sure you involve your partner in finding solutions, because fatigue can be caused or amplified by feeling isolated and overburdened. Arranging a few hours away from the kids on a regular basis can be very important. Some women find that it works best for them to get a sitter during the late afternoon and early evening rather than at night. Other women arrange for childcare at someone else's home so they can occasionally enjoy having the house to themselves. Get a sitter for a late Saturday afternoon and go with your partner to an inexpensive motel. If you take a picnic dinner, it may cost no more than going to a restaurant and a movie. When you're at the motel, start with a nap before making love. You can be back by 11:30, early enough to get your sitter home before curfew. Who says you have to go away overnight to enjoy a sexual rendezvous with your partner?

Fatigue can be physical, like sleep deprivation, or it can be emotional, like being exhausted from caring for the kids. You'll need to experiment with solutions that work for your situation.

Lack of Attraction

If you're no longer attracted to your partner, your motivation for sex has probably diminished. Lack of attraction is more complex than simply how good a person looks. Negative changes in attitude or behavior can have a far greater impact on a person's attractiveness than changes in appearance. Insensitivity, crudeness, incessant faultfinding, emotional lability, and obnoxious behavior can make a person less attractive and serve as a powerful turn-off.

If you're disgusted with your partner's behavior, have you considered telling him or her how you are feeling? Honest and open dialogue, though at first difficult, can often break down barriers. Check the resource list at the end of the book for suggested readings on improving relationships. In some cases, couples therapy can be very helpful to address resentment and communication problems in the partnership. Lack of attraction won't just "go away" on its own. Tackling the problem head-on is essential.

> "When I realized that I was getting nowhere with all my resentments, things began to change. We got into couples therapy, and I felt supported in addressing his negativity and self-absorption. He really hadn't realized how unattractive he'd become."

Relationship Problems

A troubled relationship is the most common psychological cause for the loss of a previously normal level of sexual desire. If you're angry with your partner, unable to trust, or feel betrayed, you won't be enthusiastic about jumping into bed with him or her. Strong negative emotions can override your sexual appetite even though it's a basic biological drive.

Relationship problems can impact sexual desire in different ways. Your loss of interest may be restricted to just your partner. You may still have sexual fantasies, get turned on by romantic books and movies, and masturbate. But your sexual feelings turn cold when you're confronted by the prospect of having sex with your partner. Or you may find that your disillusionment spills beyond the relationship so that all sexual interest is lost, regardless of the circumstances. In this latter case, because your partner was the center of your sex life, when he or she fell from grace, so did all of your sexual interest.

In either case, you'll need to take charge of your sex life. Can you pinpoint when you began to lose your sexual interest? Does the timing coincide with other problems occurring in your relationship? Next, review the steps you've taken to try to correct your relationship problems. Sometimes couples continue to use negative patterns of interacting with each other and don't look for, or try, new ways of relating. What strategies have you used to improve your relationship in general and sex in particular? You may benefit from concentrating on improving your relationship before addressing the sexual relationship. Take a look at the "Suggested Resources" list for self-help books that deal with relationships. If necessary, consider couples therapy. Once you feel the relationship is improving, you may want to review suggestions in Chapter 12 and the exercises in Chapter 14 for ways to reconnect sexually to each other.

INTEREST BUT NO PLEASURE

> "I used to get turned on whenever I wanted. I just had to think about sex and I'd get wet. Now I feel like the juices never flow, the heat never happens. Even though I want to be excited, I'm frustrated. I can't get a fire started."

> "I can get aroused, but it's flat, like drinking soda without the fizz."

Having Desire but No Fire

When a woman is interested in sex, wants to have sex, but doesn't find the experience pleasurable, we are most likely looking at a lack of *sexual arousal*. It's frustrating for a woman when she wants to feel arousal but can't. As one woman described it, a lack of sexual arousal is "having desire but no fire."

What is sexual arousal for women? "Turned on." "Hot pants." "Getting naked." "Wet." A woman has her own language for sexual excitement, and it tends to be highly individual. A man might equate arousal with an erection, but a woman relies on more diverse and subtle cues to signal that her body and mind are responding to sexual stimulation.

> "When I'm aroused, I feel it in my nipples. They get a little swollen and hard and I love to have them sucked. My lips and skin are sensitive. I feel like rocking my pelvis."

"Turned on is when I feel fullness in my whole crotch. My clitoris becomes sensitive to touch and my labia seem more swollen. Sometimes I get wet right away, but other times I'm aroused but not very wet."

In this section of the chapter, we will be talking about both physical arousal and mental arousal. Being sexually aroused means that not only your body but also, more important, your mind is responding to the sexual activity. As a result, you find the experience pleasurable. Sometimes, due to physical issues, the body might not respond with swelling and moistness, but the mind nevertheless gets into the sexual activity fully and enthusiastically. Feeling the "fire" is not necessarily feeling wet, but it is *always* feeling excitement and pleasure. On the other hand, sometimes the body responds to the sexual stimulation, but the mind is turned off by or indifferent to the experience. Just because a woman lubricates, for example, doesn't necessarily mean she's turned on. A woman can lubricate yet find the sexual activity unsatisfying, unpleasant, or even traumatic (Laan et al., 1994). And in some cases both the body and the mind fail to respond because of a host of possible causes such as pain, life stressors, a medical condition, medication side effect, a history of trauma, relationship problems, or other psychological issues.

When Medical Issues or Menopause Steal the Fire

"I came through a major depression, and with medication I've gotten my life back on track. Everything but my sex life, that is."

"I thought I was lucky because the only chemotherapy side effect I had was not being able to get turned on. Then one day I realized I was sick of being grateful for being alive. I wanted something more."

Rarely will a medical condition or menopause *directly* suppress a woman's ability to experience sexual pleasure. *Indirectly*, however, the pain, vaginal dryness, worry, and fatigue associated with many medical conditions can sufficiently distract a woman so that she either is unable or finds it difficult to focus on sexual cues and enjoy sexual feelings. Chapters 7 and 8 discuss the impact of illness and pain on sexual arousal and ways to minimize and overcome these challenges.

Hormonal changes due to menopause, illness, chemotherapy, medications, breast feeding, and other medical factors are one of the most common causes for decreased physical arousal during sex. Decreases in testosterone levels make the genitals less sensitive to physical stimulation. Decreases in estrogen often prevent adequate lubrication. The lubrication in your vagina and swelling in your pelvis are caused by an increased blood flow to your genitals when you're turned on. Estrogen keeps the process working smoothly by making sure that tissue stays supple and the blood supply to the genitals is steady. At menopause or with an illness or medical condition that causes estrogen deficiency, the endothelium—the tissue through which lubrication passes to the vagina—and the network of small blood vessels that provide the fluid for creating lubrication will atrophy (shrivel up).

The impact of menopause on vaginal lubrication varies dramatically among women. Although it appears that the effects of menopause are less severe for women who remain sexually active, this is not always the case. Research continues to seek explanations for why some women experience greater vaginal atrophy during menopause than others.

Table 15.1 lists the common medical conditions and drugs that decrease physical arousal (but not necessarily pleasure, at least not directly). Although these are the most likely culprits to affect arousal, they do so only rarely (except for menopause). If you have one of these illnesses or take one of these medications, chances are you don't experience any side effects at all. It's also possible that some other illness or drug could cause arousal difficulties, because some medications and medical conditions affect certain people in unique ways. So whether or not your medication or illness is listed in the table, if you're experiencing vaginal dryness or decreased genital sensitivity during sex, discuss your symptoms with your healthcare provider.

Hormone Therapy

If you have an estrogen deficiency, hormone therapy may be prescribed if you are at a low risk for developing cancer or cardiovascular problems. As an alternative for oral HT, vaginal estrogen is sometimes prescribed in the form of a cream, a suppository, or a plastic-ring insert that slowly releases the hormone. It appears that estrogen applied directly to vaginal tissue has the desired effect of reversing the effects of vaginal atrophy and improving lubrication while limiting the amount of estrogen absorbed into the bloodstream. If you are at a heightened risk for developing cancer or cardiovascular problems, there are nonprescription options that can help reduce vaginal dryness without unduly increasing health risks. Discuss with your primary care provider the possible advantages of taking black cohosh, increasing your intake of whole soy foods, or applying vitamin E oil directly to your vaginal tissue at bedtime. In Chapter 5 we discussed hormone therapy and suggested additional resources for you to consult so that you can make an informed decision on this important issue.

Lubricants

Lubricants are another remedy for vaginal dryness. Many different types of lubricants are available over the counter at your local pharmacy. You'll find them where the spermicidal jelly and condoms are kept. You can also order lubricants online (both *www.goodvibes.com* and *www.mypleasure.com* have many products to choose from). Water-based lubricants like Astroglide and K-Y have been popular for many years. There are newer silicone-based lubricants that some women like because they last longer and don't dry out and get sticky. Some women prefer vitamin E oil or vegetable oil because both are easy to find and completely natural. There are also commercial lubricants that are totally natural. Sylk, for example, is a natural extract from the kiwi fruit plant. Avoid petroleum-based lubricants (like Vaseline or Johnson's Baby Oil) because they break down the latex in condoms and can trap bacteria in your vagina, which increases the risk of irritation or infection.

Most lubricants are applied to the vulva or up into the vagina right before sexual activity. They differ in how thick, gooey, and slippery they are. Lubrin is different from most traditional lubricants because, as a vaginal suppository, it's inserted into the vagina about 30 to 60 minutes before sexual activity. It melts slowly and, mimicking the way your body works, slides down the walls of your vagina and out over your introitus. Vaginal moisturizers (e.g., Replens) are also available. Unlike traditional lubricants that are used only during or immediately before sex, products like Replens are used daily to help the vaginal walls retain moisture, which makes the tissue more resistant to irritation and damage during sexual activity.

If you are trying to conceive, chances are you are having problems with vaginal dryness. The stress of infertility, the impact of having to schedule intercourse, and the effects of fertility medications are common culprits interfering with vaginal lubrication. Unfortunately, many lubricants on the market and even good old saliva can have harmful effects on sperm viability and motility. Canola oil appears to be a natural product that provides good lubricant qualities without having a negative impact on sperm. PreSeed and ConceivEase are examples of over-the-counter lubricants designed to be fertility friendly.

You'll need to become a lubricant connoisseur and find the one that is right for you. In Chapter 4, we provided additional information about sexual response and lubrication.

Drugs for Arousal: What's Out There?

Researchers are trying to find drugs that will help women with arousal difficulties just as Viagra was successful in helping many men with erectile difficulties. Currently, there is no magic "pink" pill, but there are a number of promising developments. We'll give a brief overview of treatments currently available or in the pipeline, but we encourage you to seek the most current information from your healthcare provider.

Testosterone

We've already discussed testosterone and its relationships to sexual desire. It appears that testosterone not only prompts men and women to show more interest in sex but can also increase arousal and genital responsiveness in women. Side effects of tes- tosterone include secondary male sexual characteristics, enlargement of the clitoris, acne, weight gain, and liver damage. In the very low dosages prescribed for women, these side effects are very unlikely to occur, and if they do, they can be controlled by reducing the dosage further when necessary, taking "drug holidays," and working closely with your healthcare provider.

Viagra and Other Vasodilators

It seems reasonable to assume that vasodilators (chemicals that dilate blood ves- sels) should increase arousal by increasing pelvic blood flow during sexual stimula- tion. Because Viagra (its pharmaceutical name is sildenefil) has proven so helpful to men, it was hoped that it would have the same effect on women's arousal. So far the research has been disappointing, and though it may be helpful for some women, Viagra is certainly not the "Holy Grail" for all women with low arousal. Scientists are pursuing research on other vasodilators such as alprostadil, phentolamine, vaso- active intestinal peptide (VIP), and other chemicals as possible enhancers of sexual arousal. Because vaginal tissue is highly permeable, many of these chemicals are being developed for topical application, which will result in a more rapid response compared with medicine in pill form. Ask your healthcare provider about what med- ications are currently available.

One interesting observation on research done thus far: even when vasodilators succeed in increasing pelvic blood flow and other signs of physical arousal, research subjects are not necessarily reporting increased sexual pleasure or satisfaction. This suggests that if psychological factors are causing your lack of physical arousal, it's unlikely that any medicine by itself is going to fix the problem.

Bremelanotide

We've already discussed how this peptide increases sexual interest by acting directly in the hypothalamus of the brain. Preliminary research suggests that bremelanotide, unlike the vasodilators described above, does not directly increase vaginal blood flow, but does lead to increased satisfaction with subjective feelings of sexual arousal. As stated above, research continues.

Herbal and Other Remedies

The OTC remedies discussed earlier in this chapter for low sexual desire (Ginkgo biloba, ginseng, DHEA, *dong quai*, L-arginine, and the commercial products *ArginMax for Women* and *Zestra*) also have been reported to help with problems of low sexual arousal. As stated earlier, it's important to remember that when you're considering any OTC product, you should be cautious and educated in your decision making and be sure to discuss your decision with your healthcare provider.

Counteracting Drug Effects

If you're taking a medication that is affecting your sexual arousal, your healthcare provider may have a number of options for correcting the problem. The options discussed earlier in this chapter for low sexual desire (changing medication, decreasing the dosage, combining with an antidote, or taking a drug holiday) also apply for women with low sexual arousal. For women who experience arousal difficulties as a result of taking SSRI antidepressants (Prozac, Zoloft, Paxil, and others), the addition of Viagra may help reverse the unwanted side effect.

Gadgets

Mechanical devices for increasing sexual arousal are not new. For more than a century women have used electric vibrators to increase their arousal and frequency of orgasm. As an alternative to the direct stimulation provided by a vibrator, some women in recent years have used the EROS-CTD (clitoral therapy device), a small, hand-held device with a rubber-like cup that is placed over the clitoris and, by creating a vacuum, draws additional blood into the organ. Because of the increased blood flow, the clitoris is more sensitive to stimulation. Research data suggest that lubrication, satisfaction, and orgasm increase for many women when using this device.

Vibrators can be ordered on the Internet (see the section on "Sex Toys and Videos" in "Suggested Resources"). The EROS-CTD requires a physician's prescription.

When Your Mind Puts Out the Fire

> "It's so much work to stay tuned in to arousal that I check out. I work too hard during the week to want to work on Saturday night also. Just let me read a good book or get the laundry caught up."

> "I try to get aroused. I'll take a warm bath. I'll drink some wine. Maybe I'll feel a little twinge of turn-on, but frankly, my heart's not in it."

From time to time your ability to lubricate can be affected by worry, stress, or mental distraction. But if you experience vaginal dryness regularly, it's most likely due to medical factors. On the other hand, the lack of subjective (mental) arousal—that is, not enjoying the experience—will often be the result of psychological factors. Here are some of the most common psychological causes for a lack of mental arousal, or a lack of mental and physical arousal combined.

Where Your Head's At

One common psychological barrier to arousal is mental distraction. Focusing on the eroticism of the moment is critical for sexual arousal. Anything that distracts you from an erotic focus can prevent sexual arousal, especially your mental arousal. Examples of common distractions include:

- Tension in the relationship
- Job stress
- Financial concerns
- Health worries
- Performance pressure
- Feelings of sexual inadequacy
- Poor body image
- Demanding schedule
- Fear of being discovered or interrupted

Learning, biology, and culture influence your ability to focus on sexual cues and achieve sexual arousal. These factors appear to have a different impact on women and men. A closer look at these gender differences will help you understand common barriers to your arousal and will suggest possible steps to overcome arousal difficulties.

One important way to focus on eroticism is by tuning in to your body's response to sexual stimulation. This ability to tune in to bodily cues is not innate but largely learned. A number of writers have suggested that masturbation serves as an ideal learning opportunity for people to explore how their bodies respond to stimulation. Masturbation is a common behavior for adolescent boys that allows them to become comfortable with their genitals and sexual feelings. As we've discussed in the first part of the book, society's double standard has prevented many women from having the same opportunity to learn how to become attuned to sexual feelings. Not only are women discouraged from masturbating, but they are often taught to avoid looking at or touching their genital area except for necessary hygiene.

Whether masturbating or having sex with a partner, a man has an advantage over a woman in being aware of how his body is responding to sexual cues. He can easily feel, perhaps even see, his penis harden. There is no mistaking when his desire is becoming fire. A natural feedback loop develops. The unmistakable presence of his erection captures his attention; it draws him to the eroticism of the moment, which further increases his arousal. For you as a woman, the swelling of your labia, a feeling of fullness in your genitals, and lubrication in your vagina are much more subtle than an erection. The presence or absence of lubrication is not nearly as noticeable, unless (of course) penetration is attempted when your vagina is dry. As a result, you will find it more difficult than men to identify when you are beginning to respond physically to sexual cues. You won't have nearly as strong a feedback loop to quickly intensify your arousal.

Even when you are aware of growing sexual arousal, you may notice that it's easy to be distracted by nonsexy thoughts. You may wonder why you can't stay focused on the sexual cues around you. As we discussed in Part I, "Knowing Your Sexual Story," you were exposed to many cultural and family influences regarding your sexuality. In most cultures, there's a sexual double bind for women. From early childhood, you were warned about dangers associated with sexuality. You could be sexually exploited. You could be the victim of sexual violence. You could get pregnant by accident, and it's certain your parents warned you that you would carry the major burden of an unwanted pregnancy, whether that burden was shame, financial hardship, restricted freedom, medical risk, or physical discomfort. For all of these reasons, you developed a self-protective vigilance, a watchfulness in sexual situations. When you tune in to sex, part of your brain is still tuned in to those "be careful" messages.

For a guy, if his partner's willing and his penis is hard, life is good. For you, much more is at stake sexually. You learn to monitor for signs of danger and risk. The tendency toward vigilance can become so routine that even when you're in a trusting, loving, equal relationship, you may, through force of habit, still monitor nonerotic cues. During sex, you'll be much more likely than your male partner to notice the furnace rattling or a light coming from underneath the bedroom door.

> "I've given up trying to have sex at home. Our youngest talks in his sleep. Our oldest keeps strange hours. We get calls on the answering machine. The icemaker clunks, the water softener chugs, and somebody over on the next street must own a Harley."

> "It bothers me to have sex before I finish my lists. I can't concentrate on sexual feelings because I'm dreading having to get up early to do the things that I didn't get done before going to bed."

> "I know why women have low sexual arousal: it's called kids and work."

The Wrong Script

Not only what you think about during sex but also what you do during sex will have an important impact on your sexual arousal. Certain ways of making love can be a real turn-on, while other ways can be a turn-off or just not hit the mark. Things that usually turn men on during sex are often different from the things that turn women on. Because of how they've learned to think about sex and how their bodies respond, men see getting and keeping an erection as the essential objective for intercourse. Their script for lovemaking tends to be simple and unswerving—genital stimulation, penetration, and ejaculation. Anything else seems unnecessary.

As a woman, you may be more turned on by holding, touching, and bonding emotionally. If you're like many other women, however, you may think you're supposed to comply with a man's sexual script. Masters and Johnson (1979) demonstrated this tendency in a study in which they compared sexual behavior of heterosexual and lesbian couples. The researchers found that lesbians spent considerably more time engaging in nongenital touching and caressing during lovemaking than did heterosexual women; the heterosexual women focused more on direct genital stimulation. This finding demonstrates that when women have male sex partners, they usually go along with the male script for lovemaking.

Whether you mistakenly assume that the male sexual script is a "universal given" or your needs don't matter, you are probably cheating yourself of what turns you on. Rather than just pleasing your partner or trying to "get it over with," think about putting yourself in the sexual driver's seat. To increase arousal, you'll need to create a sexual script of your own. No time? Too much effort? It's not somebody else's responsibility to rev up your sex life, any more than it's somebody else's responsibility to pick up your kids or complete your tasks at work. Think about how you handle other parts of your life—even when you're pressed for time and burdened with responsibilities, you probably do your best to figure out how to accomplish your priorities. Making sexual arousal a priority means becoming purposeful and focused about finding ways to craft a sexual script that brings you pleasure and satisfaction.

> "I felt terrific when the last minivan pulled out of the driveway. Three kids, and every one of them at a friend's house for the night. I've got a whole night alone with my partner. If I can plan everything else in my life, I can make this happen, too."

Choosing Anger over Arousal

Some women complain and even brag to each other about how sexually unresponsive they've become since having children. They treat low sexual arousal like the red badge of courage for motherhood. If you are chronically complaining about sex being unfulfilling but do nothing to try to correct it, perhaps you need to look at your relationship with your partner. Are you relying on complaints about sex as a way of expressing dissatisfaction with your relationship or anger toward your partner? Are you choosing self-righteous anger as your arousal of choice? If you are getting back at your partner through sexual complaints and indifference, then you're giving up the pleasure of sex for the pleasure of martyrdom. If so, perhaps it's time to consider counseling. Chapter 16 explains how to find a qualified sex therapist.

Before moving to the third and final question, one last thought about arousal and pleasure. Increasing sexual arousal is not merely learning how to touch the right spots at the right time or finding the magic pill or cream that makes blood cascade into your genitals. It takes much more than a moist vagina for you to find pleasure in a sexual situation. Increasing sexual arousal requires self-knowledge, self-esteem, increased body awareness and comfort, meaningful sexual stimulation, and a relationship with your partner that works for you.

ORGASM

Question 3: When All the Circumstances Are Right (e.g., Absence of Distractions, Feeling Sensual and Aroused, Adequate Physical Stimulation), Are You Satisfied with Your Ability to Experience Orgasm?

Did you come? Was it good for you? Do you have multiple orgasms? Questions like these reflect what we call the "tyranny of the orgasm": society's insistence on placing the orgasm at the center of female, as well as male, sexuality. From an evolutionary point of view, men need to ejaculate as part of their sexual response for the purpose of procreation. Female orgasm, in contrast, is not essential for conception. Neither is a woman necessarily sexually dysfunctional if she's not orgasmic.

When we say that *sex matters*, we mean your entire sexual experience. Many women don't orgasm regularly and consider their sexual experiences to be just fine. Many don't even think that orgasm is essential for positive sexuality; instead, they value sex that is emotionally and physically satisfying. In a large magazine poll of women in the Netherlands, for example, only 20% felt that orgasm was the most important source of their sexual pleasure (de Bruijn, 1982). Because women are so different from men and because sexual satisfaction for both women and men is so subjective, we think it's a mistake to assume that orgasm—or any other single factor—is critical to positive sexuality.

In recent years, the word "satisfaction" has become an important concept in sex therapy. Rather than viewing orgasm as the gold standard for good sex, we look for a sense of satisfaction. A man or woman can become physically aroused and have a violent orgasm, yet feel unsatisfied at the end of the experience. Another person may not orgasm, but feel perfectly satisfied with the pleasure of arousal and emotional closeness that resulted from the encounter. It is satisfaction, not necessarily orgasm, that defines meaningful sex.

So when is lack of orgasm a problem? It's a problem when you consider it a problem. If you're enjoying sex unequivocally, then everything is just fine. Do you have a sexual difficulty because you've never had an orgasm? Not if you're okay with this and experience sexual satisfaction regardless. Do you have a sexual difficulty because you don't orgasm every time you have sex? We don't think so. If your partner has a bruised ego because you don't orgasm, is this your problem? It is a problem, but not yours.

We think of orgasm as a sexual choice, and it's yours to make. You have a right to make your own decision about your orgasms and when, where, and how you will have them. If you've decided that orgasms are something you'd like to have, or have more reliably, then taking steps suggested in Chapter 13 and in this chapter will help you improve your experience of orgasm. Remember, however, that this is your choice. In our experience, orgasms pursued to keep a partner happy aren't really sexual orgasms; they're just muscle spasms.

"Where Did My Orgasm Go?"

The inability to orgasm can be lifelong or can develop after a period of normal orgasmic response. Probably one out of every 10 women has never experienced an orgasm (Reinisch, 1991). Almost one out of every four American women has orgasm difficulties at some time in her life (Laumann et al., 1994). Orgasm problems can be global or situational. We call the problem global when a woman is unable to orgasm regardless of the circumstances: whether she is alone or with a partner, whether the method of stimulation is intercourse, oral sex, or a vibrator, she can't orgasm. Anorgasmia (the absence of orgasm) is situational when a woman can orgasm only under certain circumstances. For example, a woman may be able to orgasm when she masturbates but not with her partner.

A common form of situational anorgasmia is the inability to orgasm during intercourse. While some authorities have maintained that the inability to orgasm during intercourse is abnormal, the majority of experts disagree. Intercourse is highly effective in stimulating men to orgasm, but it can be inefficient in providing necessary physical stimulation for women. Depending on the position for intercourse, stimulation of the front wall of the vagina (location of the G spot) may be minimal or nonexistent. Stimulation of the clitoris, an important source of most women's arousal, is also minimal during intercourse. The total amount of clitoral stimulation during thrusting is far less than when the clitoris is stimulated directly during masturbation, oral sex, or manual stimulation. As a result, less than 30% of women report always experiencing orgasm during intercourse (Laumann et al., 1994); many of these women probably do so during intercourse only because they or their partners apply direct clitoral stimulation.

We have often had women come to our office with complaints of not being able to orgasm during intercourse, even though they were otherwise quite orgasmic and sexually satisfied. In many of these cases we found that they were seeking help because this was more of a problem for their partners than for themselves. The men mistakenly believed that it was normal for women to orgasm during intercourse. They felt sexually inadequate because their partners weren't having wild and dramatic orgasms at the time of their penile thrusting. For most of these situations, rather than trying to help the women orgasm during intercourse, we have provided education and reassurance to the couple about the normalcy of their experience.

If orgasm is not always essential for sexual satisfaction, and the inability to experience it during intercourse is not abnormal, when would an orgasm difficulty warrant a closer look?

If the inability is lifelong and global, we need to consider the possibility of a medical problem, a sexual inhibition, or a lack of critical sexual learning. If you stopped having orgasms after years of being orgasmic, a medical problem, relationship difficulties, depression, or stress may be the cause. If you can orgasm by yourself but not in the presence of your partner, you might have a sexual inhibition or relationship concern. For any of these situations, you may want to explore possible causes for the orgasm difficulty and ways to resolve it.

Could This Be a Medical Problem?

> "I stopped being able to orgasm after I took medication. I'd get very excited, feel the readiness to come, but then my body would slide right past the orgasm, like missing an exit on the highway. I'd still be aroused, but I knew I wasn't going to get off."

Normally, for an orgasm to occur your nerve impulses have to be able to travel back and forth between your genitals and spinal cord and between your spinal cord and brain. This two-way communication allows genital stimulation to register in your brain and mental activity in your brain to enhance the physical response in your genitals. When physical stimulation is sufficient and mental activity is conducive, a signal is sent to your pelvic musculature that triggers a series of pleasurable, involuntary contractions that mark the beginning of your orgasm. At the same time, a neurochemical reaction takes place in the brain that results in brief, pleasurable sensations. When a drug, injury, or medical condition interferes with the communication process along the spinal cord or the neurochemical reaction in the brain, achieving an orgasm can be difficult.

Table 15.1 lists medications and medical conditions that can inhibit orgasm. As we discussed earlier in this chapter, the information in this table is neither final nor absolute.

You may find that you continue to have orgasms after an illness or injury listed in the table. For example, even women with serious spinal cord injuries have reported experiencing orgasm. The medications and medical conditions listed in the table may not prevent orgasm but, instead, alter the physical sensations that occur with orgasm. And, of course, you can experience orgasm difficulty as a result of an illness or medication we've not listed.

If you are unable to orgasm regardless of circumstances (global anorgasmia) and you have a medical condition or take a medication listed in the table, discuss your difficulty with a healthcare professional. Even if you're in good health, if you were orgasmic in the past but are not now, and there are no psychological factors in your life to explain this loss of ability, seek a medical consultation. Sometimes the emergence of sexual symptoms can signal the early stages of a medical condition that has not yet been diagnosed.

Medical interventions may include diagnostic testing, changes in prescribed medications, the addition of medications that increase blood flow to the pelvic area, or a more aggressive management of your medical condition. Because orgasm usually requires adequate sexual arousal, the same factors that can interfere with arousal can also inhibit orgasm. Review the information about medication adjustments and devices to increase sexual arousal described earlier in the "Interest but No Pleasure" section of this chapter.

Could There Be Some Psychological Reason?

The psychological factors discussed earlier in this chapter that can inhibit sexual arousal can, by extension, inhibit orgasm. If something prevents you from getting turned on, chances are you will not orgasm. In this case, working on increasing arousal is essential to overcoming your orgasm difficulty.

On the other hand, you may find that you do get physically and emotionally aroused during sexual activity but that you reach a plateau and can't get beyond it. It may feel like some invisible barrier is preventing you from "going over the top." This can be very frustrating. Here are some common causes of, or contributors to, this barrier.

Insufficient Learning

Sexual response is natural in that everyone has the inborn potential to experience it, but learned behaviors can—and do—have an impact on it. Even though you have a natural capacity to experience orgasm, you may need to first learn how to realize this inborn potential. If not, you could experience the contractions and spasms of orgasm, perhaps weakly, but fail to interpret these feelings as signals of orgasm. As a result, you could ignore the sensations or fail to focus on them in a way that would embellish and strengthen the orgasmic response.

Culture greatly influences sexual learning. Anthropologists studying various tribes and societies around the world have noted that women coming from cultures encouraging sexual exploration and assertiveness experience orgasm more readily and with greater satisfaction than women coming from cultures that encourage modest, passive behavior. These observations highlight the importance of taking care of your sexual self: learning about your body, learning to experience sexual pleasure without shame or guilt, and learning to take responsibility for your sexual satisfaction rather than relying on your partner to take care of you.

Orgasm Watching

Even if you're aroused, obsessive self-observation can prevent you from achieving an orgasm. If you become obsessed with watching for any sign of a pending orgasm, you're likely to shut yourself down. Perhaps you feel self-conscious about taking what you feel is too long to orgasm or you may be worried that the orgasm will never come. You can get so caught up in monitoring your sexual response that you become a spectator rather than a participant in the sexual activity. At these times, your erotic focus, which is critical for heightening and sustaining arousal, is replaced by anxious vigilance. By wanting the orgasm so badly, you can end up preventing it from happening.

> "Just like Meg Ryan in *When Harry Met Sally*, I can fake my orgasm. I start out with the best of intentions. I promise myself: *not this time*. But my partner won't leave me alone till I come. Even if I've enjoyed myself and want to stop, I can't until I've done my orgasm-thing."

A common variation on orgasm-watching is your feeling pressured to have an orgasm to please your partner. Otherwise, your partner may feel that his or her sexual prowess is in doubt. If you dread disappointing your partner, you may try too hard to manufacture a response that should emerge naturally. Trying to force a natural orgasm response is like trying to force a laugh when you're under pressure—you know it's not from your heart. Orgasms require you to focus on your genuine sense of pleasure, not worry about your partner.

Fear of Losing Control

An orgasm, as brief as it may seem, is nevertheless a powerful experience. In addition to the involuntary muscular contractions in the pelvis, the body experiences sudden changes in heart rate, breathing, blood pressure, and brain-wave activity. Your body may spasm. Uncensored words and sounds may blurt out. Even the clarity of your thinking is affected for a brief moment. Researchers have suggested that one of the reasons people have difficulty accurately describing what an orgasm feels like is that at the moment of orgasm your observational thought processes are temporarily suspended.

Although for many women the brief moments of total surrender to these powerful body reactions feel like ecstasy, some women are threatened by the prospect of not being in control at all times. Women are often conditioned to be vigilant in sexual situations, to be wary of manipulation, exploitation, or violence. This wariness can be so strong that the unconscious mind will put a cap on arousal when a loss of control seems imminent.

Feeling Self-Conscious

Moaning, thrashing, and screaming may make for hot literature in romance novels, but you may balk at the prospect of such behavior for yourself. Uninhibited orgasm need not be that dramatic; orgasm can be quiet and yet intense. But you might be afraid that the gyrations of orgasm, dramatic or subtle, will make you look ridiculous. You may find it difficult to ignore your childhood lessons about acting with dignity or being a good little girl. While worrying about image and propriety, you may find it difficult, if not impossible, to throw yourself into lovemaking with abandon. If you haven't done so already, try the "An Academy Award Performance" exercise in Chapter 13; it may help you feel less self-conscious.

Holding Back Feelings

Sometimes people find it necessary to hold back intense feelings. Perhaps you harbor rage at your partner but dare not express it. Perhaps you feel grief over the death of a loved one, a grief so great you keep it buried far away from conscious thought. Efforts to hold back strong emotions can spill over into your sexual life. It's difficult to keep strong emotions submerged; the task can easily become an all-or-nothing proposition. Giving free reign to an emotion creates the risk of other emotions surfacing at the same time. In such cases, the mind becomes the jailer, conscientiously guarding against the escape of unwanted emotions. Out of self-protection, all intense emotions, including sexual feelings, become suspect; they're discouraged, denied, controlled, or avoided.

The exercises in Chapter 13 encourage you to experiment with "letting go" during sexual activity. If the exercises don't help, we encourage you to try sex therapy. If you are holding back your feelings without even realizing it, your therapist can help you unblock them in a safe and constructive way. Chapter 16 includes information on finding a qualified sex therapist.

A Battleground for Your Relationship

Sometimes the inability to orgasm is a reflection of problems in your relationship. You may be angry with your partner but haven't acknowledged it, or perhaps you don't know how or don't want to express these feelings directly. Whether unconscious or conscious, you might engage in what is called passive–aggressive behavior: you may hold back at the moment of orgasm, not wanting to give your partner the satisfaction of feeling sexually potent or competent. Conversely, your partner may engage in his or her own passive–aggressive behavior by subtly sabotaging your orgasm. By emotionally holding back or perhaps acting moody or disappointed during lovemaking, your partner can sufficiently distract you so that you don't orgasm. Your disappointment, frustration, or sense of failure would be your punishment. This holding back can be intentional and premeditated, but more often it's an example of the unconscious mind at work. At the conscious level, both partners remain puzzled; their only awareness is that a certain level of excitement is attained and then things level off and go no further. Unconsciously, however, someone is getting even.

Control issues are another example of how relationship problems can inhibit your orgasm. If you feel powerless in your relationship, you may jealously guard the few areas in which you still have control. One of those areas can be sexuality. At an unconscious level, you can find satisfaction in the fact that you, and you alone, have the power to bring yourself to orgasm. You may be reluctant to share this power with your partner, preferring instead to exert control over one of the few areas in which you have power in the relationship.

The reasoning from these two last examples may seem illogical, but remember, the unconscious mind is not governed by the normal rules of logic. As irrational as unconscious motivations may seem, they can be powerful determinants of behavior until they are explored and understood.

As you work on the self-help exercises throughout this book, you may become aware of similar relationship problems affecting your sex life. If so, this could be a valuable discovery—and hopefully you and your partner will decide to address these problems before they do serious harm to your relationship.

SIXTEEN

Seeking Help

Sex Therapy

If you develop a sexual problem, the first question you need answered is whether the symptom has a medical cause. If there is any possibility of a medical problem, always start by consulting your physician or a medical specialist. Chapter 15 offers suggestions for finding a good healthcare professional and for talking to your doctor once you do. If you discover that your symptoms aren't medical, or that in addition to medical treatment your problem requires psychological help, you may find the exercises in the preceding chapters helpful. Sometimes, though, self-help will not be enough. Many sexual problems require professional help by a clinician trained to do sex therapy.

In this final chapter, we talk about what sex therapy is and isn't, what to expect if you go into sex therapy, and how to find a qualified sex therapist.

WHAT IS SEX THERAPY?

Sex therapy, like most forms of therapy, is designed to be both a healing and a growth process. What makes it distinct from other forms of psychotherapy is that what brings the person through the office door is a sexual problem, as opposed to anxiety, depression, or stress. The client is looking for treatment that is designed specifically to correct a sexual problem. Even so, sex therapy doesn't focus solely on sex. Our sexuality is woven into our lives, making it impossible to isolate our focus on sex alone. As we discussed in Part I, "Knowing Your Sexual Story," it's impossible to have an understanding of your sexuality without taking into consideration your upbringing, religious beliefs, health, relationships, self-esteem, psychiatric status, and more. As a matter of fact, it's hard to talk about any of these topics without also talking about sex, because sex is such an important part of life.

Because sex influences so much in our lives, and so many things in our lives influence our sexuality, sex therapy usually begins with a comprehensive review of upbringing, relationships, and current level of adjustment. The sex therapist then makes suggestions about what factors may be contributing to the sexual symptom and, more important, what steps can help resolve the difficulty. In this process, most sex therapists focus on quality of life—preferring to work toward helping the client realize his or her potential to live and love most fully, as opposed to helping the client increase orgasms by 20% or have sex as frequently as the national average.

The sex therapist may treat the client individually, in a group, or, most often, together with the client's partner. In sex therapy we try to downplay the notion of illness or sickness. Instead, we approach the presenting problem as a shared opportunity for the couple to discover ways of increasing emotional and physical intimacy. The client or the couple is encouraged to find pleasure in their sexuality and to become more comfortable giving and receiving pleasure. Treatment will include identifying and examining feelings, gaining insight into reasons for maladaptive behavior, improving communication, learning new ways to approach old problems, and building on the client's or couple's inherent strengths.

WHAT TO EXPECT IN SEX THERAPY

Because sex therapy is often the subject of jokes and parodies, the public has developed many misconceptions about this valuable form of treatment. Be assured that in legitimate sex therapy you will not be asked to take off your clothes, have sex with your partner in front of the therapist, or have sex with the therapist. You should, at all times, feel that you are being treated in a professional manner and that your values and religious beliefs are respected.

The cost and length of treatment vary. Depending on where you live and your therapist's credentials, sex therapy can range from $90 to $250 a session, with most therapists charging between $100 and $175 per session. Some health insurance plans will cover the cost, or part of the cost of sex therapy. If you can afford only a limited number of visits, sex therapy can still be helpful and effective. Even a session or two can be enough to explore and correct misinformation, lead you to self-help resources, identify unrealistic expectations you may have of yourself and/or your partner, and alert you to other problems that might complicate the resolution of your symptoms.

The length of treatment can range from a couple of visits to many months of weekly sessions. If the focus of treatment expands to resolving long-standing, deep-seated problems, therapy can go on for more than a year. Your therapist should be able to give you an estimate of how many sessions will be required to accomplish your treatment goals. Here is a caution, however. Very often in therapy the problem that brings a person in may be defined differently as things move along. For example, a couple may come into therapy insisting that they have a wonderful relationship and that their only problem is that they can't agree on the frequency of sex. At first glance this may appear to be a straightforward case that shouldn't require more than a dozen sessions. But if it becomes clear during the first few sessions that there are significant relationship problems, the focus and projected length of treatment will have to change dramatically.

As we have indicated, if you are in a relationship, your therapist will probably encourage you to include your partner in treatment. If you are seen as a couple, the therapist will likely keep individual sessions to a minimum and focus on helping the two of you work through your concerns together.

Many sex therapists will use "homework assignments" to help both partners discover patterns in their sexual relationship. These assignments also provide opportunities to learn and practice new, more adaptive ways to relate. Assigned reading and the use of instructional videos are often part of treatment.

It's important to understand that, at times, you may feel uncomfortable in sex therapy. The therapist will ask you detailed questions about your sexual history. You will be encouraged to take an honest look at how you and your partner relate. The struggles you have and the ways you avoid intimacy will be discussed with the goal of helping you both grow. You and your partner will be encouraged to be honest about your needs and frustrations in the relationship.

Why, you may ask, would anyone willingly put him- or herself into such an awkward position? Usually it is because a person or couple is no longer willing to accept the status quo and honestly wishes to change things for the better. They accept that meaningful growth doesn't come easily and that if they can tolerate the momentary discomfort that comes from the process of growing, they can achieve deeper passion and intimacy.

FINDING A SEX THERAPIST

Because a therapist is a social worker, psychiatrist, psychologist, or nurse does not guarantee that she or he has the expertise to treat sexual disorders. When considering sex therapy, you will want to look for a skilled mental health professional who has additional training and experience in the area of human sexuality.

With less than an hour of research, you should be able to find qualified sex therapists in your community. The American Association of Sexuality Educators, Counselors, and Therapists (AASECT) is a national organization that certifies sex therapists. You can obtain a list of certified sex therapists in your area by visiting AASECT's website at *www.aasect.org*. There are also many excellent sex therapists who do not have formal certification but are well trained and highly experienced in treating sexual problems. Ask your healthcare provider if he or she can recommend a qualified sex therapist. If you live near a university, contact the psychology or social work department and ask for recommendations. If you live in the United States, try calling your state psychological association, psychiatric association, or the state office for the National Association of Social Workers (NASW) for recommendations. Check the Yellow Pages under *Psychologists; Counselors;* or *Marriage, Family, Child, and Individual Counselors* and look for therapists who specialize in treating sexual problems. If you live in another part of the world, look at the Resources section at the end of this book for suggestions, or you can go to any one of the popular Internet search engines and type in "sex therapy" and the name of your country.

Once you have the name of a therapist, call and ask questions before scheduling your first appointment. Find out about the therapist's training and experience in treating sexual problems. Ask about the cost of therapy and whether the therapist accepts insurance. If the therapist is unwilling to answer these basic questions, you may want to keep searching. As a consumer, you have the right to know what kind of services you're purchasing.

Besides competence, what other characteristics should you look for in a sex therapist? People sometimes wonder whether they should see a female or male therapist. Research shows that sex therapy can be effective regardless of the therapist's gender. What is far more important than gender is your comfort level with the therapist. You need to be able to trust your therapist and believe that he or she is concerned about your well-being and is respectful of your circumstances, feelings, and beliefs.

If you don't think you have a comfortable rapport with your therapist after a few sessions, discuss your concerns. If you still feel uncomfortable, consider transferring to another therapist. But be careful that by changing therapists you're not "shooting the messenger." As we discussed earlier, to grow you will likely have to face things that will make you feel uncomfortable. It can be tempting to blame the therapist for this discomfort rather than asking what it is about yourself, your background, or your relationship that might be creating this discomfort. If you want to change therapists, be sure that you're reacting to "bad chemistry" and not to the pain and embarrassment that are coming from the truth.

CONCLUSION

If your car's engine breaks down, you'll repair it. If your car still has a cigarette lighter and it breaks, even if you're a smoker, you'll probably let it slide. Far too many people view their sexuality like the cigarette lighter, an accessory they can live without. We hope that throughout this book we have made a case for just the opposite. Sexuality should be considered as important as a car's air-conditioner in the middle of summer or a car's heater in the frigid months of winter. You can get around without them, but they sure make the ride more pleasurable.

Sexual problems should not be ignored. They can harm our self-esteem, place a strain on our relationships, and, in some cases, serve as a warning for undiagnosed medical problems. For these reasons, if you develop a sexual problem, you should not suffer silently. Medical and psychological help are available and highly effective. When in need, make use of them.

Reading this book can be an important step in overcoming a sexual problem. We encourage you to take as many additional steps as necessary to continue your journey to sexual health and satisfaction.

Suggested Resources

ANXIETY

Burns, D. (2007). *When panic attacks: The new drug-free therapy that can change your life*. New York: Three Rivers Press.

Stahl, B., & Goldstein, E. (2010). *A mindfulness-based stress reduction workbook*. Oakland, CA: New Harbinger.

Wilson, R. (1996). *Don't panic revised edition: Taking control of anxiety attacks*. New York: Harper Paperbacks.

BODY IMAGE

Brumberg, J. J. (1997). *The body project: An intimate history of American girls*. New York: Random House.

Cash, T. (1997). *The body image workbook: An 8-step program for learning to like your looks*. Oakland, CA: New Harbinger.

Erdman, C. K. (1996). *Nothing to lose: A guide to sane living in a large body*. San Francisco: HarperOne.

Hirschmann, J. R., & Munter, C. H. (1995). *When women stop hating their bodies: Freeing yourself from food and weight obsession*. New York: Fawcett Columbine.

Northrup, C. (2010). *Women's bodies, women's wisdom: Creating physical and emotional health and healing*. New York: Bantam Books.

Pipher, M., & Ross, R. (2005). *Reviving Ophelia: Saving the selves of adolescent girls*. New York: Ballantine Books.

Wolf, N. (2002). *The beauty myth*. New York: Anchor.

COUPLES COMMUNICATION AND INTIMACY

Barbach, L. (1984, 2001). *For each other: Sharing sexual intimacy*. New York: New American Library.

Barbara, M. (2008). *Bring yourself to love: How couples turn disconnection into intimacy.* Providence, RI: Dos Monos Press.

Berman, L. (2010). *It's not him, it's you!: How to take charge of your life and create the love and intimacy you deserve.* New York: DK.

Brown, E. (2001). *Patterns of infidelity and their treatment.* New York: Routledge.

Fisher, H. (2004). *Why we love: The nature and chemistry of romantic love.* New York: Holt.

Glass, S. (2002). *Not "just friends": Protect your relationship from infidelity and heal the trauma of betrayal.* New York: Free Press.

Gottman, J., & Silver, N. (2004). *The seven principles for making marriage work.* New York: Crown.

Hendricks, G., & Hendricks, K. (2002). *Conscious loving: The journey to co-commitment.* New York: Bantam Books.

Hendrix, H. (2007). *Getting the love you want: A guide for couples.* New York: HarperPerennial.

Love, P. (2001). *The truth about love: The highs, lows, and how you can make it last forever.* New York: Fireside Press.

McCarthy, B., & McCarthy, E. (2003). *Rekindling desire: A step-by-step program to help low-sex and no-sex marriages.* New York: Taylor & Francis.

Mitchell, S. (2003). *Can love last? The fate of romance over time.* New York: Norton.

Schnarch, D. (1997). *Passionate marriage: Sex, love and intimacy in emotionally committed relationships.* New York: Norton.

Schnarch, D. (2002). *Resurrecting sex: Resolving sexual problems in your relationship.* New York, HarperCollins.

Siegel, D. (2008). *The neurobiology of "we": How relationships, the mind, and the brain shape who we are* [Audio CD]. Louisville, CO: Sounds True.

Snyder, D. K., Baucom, D. H., & Gordon, K. C. (2007). *Getting past the affair: A program to help you cope, heal, and move on—together or apart.* New York: Guilford Press.

Spring, J. A. (1996). *After the affair: Healing the pain and rebuilding trust when a partner has been unfaithful.* New York: HarperCollins.

Spring, J. A. (2005). *How can I forgive you? The courage to forgive, the freedom not to.* New York: Harper.

Stanley, S., Blumberg, S., Markman, H., & Edell, D. (2010). *Fighting for your marriage.* San Francisco: Jossey-Bass.

Subotnik, R., & Harris, G. (2005). *Surviving infidelity: Making decisions, recovering from the pain* (3rd ed.). Avon, MA: Adams Media.

Vaughn, P. (2003). *The monogamy myth: A personal handbook for recovering from affairs.* New York: Newmarket Press.

Zoldbrod, A., & Dockett, L. (2002). *Sex talk: Uncensored exercises for exploring what really turns you on.* Oakland, CA: New Harbinger.

DESIRE AND AROUSAL

Golden, G. (2009). *In the grip of desire: A therapist at work with sexual secrets.* New York: Routledge.

Hall, K. (2004). *Reclaiming your sexual self.* Hoboken, NJ: Wiley.

Meston, C., & Buss, D. (2009). *Why women have sex: Understanding sexual motivations from adventure to revenge (and everything in between).* New York: Times Books.

Weiner-Davis, M. (2003). *The sex-starved marriage: A couple's guide to boosting their marital libido.* New York: Simon & Schuster.

DISABILITY AND ILLNESS

Books

Alderowitz, R. (2004). *Intimacy with impotence: The couple's guide to better sex after prostate disease.* Cambridge, MA: Da Capo Press.

Brownworth, V. A., & Raffo, S. (Eds.). (1999). *Restricted access: Lesbians on disability.* Berkeley, CA: Seal Press.

Chapunoff, E. (2007). *Answering your questions about heart disease and sex.* Long Island City, NY: Hatherleigh Press.

Katz, A. (2009). *Woman Cancer Sex.* Pittsburgh, PA: Hygeia Media.

Kaufman, M., Silverberg, C., & Odette, F. (2003). *The ultimate guide to sex and disability: For all of us who live with disabilities, chronic pain and illness.* San Francisco: Cleis Press.

Kayser, K., & Scott, J. L. (2010). *Helping couples cope with women's cancers.* Springer Science and Business Media.

Kroll, K., & Klein, E. L. (1992). *Enabling romance: A guide to love, sex, and relationships for people with disabilities.* Horsham, PA: No Limits Communications.

Laken, V., & Laken, K. (2002). *Making love again: Hope for couples facing loss of sexual intimacy.* Sandwich, MA: Ant Hill Press.

Rozler, J., & Rice, D. (2007). *Sex and diabetes.* Alexandria, VA: American Diabetes Association.

Schover, L. (1997). *Sexuality and fertility after cancer.* New York: Wiley.

Sipski, M., & Alexander, C. (1997). *Sexual function in people with disability and chronic illness: A health professional's guide.* Frederick, MD: Aspen.

Organizations and Websites

United States

American Association on Intellectual and Developmental Disabilities (formerly the AAMR)
www.aamr.org or *www.aaidd.org*

American Cancer Society
www.cancer.org

The Arc: For People with Intellectual and Developmental Disabilities
www.thearc.org

Autism Society of America
www.autism-society.org

Disability Resources (DRM WebWatcher)
www.DisabilityResources.org

Aspires (online resource for partners and family members of individuals on the autistic spectrum)
www.aspires-relationships.com

Association of Cancer Online Resources (ACOR)
www.acor.org

National Alliance on Mental Illness (NAMI)
www.nami.org

National Down Syndrome Society
www.ndss.org

Sexual Health Network
www.sexualhealth.com

United Cerebral Palsy
www.ucp.org

Australia

Cancer Council Australia
www.cancer.org.au

People with Disability
www.pwd.org.au

Canada

Canadian Cancer Society/Société Canadienne du Cancer
www.cancer.ca

Canadian Mental Health Association (CMHA)
www.cmha.ca

DisAbled Women's Network (DAWN)
www.dawncanada.net

Great Britain

British Council of Disabled People (BCODP)
www.bcodp.org.uk

CancerHelp UK
www.cancerhelp.org.uk

Cerebral Palsy Register for Scotland
www.napier.ac.uk/cprs

National Autistic Society
www.autism.org.uk

Scope (cerebral palsy)
www.scope.org.uk

Ireland

Enable Ireland (formerly Cerebral Palsy Ireland)
www.enableireland.ie

Irish Cancer Society
www.cancer.ie

New Zealand

Cancer Society of New Zealand
www.cancernz.org.nz

EROTIC POWER PLAY (SAFE, SANE, AND CONSENSUAL)

Easton, D., & Liszt, C. A. (1998). *The bottoming book: How to get terrible things done to you by wonderful people.* Emeryville, CA: Greenery Press.

Easton, D., & Liszt, C. A. (1998). *The topping book: Or getting good at being bad.* Emeryville, CA: Greenery Press.

Green, L. (1998). *The sexually dominant woman: A workbook for nervous beginners.* Emeryville, CA: Greenery Press.

Moser, C., & Madeson, J. J. (1998). *Bound to be free: The SM experience.* New York: Continuum.

Wiseman, J. (1998). *SM 101: A realistic introduction.* San Francisco, CA: Greenery Press.

EROTICA AND FANTASY

Bader, M. (2003). *Arousal: The secret logic of sexual fantasies.* New York: St. Martin's/Griffen.

Bright, S. (Ed.). (2008). *Best American erotica 2008.* New York: Touchstone Books.

Kudaka, G. (Ed.). (1995). *On a bed of rice: An Asian American erotic feast.* New York: Anchor.

Martin, R. (Ed.). (1999). *Dark Eros: Black erotic writings.* New York: St. Martin's Press.

Queen, C., & Davis, J. (Eds.). (1997). *Sex spoken here: Good vibrations erotic reading circle selections.* San Francisco: Down There Press.

Taormino, T. (1996–2000). *Best lesbian erotica.* San Francisco: Cleis Press.

G SPOT

Ladas, A., Whipple, B., & Perry, J. (2005). *The G spot: And other discoveries about human sexuality.* New York: Holt/Owl.

Winks, C. (1998). *The good vibrations guide to the G-spot.* San Francisco: Down There Press.

GENERAL SEXUALITY INFORMATION

Books

Anderson, D. (2008). *Sex tips for straight women from a gay man.* New York: HarperCollins.

Angier, N. (1999). *Woman: An intimate geography.* New York: Houghton Mifflin.

Barbach, L. (2001). *For each other: Sharing sexual intimacy.* New York: New American Library.

Berman, L. (2010). *Real sex for real women: Intimacy, pleasure, and sexual well-being.* New York: DK.

Boston Women's Health Book Collective. (2005). *Our bodies, ourselves: For the new century.* New York: Touchstone.

Daniluk, J. C. (2003). *Women's sexuality across the lifespan: Challenging myths, creating meanings.* New York: Guilford Press.

Hutcherson, H. (2003). *What your mother never told you about sex.* New York: Perigee.

Hutcherson, H. (2006). *Pleasure: A woman's guide to getting the sex you want, need, and deserve.* New York: Perigee Trade.

Joannides, P., & Gross, D. (2009). *The guide to getting it on: The universe's coolest and most informative book about sex* (6th ed.). West Hollywood, CA: Goofy Foot Press.

Komisaruk, B., Beyer-Flores, C., & Whipple, B. (2006). *The science of orgasm.* Baltimore: Johns Hopkins University Press.

Love, P., & Robinson, J. (1995). *Hot monogamy: Essential steps to more passionate, intimate lovemaking.* New York: Plume/Penguin.

McCarthy, B., & McCarthy, E. (1998). *Couple sexual awareness: Building sexual happiness.* New York: Carroll & Graf.

Michael, R. T., Ganon, J. H., Laumann, E. O., & Kolata, G. (1994). *Sex in America: A definitive survey.* New York: Warner Books.

Morin, J. (1998). *Anal pleasure and health: A guide for men and women.* San Francisco: Down There Press.

Ogden, G. (1999). *Women who love sex: An inquiry into the expanding spirit of women's erotic experience.* Cambridge, MA: Womanspirit Press.

Ogden, G. (2008). *The return of desire: A guide to rediscovering your sexual passion.* Boston: Trumpeter.

Paget, L. (2000). *How to give her absolute pleasure: Totally explicit techniques every woman wants her man to know.* New York: Bantam Doubleday Dell.

Penner, C., & Penner, J. (2003). *The gift of sex: A guide to sexual fulfillment.* Nashville, TN: Word Books.

Perel, E. (2007). *Mating in captivity: Unlocking erotic intelligence.* New York: Harper.

Schwartz, P., & Lever, J. (2000). *The great sex weekend: A 48-hour guide to rekindling sparks for bold, busy, or bored lovers.* New York: Perigee/Penguin.

Stewart, E. (2002). *The V book: The doctor's guide to complete vulvovaginal health.* New York: Bantam Books.

Taormino, T. (2006). *The ultimate guide to anal sex for women.* San Francisco: Cleis Press.

Tiefer, L. (1994). *Sex is not a natural act and other essays.* New York: Westview Press.

Winks, C., & Semans, A. (1997). *The new good vibrations guide to sex: How to have safe, fun sex.* San Francisco: Cleis Press.

Zoldbrod, A. (1998). *Sex smart: How your childhood shaped your sexual life and what to do about it.* Oakland, CA: New Harbinger.

Organizations, Sex Therapy Associations, and Websites

United States

AASECT (American Association of Sexuality Educators, Counselors, and Therapists)
www.aasect.org

Association of Reproductive Health Professionals
www.arhp.org/publications-and-resources

Columbia University's Health Education Program
www.goaskalice.columbia.edu

Kinsey Institute for Research in Sex, Gender, and Reproduction
www.kinseyinstitute.org

Planned Parenthood
www.plannedparenthood.org

Sallie Foley
www.salliefoley.com

Sexuality Information and Education
Council of the United States (SIECUS)
www.siecus.org

Society for Human Sexuality
www.sexuality.org

Australia

Australian Counselling Association
www.theaca.net.au

Australian Society for Sex Educators,
Researchers and Therapists
www.assertnational.org.au

Canada

American Association of Sexuality
Educators, Counselors, and Therapists
www.aasect.org

BESTCO (sex therapists in Ontario)
www.bestco.info/index.html

Options for Sexual Health (sexual health
services and support for British Columbia)
www.optionsforsexualhealth.org

Sex Information and Education Council of
Canada (SIECCAN)
www.sieccan.org

Sexuality and U
www.sexualityandu.ca/en

Great Britain

British Association for Sexual Health and
HIV
www.bashh.org

College of Sexual and Relationship
Therapists (formerly the British Association
for Sexual and Relationship Therapy
[BASRT])
www.cosrt.org.uk

Family Planning Association (sexual
health)
www.fpa.org.uk

Relate (relationship counseling and sex
therapy resources)
www.relate.org.uk/home/index.html

Sexual Health Scotland
*www.sexualhealthscotland.co.uk/get-help/
directory-of-local-and-national-services*

New Zealand

Family planning, sexual health, sex
therapist referrals
www.familyplanning.org.nz

Sex Therapy New Zealand
www.sextherapy.co.nz/homepage.html

INFERTILITY

Domar, A. D., & Dreher, H. (1997). *Healing mind, healthy woman: Using the mind-body connection to manage stress and take control of your life.* New York: Holt.

Zoldbrod, A. (1990). *Getting around the boulder in the road: Using imagery to cope with fertility problems.* Lexington, MA: Center for Reproductive Problems. (Available from author: 12 Rumford Road, Lexington, MA 02420)

Zoldbrod, A. (1992). *Men, women, and infertility: Intervention and treatment strategies.* New York: Lexington Books.

LESBIAN, BISEXUAL, TRANSGENDER, QUEER, AND INTERSEX

Books

Berzon, B. (2004). *Permanent partners: Building gay and lesbian relationships that last.* New York: Plume.

Bright, S. (1999). *Susie sexpert's lesbian sex world.* San Francisco: Cleis Press.

Caster, W. (2008). *The new lesbian sex book* (3rd ed.). Boston: Alyson.

Clunis, D. M. (2004). *Lesbian couples: A guide to creating healthy relationships.* Seattle, WA: Seal Press.

Devor, H. (1999). *FTM: Female-to-male transsexuals in society.* Bloomington: Indiana University Press.

Diamond, L. (2008). *Sexual fluidity: Understanding women's love and desire.* Cambridge, MA: Harvard University Press.

Dreger, A. (1999). *Intersex in the age of ethics.* Hagerstown, MD: University Publishing Group.

Huegel, K. (2003). *GLBTQ: The survival guide for queer and questioning teens.* Minneapolis, MN: Free Spirit Press.

Hutchins, L., & Ka'ahumanu, L. (1991). *Bi any other name: Bisexual people speak out.* Boston: Alyson.

Makadon, H. J., Mayer, K. H., Potter, J., & Goldhammer, H. (Eds.). (2007). *The Fenway guide to lesbian, gay, bisexual and transgender health.* Philadelphia: American College of Physicians.

Morris, K. E. (2000). *Speaking in whispers.* Chicago: Third Side Press. (African American lesbian erotica)

Newman, F. (2004). *The whole lesbian sex book: A passionate guide for all of us.* San Francisco: Cleis Press.

Samons, S. L. (2009). *When someone of the opposite sex isn't: Sexual orientation in male-to-female transgender people.* New York: Routledge.

Schell, J. (2008). *Lesbian sex: 101 lovemaking positions.* Berkeley, CA: Celestial Arts.

Stendhal, R. (2003). *True secrets of lesbian desire: Keeping sex alive in long-term relationships.* Berkeley, CA: North Atlantic Books.

Organizations and Websites

United States

Accord Alliance (replaces Intersex Society of North America)
www.accordalliance.org

Bisexual Resource Center
www.biresource.net

Gay.com
www.gay.com

Gay and Lesbian Medical Association
www.glma.org

Gender Education and Advocacy
www.gender.org

Human Rights Campaign
www.hrc.org

International Foundation for Gender Education (IFGE)
www.ifge.org

Lesbian.org: Resources for Lesbian and Bisexual Women
www.lesbian.org

National Gay and Lesbian Task Force
www.ngltf.org

Parents, Families and Friends of Lesbians and Gays (PFLAG)
www.pflag.org

Queer Net
www.queernet.org

World Professional Association for Transgender Health (WPATH)
www.wpath.org

Australia

ACON (Australia's largest community-based GLBT health and HIV/AIDS organization)
www.acon.org.au

Coming Out Australia (support line and national resources)
www.comingout.com.au

Gay and Lesbian Community Services (Western Australia community resources)
www.glcs.org.au

National LGBTI Health Alliance (GLBT and intersex national health alliance)
www.lgbthealth.org.au

Not So Straight (national resources)
www.notsostraight.com.au/links

Canada

Canadian Rainbow Health Coalition
www.rainbowhealth.ca

GayCanada
www.gaycanada.com

PFLAG Canada
www.pflagcanada.ca

Vancouver Coastal Health (transgender health resources)
transhealth.vch.ca/resources/links

Youthline (LGBT youth hotline and support site)
www.youthline.ca

Great Britain

Family and Friends of Lesbians and Gays
www.fflag.org.uk

Gay in the United Kingdom (social support group for LGBT asylum seekers/refugees to United Kingdom)
e-mail: *lgbtisocial@yahoo.co.uk*

GLBTQ (support, counseling for immigrants to United Kingdom)
www.uklgig.org.uk

Lesbian and Gay Christian Movement (LGCM)
www.lgcm.org.uk
e-mail: *lgcm@lgcm.org.uk*
Hotline: 020-7613-1095 (support, especially for Christian homophobia)

Lesbian and Gay Foundation
www.lgf.org.uk

LGBT Youth Scotland
www.lgbtyouth.org.uk

London Friend (support and counseling for residents of the United Kingdom)
www.londonfriend.org.uk

London Lesbian and Gay Switchboard
www.llgs.org.uk

Love Exiles (links LGBT individuals throughout UK for information, support)
www.loveexiles.org

Scottish Transgender Alliance
www.scottishtrans.org

United Kingdom transgender resources
www.transgenderzone.com

New Zealand

Gay and Lesbian Health Victoria
www.glhv.org.au

Gay Line Wellington (gay, lesbian, bisexual, transgender, *takatāpui* [GLBTT] support site for Wellington)
www.gayline.gen.nz

GayNZ
www.gaynz.com

Gender Bridge (transgender support site)
www.genderbridge.org

Intersex Awareness New Zealand
www.ianz.org.nz

OUTLine NZ (support and crisis line and resources)
www.outlinenz.com

PFLAG South
www.pflag.org.nz

Auckland Pride Centre (information and support)
www.pride.org.nz

Queer Resources Aotearoa
www.qrd.org.nz

Rainbow Youth (Aukland youth support site)
www.rainbowyouth.org.nz

Rainbow Wellington (information and support)
www.rainbowwellington.org.nz

Transgender (trans individuals' clinical resources)
www.transgender.co.nz/nz_health_medical. php

MASTURBATION

Dodson, B. (1996). *Sex for one: The joy of self-loving.* New York: Three Rivers Press.

MENOPAUSE AND AGING

Anderson, C. M., & Stewart, S. (1995). *Flying solo: Single women in midlife.* New York: Norton.

Barbach, L. (2000). *The pause: Positive approaches to menopause.* New York: Plume/Penguin.

Block, J. (2008). *Sex over 50 (Updated and expanded).* New York: Prentice Hall.

Foley, S. (2005). *Love and sex for grown-ups: A no-nonsense guide to a life of passion.* New York: Sterling Press. (Released in paperback in 2006 as *Modern love: A no-nonsense guide to a life of passion.*)

Friedan, B. (2006). *The fountain of age.* New York: Simon & Schuster.

Gordon, S., & Shimberg, E. (2004). *Another chance for love: Finding a partner later in life.* New York: Adams Media.

Levine, S. (2004). *Sexuality in mid-life.* New York: Plenum Press.

Northrup, C. (2007). *The wisdom of menopause journal: Your guide to creating vibrant health and happiness in the second half of your life.* New York: Hay House.

Rako, S. (1999). *The hormone of desire: The truth about testosterone, sexuality, and menopause.* New York: Three Rivers Press.

Siegal, D. L., Doress-Worters, P. B., & Sanford, W. (1994). *The new ourselves, growing older: Women aging with knowledge and power.* New York: Touchstone/Simon & Schuster.

MEN'S SEXUALITY

Castleman, M. (2004). *Great sex: A man's guide to the secret principles of total body sex.* Emmaus, PA: Rodale Press.

Levine, L. (2008). *Understanding Peyronie's disease: A treatment guide for curvature of the penis.* Omaha, NE: Addicus Books.

McCarthy, B., & Metz, M. (2008). *Men's Sexual Health.* New York: Routledge.

Metz, M., & McCarthy, B. (2003). *Coping with premature ejaculation: How to overcome PE, please your partner and have great sex.* Oakland, CA: New Harbinger.

Metz, M., & McCarthy, B. (2004). *Coping with ED: How to regain confidence and enjoy great sex.* Oakland, CA: New Harbinger.

Milstein, R., & Slowinski, J. (2000). *The sexual male: Problems and solutions.* New York: Norton.

Zilbergeld, B. (1999). *The new male sexuality: A guide to sexual fulfillment.* New York: Bantam Doubleday Dell.

MINDFULNESS

Hanh, T. (2009). *Happiness: Essential mindfulness practices.* Berkeley, CA: Parallax Press.

Kabat-Zinn, J. (2005). *Guided mindfulness meditation* [Audio CD]. Louisville, CO: Sounds True.

Kabat-Zinn, J. (2006). *Mindfulness for beginners* [Audio CD]. Louisville, CO: Sounds True.

Kabat-Zinn, J. (2006). *Wherever you go, there you are.* New York: Hyperion.

Sarno, J. (1999). *The mindbody prescription: Healing the body, healing the pain.* New York: Warner Books.

Siegel, D. (2008). *The neurobiology of "we": How relationships, the mind, and the brain interact to shape who we are* [Audio CD]. Louisville, CO: Sounds True.

Siegel, D. (2010). *Mindsight: The new science of personal transformation.* New York: Bantam Books.

ORGASM

Books

Barbach, L. (2000). *For yourself: The fulfillment of female sexuality.* New York: New American Library.

Heiman, J., & LoPiccolo, J. (1988). *Becoming orgasmic: A sexual growth program for women.* New York: Simon & Schuster.

Solot, D., & Miller, M. (2007). *I love female orgasm: An extraordinary orgasm guide.* Cambridge, MA: Da Capo Press.

Swift, R. (2005). *How to have an orgasm—As often as you want.* New York: Carroll & Graf.

Video

Becoming Orgasmic
Sinclair Intimacy Institute
Available from *www.bettersex.com*

PAIN

Books

Catalano, E., Hardin, K., & Tupper, S. (1996). *The chronic pain workbook: A step by step guide for coping with and overcoming pain.* Oakland, CA: New Harbinger.

Goldstein, A., Pukall, C., & Goldstein, I. (2011). *When sex hurts: A woman's guide to banishing sexual pain.* Jackson, TN: Da Capo Press.

Goodwin, A. J., & Agronin, M. (1997). *A woman's guide to overcoming sexual fear and pain.* Oakland, CA: New Harbinger.

Organizations and Websites

United States

International Pelvic Pain Society
www.pelvicpain.org

National Vulvodynia Association (NVA)
www.nva.org

University of Michigan Center for Vulvar Disease
www.med.umich.edu/obgyn/cvd/ref_phys.htm

The VP Society
www.vulvalpainsociety.org

Vulvar Pain Foundation
www.vulvarpainfoundation.org

Australia

Australian and New Zealand Vulvovaginal Society
www.anzvs.org/index.html

Gynaecological Awareness Information Network
www.gain.org.au

Canada

Island Sexual Health Society (Vancouver and national sexual health resources)
www.islandsexualhealth.org/resources/links

Women's Health Matters
www.womenshealthmatters.ca/health-resources/pelvic_health/vulvodynia

Great Britain

Gynaecologics and vulvodynia treatment
www.gynaecologists.co.uk/vulvodynia.html

Vulval Pain Society
www.vulvalpainsociety.org

New Zealand

Australian and New Zealand Vulvovaginal Society
www.anzvs.org/index.html

Auckland Sexual Health Services (Directory of clinics specializing in sexual health problems, pain)
www.ashs.org.nz/services.html

Healthpoint (Clinic specializing in vulvar pain)
www.healthpoint.co.nz/default,151341.sm

Vulvodynia Support NZ (national resource site)
www.vulvodynia.org.nz/home

Polyamory

Easton, D., & Hardy, J. (2009). *The ethical slut: A practical guide to polyamory, open relationships, and other adventures.* San Francisco, CA: Celestial Arts.

Taormino, T. (2008). *Opening up: A guide to creating and sustaining open relationships.* San Francisco: Cleis Press.

Pregnancy

Murkoff, H., & Mazel, S. (2008). *What to expect when you're expecting* (4th ed.). New York: Workman.

Pepper, R. (2005). *The ultimate guide to pregnancy for lesbians: Tips and techniques from conception to birth—How to stay sane and care for yourself.* San Francisco: Cleis Press.

RACE, ETHNICITY, AND SEXUALITY

Books

Villarosa, L. (Ed.). (2003). *Body and soul: The black woman's guide to physical health and emotional well-being.* New York: HarperPerennial.

White, E. C. (Ed.). (2006). *The black woman's health book: Speaking for ourselves.* Seattle, WA: Seal Press.

Organizations and Websites

Cultural Diversity in Sexuality (website links for African American, Latina, Asian, and Native American peoples, sponsored by the Society for the Scientific Study of Sexuality [SSSS]) *www.pages.prodigy.net/sixx/links.htm*

SEX EDUCATION FOR CHILDREN AND TEENS

Books

Ashton, J. (2009). *The body scoop for girls: A straight-talk guide to a healthy beautiful you.* New York: Avery/Penguin.

Bass, E., & Kaufman, K. (1996). *Free your mind: The book for gay, lesbian, and bisexual youth and their allies.* New York: HarperCollins.

Columbia University Staff. (1998). The *'Go ask Alice' book of answers: A guide to good physical, sexual, and emotional health.* New York: Holt Press.

Corinna, H. (2007). *S.E.X.: The all-you-need-to-know progressive sexuality guide to get you through high school and college.* Cambridge, MA: Da Capo Press.

Drill, E. (1999). *Deal with it: A whole new approach to your body, brain, and life as a gURL.* New York: Pocket.

Gravelle, K., Gravelle, J., & Palen, D. (2006). *The period book: Everything you don't want to ask but need to know.* New York: Walker.

Haffner, D. (2004). *From diapers to dating: A parent's guide to raising sexually healthy children—from infancy to middle school.* New York: Newmarket Press.

Harris, R. (1994). *It's perfectly normal: A book about changing bodies, growing up, sex and sexual health.* Somerville, MA: Candlewick Press.

Harris, R. (1999). *It's so amazing! A book about eggs, sperm, birth, babies, and families.* Somerville, MA: Candlewick Press.

Harris, R., & Emberly, M. (2008). *It's not the stork: A book about girls, boys, bodies, families and friends.* Somerville, MA: Candlewick Press. (Also in Spanish: *No es la ciguena.*)

Levy, B. (2006). *In love and in danger: A teen's guide to breaking free of abusive relationships.* Seattle, WA: Seal Press.

Loulan, J., & Worthen, B. (2001). *Period.: A girl's guide.* Volcano, CA: Volcano Press.

Madaras, L. (2000). *What's happening to my body? Book for boys: A growing up guide for parents and sons.* New York: Newmarket Press.

Madaras, L. (2003). *Ready, set, grow!: A what's happening to my body? book for younger girls.* New York: Newmarket Press.

Madaras, L. (2007). *The "What's happening to my body" book for girls* (Rev., 3rd ed.). New York: Newmarket Press.

Mayle, P. (2000). *Where did I come from?* Secaucus, NJ: Carol Publishing Group.

Miron, C., & Miron, A. (2001). *How to talk to teens about love, relationships, and S-E-X: A guide for parents.* Minneapolis, MN: Free Spirit Press.

Resh, E. (2009). *The secret lives of teen girls: What your mother wouldn't talk about but your daughter needs to know.* Carlsbad, CA: Hay House.

Roffman, D. (2000). *The thinking parent's guide to talking sense about sex.* Cambridge & Berkeley, CA: Perseus.

Schoen, M. (2008). *Belly buttons are navels.* Buffalo, NY: Prometheus.

Weill, S. (2005). *The real truth about teens and sex.* New York: Perigee.

Organizations and Websites

United States

TEENS GENERAL

Advocatesforyouth.org
www.advocatesforyouth.org

kidshealth.org
www.kidshealth.org

Answer.rutgers.edu
www.answer.rutgers.edu/page/sexetc_website/

Sexetc.org
www.sexetc.org

Great Britain

LGBT YOUTH

Queer Youth Network
www.queeryouth.org.uk

SEXUALITY, SPIRITUALITY, AND TOUCH

Books

Gach, M. R. (1997). *Acupressure for lovers: Secrets of touch for increasing intimacy.* New York: Bantam Doubleday Dell.

Lacroix, N. (2006). *The art of tantric sex.* New York: DK Adult.

Stubbs, K. R. (1999). *Erotic massage: The tantric touch of love.* New York: Tarcher.

Organizations and Websites

Tantra.com
www.tantra.com

SEX TOYS AND VIDEOS

Books

Blank, J. (2000). *Good vibrations: The complete guide to vibrators.* San Francisco: Down There
    Press.

Mail Order

United States

Adam and Eve
PO Box 800
Carrboro, NC 27510
800-293-4654
www.adameve.com

Blowfish
PO Box 411290
San Francisco, CA 94141-1290
415-252-4340
800-325-2569
www.blowfish.com

Condomania
Attention: Mail Order
1009 North Orange Drive
Los Angeles, CA 90038
800-926-6366
www.secure.condomania.com

Drugstore.com
www.drugstore.com

Eve's Garden
147 Summit Street, Building 3B
Peabody, MA 01960
800-848-3837
www.evesgarden.com

Good Vibrations/Passion Press/Sex Positive
Productions (Open Enterprises)
934 Howard Street
San Francisco, CA 94103
415-974-8990
800-289-8423
www.goodvibes.com

Grand Opening!
126 SW 148th Street, #c100
PMB 3407
Burien, WA 98166
617-666-7826
www.grandopening.com

Libida
www.libida.com

MyPleasure
866-697-5327
www.mypleasure.com

Pure Romance
www.pureromance.com

Sinclair Intimacy Institute
PO Box 8865
Chapel Hill, NC 27515
800-955-0888
www.bettersex.com

Stormy Leather
2807 West Sunset Boulevard
Los Angeles, CA 90026
415-626-1672
800-486-9650
www.stormyleather.com

Toys in Babeland
707 East Pike Street
Seattle, WA 98122
206-328-2914
800-658-9119
www.babeland.com

Australia

Femplay (sex toys for women)
www.femplay.com.au

D.vice
www.dvice.com.au

Wild Secrets
www.wildsecrets.com.au

Sex Toys 247
www.sextoys247.com.au

Adult Sex Toys
www.adultsextoys.com.au

Canada

Adult Sensations
www.adultsensations.ca

Lovedreamer
www.lovedreamer.com

Come As You Are
www.comeasyouare.com

Sex Shop Canada
www.sexshopcanada.com

Great Britain

Adult World
www.adultworld.co.uk

Sex Toys
www.sextoys.co.uk

Bedroom Pleasures
www.bedroompleasures.co.uk

Sexshop365
www.sexshop365.co.uk

Lovehoney
www.lovehoney.co.uk

New Zealand

D.vice
www.dvice.co.nz

Sex Gear
www.sexgear.co.nz

Femplay
www.femplay.co.nz

Sex.co.nz
www.sex.co.nz

NZ Adult Toys
www.nzadulttoys.co.nz

Wild Secrets
www.wildsecrets.co.nz/pages/show/118-postage-handling

SEXUALLY TRANSMITTED INFECTIONS (STIs) AND SAFER SEX

Ebel, C., & Wald, A. (2007). *Managing herpes: Many living and loving with HSV.* Research
   Triangle Park, NC: American Social Health Association.

Organizations and Websites

United States

American Social Health Association (STI
resource center hotline)
www.ashastd.org

Centers for Disease Control and Prevention
National STD hotline: 800-227-8922
www.cdc.gov

HIV/AIDS Information and Resources
www.thebody.com

National HIV/AIDS Hotline
English: (800) 342-2437 (24 hours a day)
Spanish: (800) 344-7432

Australia

Health Insite
www.healthinsite.gov.au/topics/Sexually_Transmitted_Infections

Canada

Canadian AIDS Society
www.cdnaids.ca

Public Health Agency of Canada
www.phac-aspc.gc.ca/std-mts/index-eng.php

Great Britain

British Association for Sexual Health
and HIV
www.bashh.org

England's National Health Service
*www.nhs.uk/Conditions/Sexually-transmitted-
infections/Pages/Introduction.aspx*

United Kingdom–based International HIV
and AIDS Charity
www.avert.org

New Zealand

STIs

Health Ed
*www.healthed.govt.nz/resources/search-
resources.aspx?id=18*

New Zealand Ministry of Health
www.moh.govt.nz/sexualhealth

TRAUMA

Books

Carter, C. (1997). *The other side of silence: Women tell about their experience with date rape.* Gilsum, NH: Avocus.

Cohn, R. (2011). *Coming home to passion: Restoring loving sexuality in couples with histories of childhood trauma and neglect.* Santa Barbara, CA: Praeger.

Haines, S. (1999). *The survivor's guide to sex: How to have an empowered sex life after child sexual abuse.* San Francisco: Cleis Press.

Haines, S. (2007). *Healing sex: A mind-body approach to healing sexual trauma.* San Francisco: Cleis Press

Herman, J. (1997). *Trauma and recovery: The aftermath of violence—from domestic abuse to political terror.* New York: Basic Books.

Knauer, S. (2002). *Recovering from sexual abuse, addiction, and compulsive behaviors: "Numb Survivors."* New York: Haworth Press.

Levine, P., & Frederick, A. (1997). *Waking the tiger: Healing trauma—The innate capacity to transform overwhelming experiences.* Berkeley, CA: North Atlantic Books.

Maltz, W. (2001). *The sexual healing journey: A guide for survivors of sexual abuse.* New York: HarperPerennial.

Maltz, W., & Holman, B. (1991). *Incest and sexuality: A guide to understanding and healing.* Lexington, MA: Lexington Books.

Naparstek, B. (2004). *Invisible heroes: Survivors of trauma and how they heal.* New York: Bantam Books.

Nicarthey, G. (2004). *Getting free: You can end abuse and take back your life.* Seattle, WA: Seal Press.

Pierce-Baker, C. (2000). *Surviving the silence: Black women's stories of rape.* New York: Norton.

Rothschild, B. (2000). *The body remembers: Psychophysiology and trauma treatment.* New York: Norton.

Stone, R. (2005). *No secrets, no lies: How Black families can heal from sexual abuse.* New York: Broadway.

Warshaw, R. (1994). *I never called it rape: The Ms. report on recognizing, fighting and surviving date and acquaintance rape.* New York: HarperPerennial.

Wiehe, V. R., & Richards, A. L. (1995). *Intimate betrayal: Understanding and responding to the trauma of acquaintance rape.* Thousand Oaks, CA: Sage.

Williams, M., & Poijula, S. (2002). *The PTSD workbook: Simple, effective techniques for overcoming traumatic stress symptoms.* Oakland, CA: New Harbinger.

Organizations and Websites

United States

Jim Hopper Child Sexual Abuse Resource Page
www.jimhopper.com

Trauma Center
www.traumacenter.org

Great Britain

Women's Aid Federation of England
www.womensaid.org.uk

References

Administration on Aging, U.S. Department of Health and Human Services. (2000). *A profile of older Americans: 2000*. Washington, DC: Author.

Albert, B. (2010). *With one voice 2010: America's adults and teens sound off about teen pregnancy*. Washington, DC: The National Campaign to Prevent Teen and Unplanned Pregnancy.

Allen, K., & Goldberg, A. (2009). Sexual activity during menstruation: A qualitative study. *Journal of Sex Research, 46*(6), 535–545.

American Association of Retired Persons. (2010). *Sex, romance, and relationships: AARP survey of midlife and older adults*. Washington, DC: AARP.

American Society of Plastic Surgeons (ASPS). (2007, March 9). *11 Million Cosmetic Plastic Surgery Procedures in 2006—up 7%* [Press release]. Retrieved June 6, 2011, from *www.archivenewsmax.com/archives/articles/2007*.

Angier, N. (1999). *Woman: An intimate geography*. New York: Houghton Mifflin.

Anticević, V., & Britvić, D. (2008). Sexual functioning in war veterans with posttraumatic stress disorder. *Croatian Medical Journal, 49*, 499–505.

Atkinson, B. J. (2005). *Emotional intelligence in couples therapy: Advances from neurobiology and the science of intimate relationships*. New York: Norton.

Atwood, J. D., & Schwartz, L. (2002). Cyber-sex: The new affair treatment considerations. *Journal of Couple & Relationship Therapy, 1*(3), 37–56.

Austin, J. H. (1998). *Zen and the brain*. Cambridge, MA: MIT Press.

Bacon, C. G., Mittleman, M. A., Kawachi, I., Giovannucci, E., Glasser, D. B., & Rimm, E. B. (2003). Sexual function in men older than 50 years of age: Results from the Health Professionals Follow-up Study. *Annals of Internal Medicine, 139*, 161–168.

Bancroft, J., Loftus J., & Long, J. S. (2003). Distress about sex: A national survey of women in heterosexual relationships. *Archives of Sexual Behavior, 32*, 193–208.

Bancroft, J., Sherwin, B., Alexander, G., Davidson, D., & Walker, A. (1991). Oral contraception, androgens, and the sexuality of young women: I. A comparison of sexual experience, sexual attitudes, and gender role in oral contraceptive users and nonusers. *Archives of Sexual Behavior, 20*(2), 105–120.

Basson, R. (1998). Sexual health of women with disabilities. *Canadian Medical Association Journal, 159*(4), 359–362.

Basson, R. (2005). Women's sexual dysfunction: Revised and expanded definitions. *Canadian Medical Association Journal, 172*(10), 1327–1333.

Berne, E. (1964). *Games people play.* New York: Grove Press.

Binik, Y. M. (2010). The DSM diagnostic criteria for vaginismus. *Archives of Sexual Behavior, 39,* 278–291.

Binik, Y. M., Reissing, E., Pukall, C., Flory, N., Payne, K. A, & Khalifé, S. (2002). The female sexual pain disorders: Genital pain or sexual dysfunction? *Archives of Sexual Behavior, 31*(5), 425–429.

Bogaert, A. F. (2004). Asexuality: Prevalence and associated factors in a national probability sample. *Journal of Sex Research, 41*(3), 279–287.

Brotto, L. A., Basson, R., & Luria, M. (2008). A mindfulness-based group psychoeducational intervention targeting sexual arousal disorder in women. *Journal of Sexual Medicine, 5*(7), 1646–1659.

Brown, D. W., Anda, R. F., Tiemeier, H., Felitti, V. J., Edwards, V. J., Croft, J. B., & Giles, W. H. (2009). Adverse childhood experiences and the risk of premature mortality. *American Journal of Preventive Medicine, 37*(5), 389–396.

Browne, J., & Russell, S. (2005). My home, your workplace: People with physical disability negotiate their sexual health without crossing professional boundaries. *Disability and Society, 20*(4), 375–388.

Brumberg, J. (1997). *The body project: An intimate history of American girls.* New York: Random House.

Burchell, A. N., Winer, R. L., de Sanjosé, S., & Franco, E. L. (2006). Chapter 6: Epidemiology and transmission dynamics of genital HPV infection. *Vaccine, 24*(Suppl. 3), 52–61.

Burns, D. (1999). *The feeling good handbook* (Rev. ed.). New York: Plume.

Butrick, C. W. (2009). Pelvic floor hypertonic disorders: Identification and management. *Obstetrics and Gynecology Clinics of North America, 36,* 707–722.

Carballo-Diéguez, A., Bauermeister, J. A., Ventuneac, A., Dolezal, C., Balan, I., & Remien, R. H. (2008). The use of rectal douches among HIV-uninfected and infected men who have unprotected receptive anal intercourse: Implications for rectal microbicides. *Aids and Behavior, 12,* 860–866.

Caruso, S., Agnello, C., Intelisano, G., Farina, M., DiMari, L., & Cianci, A. (2004). Sexual behavior of women taking low-dose oral contraceptive containing 15 ug ethinylestradio/60 ug gestodene. *Contraception, 69,* 237–240.

Castleman, M. (2004). *Great Sex: A man's guide to the secret principles of total body sex.* Emmaus, PA: Rodale Press.

Centers for Disease Control and Prevention (CDC). (n.d.). STD FAQs and basic facts. Retrieved April 28, 2010, from *www.cdcnpin.org/scripts/std/faq.asp.*

Chudakov, B., Cohen, H., Matar, M. A., & Kaplan, S. (2008). A naturalistic prospective open study of the effects of adjunctive therapy of sexual dysfunction in chronic PTSD patients. *Israeli Journal of Psychiatry Relationship Science, 25*(1), 26–32.

Connor, J. J., Robinson, B., & Wieling, E. (2008). Vulvar pain: A phenomenological study of couples in search of effective diagnosis and treatment. *Family Process, 47*(2), 139–155.

Crepaz, N., Marshall, K. J., Aupont, L. W., Jacobs, E. D., Mizuno, Y., Kay, L. S., & O'Leary, A. (2009). The efficacy of HIV/STI behavioral interventions for African American females in the United States: A meta-analysis. *American Journal of Public Health, 99*(11), 2069–2078.

Davidson, R. J., Kabat-Zinn, J., Schumacher, J., Rosenkranz, M., Muller, D., Santorelli, S. F., & Sheridan, J. F. (2003). Alterations in brain and immune function produced by mindfulness meditation. *Psychosomatic Medicine, 65,* 564–570.

Davis, H. J., & Reissing, E. D. (2007). Relationship adjustment and dyadic interaction in couples with sexual pain disorders: A critical review of the literature. *Sexual and Relationship Therapy, 22*(2), 245–254.

de Bruijn, G. (1982). From masturbation to orgasm with a partner: How some women bridge the gap—and why others don't. *Journal of Sex and Marital Therapy, 8,* 151–167.

Dennerstein, L., Dudley, E., & Burger, H. (2001). Are changes in sexual functioning during midlife due to aging or menopause? *Fertility and Sterility, 76*(3), 456–460.

Dennerstein, L., Lehert, P., & Burger, H. (2005). The relative effects of hormones and relationship factors on sexual function of women through the natural menopause transition. *Fertility and Sterility, 84*(1), 174–180.

Desrosiers, M., Bergeron, S., Meana, M., Leclerc, B., Binik, Y. M., & Khalifé, S. (2008). Psychosexual characteristics of vestibulodynia couples: Partner solicitousness and hostility are associated with pain. *Journal of Sexual Medicine, 5*(2), 418–427.

Diamond, L. (2005). A new view of lesbian subtypes: Stable versus fluid identity trajectories over an 8-year period. *Psychology of Women Quarterly, 29,* 119–128.

Diamond, L. (2008). *Sexual fluidity: Understanding women's love and desire.* Cambridge, MA: Harvard University Press.

Dove, N. L., & Wiederman, M. W. (2000). Cognitive distraction and women's sexual functioning. *Journal of Sex and Marital Therapy, 26,* 67–78.

Edwards, G., & Barber, G. (2010). Women may underestimate their partners' desires to use condoms: Possible implications for behavior. *Journal of Sex Research, 47*(2), 59–65.

Ehrström, S., Kornfeld, D., Rylander, E., & Bohm-Starke, N. (2009). Chronic stress in women with localized provoked vulvodynia. *Journal of Psychosomatic Obstetrics and Gynecology, 30*(1), 73–79.

Esposito, K., Giugliano, F., Ciotola, M., De Sio, M., D'Armiento, M., & Giugliano, D. (2008). Obesity and sexual dysfunction, male and female. *International Journal of Impotence Research, 20,* 358–365.

Feldman, H. A., Goldstein, I., Hatzichristou, D. G., Krane, R. J., & McKinlay, J. B. (1994). Impotence and its medical and psychosocial correlates: Results of the Massachusetts Male Aging Study. *Journal of Urology, 151,* 54–61.

Fisher, H. (2004). *Why we love: The nature and chemistry of romantic love.* New York: Holt.

Fisher, H. (2009). *Why him? Why her? How to find and keep lasting love.* New York: Holt.

Foley, S. (2005). *Sex and love for grownups: A no-nonsense guide to a life of passion.* New York: AARP/Sterling.

Frankel, V. (2005, February). Sex after 40, 50 and beyond. *More,* 74–77.

Freeman, D. (2009). Life cycle of a penis: Experts explain how a penis changes in size, appearance, and sexual function as a man ages. *WebMD.* Retrieved May 9, 2010, from *www.men.webmd.com/features/life-cycle-of-a-penis.*

Friedan, B. (1994). *The fountain of age.* New York: Simon & Schuster.

Gerressu, M., Mercer, C. H., Graham, C. A., Wellings, K., & Johnson, A. M. (2008). Prevalence of masturbation and associated factors in a British national probability survey. *Archives of Sexual Behavior, 37*(2), 266–278.

Goggin, K., Engelson, E. S., Rabkin, J. G., & Kotler, D. P. (1998). The relationship of mood, endocrine, and sexual disorders in human immunodeficiency virus positive (HIV+) women: An exploratory study. *Psychosomatic Medicine, 60*, 11–16.

Goldmeier, D. (2001). Female low sexual desire and sexually transmitted infections. *Sexually Transmitted Infections, 77*, 293–294.

Gossmann, I., Mathieu, M., Julien, D., & Chartrand, E. (2003). Determinants of sex initiation frequencies and sexual satisfaction in long-term couples' relationships. *Canadian Journal of Human Sexuality, 12*(3–4), 169–181.

Gottman, J. (1994). *Why marriages succeed or fail: And how you can make yours last*. New York: Simon & Schuster.

Gottman, J. (1999). *The seven principles for making marriage work*. New York: Crown.

Graham, C., Ramos, R., Bancroft, J., Maglaya, C., & Farley, T. (1995). The effects of steroidal contraceptives on the well-being and sexuality of women: A double-blind placebo controlled, two-centre study of combined and progestogen-only methods. *Contraception, 52*(6), 363–369.

Greene, B., & Winfrey, O. (1996). *Make the connection: Ten steps to a better body and a better life*. New York: Hyperion.

Greenspan, J. R., & Nakashima, A. K. (1994). *Sexually transmitted disease surveillance, 1993*. Atlanta, GA: Centers for Disease Control and Prevention.

Grunbaum, J. A., Kann, L., Kinchen, S., Ross, J., Hawkins, J., Lowry, R., Collins, J. (2004). Youth risk behavior surveillance. United States, 2003. *MMWR. Surveillance Summaries: Morbidity and Mortality Weekly Report. Surveillance Summaries/CDC, 53*(2),1–96.

Haavio-Mannila, E., & Kontula, O. (1997). Correlates of increased sexual satisfaction. *Archives of Sexual Behavior, 26*(4), 399–419.

Haefner, H. (2000). Critique of new gynecologic surgical procedures: Surgery for vulvar vestibulitis. *Clinical Obstetrics and Gynecology, 43*(3), 689–700.

Haines, S. (1999). *The survivor's guide to sex: How to have an empowered sex life after child sexual abuse*. San Francisco: Cleis Press.

Hales, D., & Hales, R. (1996). *Caring for the mind: The comprehensive guide to mental health*. New York: Bantam Books.

Hanh, T. N. (1996). *The miracle of mindfulness: A manual on meditation*. Boston: Beacon Press.

Heiman, J., & LoPiccolo, J. (1988). *Becoming orgasmic: A sexual and personal growth program for women*. New York: Simon & Schuster.

Hemingway, E. (1929). *A farewell to arms*. New York: Simon & Schuster.

Hendrix, H. (1988). *Getting the love you want: A guide for couples*. New York: Harper & Row.

Herbenick, D., Reece, M., Sanders, S. A., Dodge, B., Ghassemi, A., & Fortenberry, J. D. (2009). Prevalence and characteristics of vibrator use by women in the United States: Results from a nationally representative study. *Journal of Sexual Medicine, 6*, 1857–1866.

Hockenbury, S., & Hockenbury, D. (2003). *Psychology* (3rd ed.). New York: Worth.

Hormes, J. M., Lytle, L. A., Gross, C. R., Ahmed, R. L., Troxel, A. B., & Schmitz, K. H. (2008). The body image and relationships scale: Development and validation of a measure of body image in female breast cancer survivors. *Journal of Clinical Oncology, 8,* 1269–1274.

Kabat-Zinn, J. (2005). *Wherever you go, there you are.* New York: Hyperion.

Kabat-Zinn, J. (2006). *Mindfulness for beginners* [Audio CD]. Louisville, CO: Sounds True.

Kaplan, H. S. (1979). *Disorders of sexual desire.* New York: Brunner/Mazel.

Kaplow, J., & Widom, C. (2007). Age of onset of child maltreatment predicts long-term mental health outcomes. *Journal of Abnormal Psychology, 116*(1), 176–187.

Katz, A. (2005). The sounds of silence: Sexuality information for cancer patients. *Journal of Clinical Oncology, 23*(1), 238–241.

Kawana, K., Yasugi, T., & Taketani, Y. (2009). Human papillomavirus vaccines: Current issues and future. *Indian Journal of Medical Research, 130,* 341–347.

Kelly, L. (2007). Lesbian body image perceptions: The context of body silence. *Qualitative Health Research, 177*(7), 873–883.

Kenney, J. W., Reinholtz, C., & Angelini, P. J. (1998). Sexual abuse, sex before age 16, and high-risk behaviors of young females with sexually transmitted diseases. *Journal of Obstetric, Gynecologic, and Neonatal Nursing, 27*(1), 54–63.

Kitzinger, S. (1985). *The complete book of pregnancy and childbirth.* New York: Knopf.

Koch, P. B., Mansfield, P. K., Thurau, D., & Carey, M. (2005). "Feeling frumpy": The relationships between body image and sexual response changes in mid-life women. *Journal of Sex Research, 42*(3), 215–223.

Komisaruk, B. R., Beyer-Flores, C., & Whipple, B. (2006). *The science of orgasm.* Baltimore: Johns Hopkins University Press.

Komisaruk, B. R., Whipple, B., Nasserzadeh, S., & Beyer-Flores, C. (2010). *The orgasm answer guide.* Baltimore: Johns Hopkins University Press.

Krychman, M., Pereira, L., Carter, J., & Amsterdam, A. (2006). Sexual oncology: Sexual health issues in women with cancer. *Oncology, 71,* 18–25.

Laan, E., Everaerd, W., Bellen, G., & Hanewald, G. (1994). Women's sexual and emotional responses to male- and female-produced erotica. *Archives of Sexual Behavior, 23,* 153–170.

Ladas, A. K., Whipple, B., & Perry, J. D. (2005). *The G spot and other discoveries about human sexuality.* New York: Holt/Owl.

Lancaster, L., & Stillman, D. (2010). *The M-factor: How the millennial generation is rocking the workplace.* New York: Harper.

Laumann, E. O., Gagnon, J., Michael, R., & Michaels, S. (1994). *The social organization of sexuality.* Chicago: University of Chicago Press.

Laumann, E. O., Nicolosi, A., Glasser, D. B., Paik, A., Gingell, C., Moreira, E., & Wang, T. (2005). Sexual problems among women and men aged 40–80 y: Prevalence and correlates identified in the Global Study of Sexual Attitudes and Behaviors. *International Journal of Impotence Research, 17,* 39–57.

Laumann, E. O., Paik, A., & Rosen, R. C. (1999). Sexual dysfunction in the United States: Prevalence and predictors. *Journal of the American Medical Association, 281*(6), 537–544.

Legenbauer, T., Vocks, S., Schäfer, C., Schütt-Strömel, S., Hiller, W., Wagner, C., & Vögele. C. (2009). Preference for attractiveness and thinness in a partner: Influence of internalization of the thin ideal and shape/weight dissatisfaction in heterosexual women, heterosexual men, lesbians, and gay men. *Body Image, 6,* 228–234.

Leiblum, S. R., Koochaki, P. E., Rodenberg, C. A., Barton, I. P., & Rosen, R. C. (2006). Hypoactive sexual desire disorder in postmenopausal women: U.S. results from the Women's International Study of Health and Sexuality (WISHeS). *Menopause, 13*, 46–56.

Leiblum, S., & Rosen, R. (Eds.). *Principles and practices of sex therapy* (3rd ed.). New York: Guilford Press.

Lemieux, L., Kaiser, S., Pereira, J., & Meadows, L. M. (2004). Sexuality in palliative care: Patient perspectives. *Palliative Medicine, 18*(7), 630–637.

Lever, J., Frederick, D. A., & Peplau, L. A. (2006). Does size matter?: Men's and women's views on penis size across the lifespan. *Psychology of Men & Masculinity, 7*(3), 129–143.

Lief, H. I. (Ed.). (1981). *Sexual problems in medical practice.* Monroe, WI: American Medical Association.

Lindh-Astrand, L., Hoffmann, M. I., Hammar, M., & Kjellgren, K. (2007). Women's conception of the menopausal transition: A qualitative study. *Journal of Clinical Nursing, 16*, 509–517.

Lindley, L. L., Barnett, C. L., Brandt, H. M., Hardin, J. W., & Burcin, M. (2008). STDs among sexually active female college students: Does sexual orientation make a difference? *Perspectives on sexual and reproductive health, 40*(4), 212–217.

Lloyd, E. A. (2005). *The case of the female orgasm: Bias in the science of evolution.* Cambridge, MA: Harvard University Press.

Lowenstein, L., Gruenwald, I., Gartman, I., & Vardi, Y. (2010). Can stronger pelvic muscle floor improve sexual function? *International Urogynecology Journal, 21*(5), 553–556.

Madrid-Marina, V., Torres-Poveda, K., López-Toledo, G., & García-Carrancá, A. (2009). Advantages and disadvantages of current prophylactic vaccines against HPV. *Archives of Medical Research, 40*, 471–477.

Maltz, W. (2001). *The sexual healing journey: A guide for survivors of sexual abuse* (rev ed.). New York: HarperCollins.

Marrazzo, J. M., Coffey, P., & Bingham, A. (2005). Sexual practices, risk perception and knowledge of sexually transmitted disease risk among lesbian and bisexual women. *Perspectives on Sexual and Reproductive Health, 37*(1), 6–12.

Marrazzo, J. M., Thomas, K. K., Agnew, K., & Ringwood, K. (2010). Prevalence and risks for bacterial vaginosis in women who have sex with women. *Sexually Transmitted Diseases, 37*(5), 335–339.

Masters, W., & Johnson, V. (1966). *Human sexual response.* Boston: Little, Brown.

Masters, W., & Johnson, V. (1979). *Homosexuality in perspective.* Boston: Little, Brown.

McCarthy, B., & McCarthy, E. (2009). *Discovering your couple sexual style: Sharing desire, pleasure, and satisfaction.* New York: Routledge.

McCullough, D. (2001). *John Adams.* New York: Simon & Schuster.

McGowan, I. (2008). Rectal microbicides. *Sexually Transmitted Infections, 84*, 413–417.

McKinlay, J. B. (2000). The worldwide prevalence and epidemiology of erectile dysfunction. *International Journal of Impotence Research, 12*(Suppl. 4), S6–S11.

Meadow, R., & Weiss, L. (1992). *Good girls don't eat dessert: Women's conflict about eating and sexuality.* New York: Harrington Park Press.

Meana, M., & Lykins, A. (2009). Negative affect and somatically focused anxiety in young women reporting pain with intercourse. *Journal of Sex Research, 46*(1), 80–88.

Meana, M., & Nunnink, S. E. (2006). Gender differences in the content of cognitive distraction during sex. *Journal of Sex Research, 43*(1), 59–67.

Molloy, B. L., & Herzberger, S. D. (1998). Body image and self-esteem: A comparison of African American and Caucasian women. *Body Image, 38*(7/8), 631–643.

Nappi, R. E., Ferdeghini, F., Abbiati, I., Vercesi, C., Farina, C., & Polatti, F. (2003). Electrical stimulation (ES) in the management of sexual pain disorders. *Journal of Sex and Marital Therapy, 29*(Suppl. 1), 103–110.

National Campaign to Prevent Teen Pregnancy. (2000). Not just another thing to do. Retrieved June 30, 2000, from *www.teenpregnancy.org.*

National Center for Health Statistics, U.S. Dept. of Health and Human Services. (2004). National survey of family growth, Cycle VI, 2002 [Computer file]. Ann Arbor, MI: Institute for Social Research.

Nichols , M. (2000). Therapy with sexual minorities. In S. Leiblum & R. Rosen (Eds.), *Principles and practices of sex therapy* (3rd ed., pp. 335–367). New York: Guilford Press.

Northrup, C. (2010). *Women's bodies, women's wisdom: Creating physical and emotional health and healing.* New York: Bantam Books.

Pacik, T. (2009). Viewpoint: Botox treatment for vaginismus. *Plastic and Reconstructive Surgery, 124*(6), 455e–456e.

Panzer, C., Wise, S., Fantini, G., Kang, D., Munarriz, R., Guay, A., & Goldstein, I. (2006). Impact of oral contraceptives on sex hormone-binding globulin and androgen levels: A retrospective study in women with sexual dysfunction. *Journal of Sexual Medicine, 3*(1), 104–113.

Perel, E. (2007). *Mating in captivity: Unlocking erotic intelligence.* New York: HarperCollins.

Perry, J. D., & Whipple, B. (1981). Pelvic muscle strength of female ejaculators: Evidence in support of a new theory of orgasm. *Journal of Sex Research, 17*(1), 22–39.

Pfeiffer, E., Verwoerdt, A., & Davis, G. C. (1972). Sexual behavior in middle life. *American Journal of Psychiatry, 128 ,* 1262–1267.

Pujols, Y., Meston, C. M., & Seal, B. N. (2010). The association between sexual satisfaction and body image in women. *Journal of Sexual Medicine, 7,* 905–916.

Reed, B. D., Haefner, H. K., & Edwards, L. (2008). A survey on diagnosis and treatment of vulvodynia among vulvodynia researcher and members of the International Society for the Study of Vulvovaginal Disease. *Journal of Reproductive Medicine, 53*(12), 921–929.

Reinisch, J. M. (1991). *The Kinsey Institute new report on sex: What you must know to be sexually literate.* New York: St. Martin's Press.

Rostosky, S., Riggle, E., Dudley, M., & Comer Wright, M. (2006). Commitment in same-sex relationships: A qualitative analysis of couples' conversations. *Journal of Homosexuality, 51*(3), 199–222.

Sanchez, D. T., & Kiefer, A. K. (2007). Body concerns in and out of the bedroom: Implications for sexual pleasure and problems. *Archives of Sexual Behavior, 36,* 808–820.

Sarno, J. (1999). *The mindbody prescription: Healing the body, healing the pain.* New York: Warner Books.

Schaffir , J. (2006). Hormonal contraception and sexual desire: A critical review. *Journal of Sex and Marital Therapy, 32,* 305–314.

Schnarch, D. (2000). Desire problems: A systemic approach. In S. Leiblum & R. Rosen (Eds.), *Principles and practices of sex therapy* (3rd ed., pp. 17–56). New York: Guilford Press.

Schnurr, P., Lunney, C. A., Forshay, E., Thurston, V. L., Chow, B. K., Resick, P. A., & Foa, E. B. (2009). Sexual function outcomes in women treated for posttraumatic stress disorder. *Journal of Women's Health, 18*(10), 1549–1557.

Schooler, D., Ward, L. M., Merriweather, A., & Caruthers, A. (2005). Cycles of shame: Menstrual shame, body shame, and sexual decision-making. *Journal of Sex Research, 42*(4), 324–334.

Schubiner, H., & Betzold, M. (2010). *Unlearn your pain.* Pleasant Ridge, MI: Mind Body.

Seal, B. N., & Meston, C. M. (2007). The impact of body awareness on sexual arousal in women with sexual dysfunction. *Journal of Sexual Medicine, 4,* 990–1000.

Siegel, D. (2007). The mindful brain: Reflection and attunement in the cultivation of well-being. New York: Norton.

Siegel, D. (2008). *The neurobiology of "we": How relationships, the mind, and the brain interact to shape who we are* [Audio CD]. Louisville, CO: Sounds True.

Siegel, D. (2010). *Mindsight: The new science of personal transformation.* New York: Bantam Books.

Soet, J., Dudley, W., & Dilorio, C. (1999). The effects of ethnicity and perceived power on women's sexual behavior. *Psychology of Women Quarterly, 23*(4), 707–723.

Strauch, B. (2010). *The secret life of the grown-up brain: The surprising talents of the middle-aged mind.* New York: Viking.

Strong, B., & DeVault, C. (1988). *Understanding our sexuality.* New York: West Group.

Stubbs, M., & Costos, D. (2004). Negative attitudes toward menstruation: Implications for disconnection within girls and between women. In J. C. Chrisler (Ed.), *From menarche to menopause: The female body in feminist therapy* (pp. 37–54). New York: Haworth Press.

Sugrue, D. P., & Whipple, B. (2001). The Consensus-based classification of female sexual dysfunction: Barriers to universal acceptance. *Journal of Sex and Marital Therapy, 27*(2), 221–226.

Suschinsky, K. D., Lalumière, M. L., & Chivers, M. L. (2009). Sex differences in patterns of genital arousal: Measurement artifact or true phenomena? *Archives of Sexual Behavior, (38)*4, 559–573.

Taylor, C. (2001, May 11). Who goes there and how?: Lesbians and disability. *Women Writers: A Zine.* Retrieved March 13, 2011, from *www.womenwriters.net/may2001/taylor.htm.*

Tepper, M. (2009, January 20). Facilitated sex: The next frontier in sexuality? *Sexual Health. com.* Retrieved March 13, 2011, from *www.sexualhealth.com/article/read/disability-illness/ rediscovering-sex-after-disability-illness-trauma/8.*

ter Kuile, M. M., & Weijenborg, P. T. (2006). A cognitive/behavioral group program for women with vulvar vestibulitis syndrome (VVS): Factors associated with treatment success. *Journal of Sex and Marital Therapy, 32,* 199–213.

United Nations Population Fund. (n.d.). Reproductive health: Breaking the cycle of sexually transmitted infections. Retrieved April 28, 2010, from *www.unfpa.org/rh/stis.htm.*

Verschuren, J., Enzlin, P., Dijkstra, P., Geertzen, J., & Dekker, R. (2010). Chronic disease and sexuality: A generic conceptual framework. *Journal of Sex Research, 47*(2–3), 153–170.

von Soest, T., Kvalem, I. L., Roald, H. E., & Skolleborg, K. C. (2009). The effects of cosmetic surgery on body image, self-esteem and psychological problems. *Journal of Plastic, Reconstructive and Aesthetic Surgery, 62*(10), 1238–1244.

Vozina, C., & Steben, M. (2001). Genital herpes: Psychosexual impacts and counseling. *Canadian Journal of Continuing Medical Education. 13,* 125–134.

Wallwiener , C., Wallwiener, L. M., Seeger, H., Muck, A., Bitzer, J., & Wallwiener, M. (2010). Prevalence of sexual dysfunction and impact of contraception in female German medical students. *Journal of Sexual Medicine, 7*(6), 2139–2148.

Walsh, F. (1991). Promoting healthy functioning in divorced and remarried families. In A. Gurman and D. Kniskern (Eds.), *Handbook of family therapy* (Vol. 2, pp. 525–545). New York: Brunner/Mazel.

Webbe, S. A., Fariello, J. Y., & Whitmore, K. (2010). Minimally invasive therapies for chronic pelvic pain syndrome. *Current Urology Reports, 11*(4), 276–285.

Weijmar-Schultz, W., Basson, R., Binik, Y., Eschenbach, D., Wesselmann, U., & Van Lankveld, J. (2005). Women's sexual pain and its management. *Journal of Sexual Medicine, 2,* 301–316.

Whipple, B., & Brash-McGreer, K. (1997). Management of female sexual dysfunction. In M. L. Sipski & C. J. Alexander (Eds.), *Sexual function in people with disability and chronic illness: A health professional's guide* (pp. 509–534). Gaithersburg, MD: Aspen.

Whipple, B., Gerdes, C., & Komisaruk, B. (1996). Sexual response to self-stimulation in women with complete spinal cord injury. *Journal of Sex Research, 33*(3), 231–240.

Wienke, C., & Hill, G. J. (2009). Does the "marriage benefit" extend to partners in gay and lesbian relationships?: Evidence from a random sample of sexually active adults. *Journal of Family Issues, 30*(2), 259–289.

Wingood, G. M., DiClemente, R. J., Harrington, K., & Davies, S. L. (2002). Body image and African American females' sexual health. *Journal of Women's Health and Gender-Based Medicine, 11*(5), 433–439.

Worden, J. W. (2002). *Grief counseling and grief therapy* (3rd ed.). New York: Springer.

World Health Organization (WHO). (2007, October). Sexually transmitted infections: Fact sheet No. 110. Retrieved March 20, 2011, from *www.who.int/mediacentre/factsheets/fs110/en/index.html*.

Zoldbrod, A. (1993). *Men, women and infertility: Intervention and treatment strategies.* New York: Lexington Books.

Zoldbrod, A. (1998). *Sex smart: How your childhood shaped your sexual life and what to do about it.* Oakland, CA: New Harbinger.

Zoldbrod, A., & Dockett, L. (2002). *Sex talk: Uncensored exercises for exploring what really turns you on.* Oakland, CA: New Harbinger.

Index

About the Authors

Sallie Foley, MSW, a faculty member at the University of Michigan School of Social Work, is Director of the University of Michigan Sexual Health Certificate Program and founder and former director of the University of Michigan Health System's Center for Sexual Health. She has a private practice in Ann Arbor, Michigan. She and her husband have three grown children. Her website is *www.salliefoley.com.*

Sally A. Kope, MSW, is in private practice in Ann Arbor, Michigan, and is the former program director of the University of Michigan's Sexual Health Counseling Services. She and her husband are the parents of four and grandparents of six.

Dennis P. Sugrue, PhD, is on the faculty of the Department of Psychiatry at the University of Michigan Medical School and has a private practice in Bloomfield Hills, Michigan. He is the founder and former codirector of the Henry Ford Center for Human Sexuality and past president of the American Association of Sexuality Educators, Counselors, and Therapists. He and his wife have two grown sons.